W9-CCY-687

Developments in Cardiovascular Medicine

Previous volumes are still available

PREVENTION OF CORONARY HEART DISEASE
DIET, LIFESTYLE AND RISK FACTORS
IN THE SEVEN COUNTRIES STUDY

Editors:

Daan Kromhout
Professor
Director Nutrition and Consumer Safety Division
National Institute of Public Health and the Environment
P.O.Box 1, 3720 BA Bilthoven
The Netherlands

Alessandro Menotti
Professor
Association for Cardiac Research
Cardioricerca
Via Adda 87
Rome 00198
Italy

Henry Blackburn
Mayo Professor Emeritus
Division of Epidemiology
School of Public Health
University of Minnesota
1300 South Second Street,
Minneapolis, MN 55454-1015,
U.S.A.

Kluwer Academic Publishers

Distributors for North, Central and South America:
Kluwer Academic Publishers
101 Philip Drive
Assinippi Park
Norwell, Massachusetts 02061 USA
Telephone (781) 871-6600
Fax (781) 681-9045
E-Mail: kluwer@wkap.com

Distributors for all other countries:
Kluwer Academic Publishers Group
Post Office Box 322
3300 AH Dordrecht, THE NETHERLANDS
Telephone 31 786 576 000
Fax 31 786 576 474
E-Mail: services@wkap.nl

 Electronic Services <http://www.wkap.nl>

Library of Congress Cataloging-in-Publication Data

A C.I.P. Catalogue record for this book is available
from the Library of Congress.

Prevention of coronary heart disease
Diet, lifestyle and risk factors
in the Seven Countries Study

Daan Kromhout, Alessandro Menotti, Henry Blackburn (Editors)

Dedicated to Ancel Keys,
distinguished scientist, who
conceived, organized, and for
many collegial years directed
the Seven Countries Study

Contents

Preface

In the 1940s I was struck by reports about many apparently healthy middle-aged men who dropped dead instantly from heart attacks. The causes of these sudden deaths were unknown. I was interested to discover physio-chemical characteristics of individuals with predictive value for the occurrence of these fatal heart attacks. The discovery of preventive variables would point ways to prevent this disease.

In order to find relationships between mode of life and susceptibility to heart disease contrasting populations had to be studied. Variety - not a high degree of homogeneity in culture and habits - must be sought. After exploratory surveys in countries with supposed differences in dietary patterns, lifestyle and heart disease rates in the early 1950s, the Seven Countries Study took off in 1958. This study established relationships between risk factors and development of heart disease in middle-aged men in health examined in countries with cultures we demonstrated to contrast in diet and lifestyle. The results obtained in the Seven Countries Study from its inception till now are presented in this book entitled: "Prevention of coronary heart disease. Diet, lifestyle and risk factors in the Seven Countries Study."

Long ago I realized that our concern should not be restricted to the prevention of coronary heart disease but should be extended to all diseases and premature death. It is therefore necessary that characteristics of people were recorded and the follow-up of populations continued until there was a change of vital status, providing the data to associate conditions in health with changes in that vital status. The first application of that idea was a prospective study of 283 men in Minnesota who were first examined in 1947. The follow-up showed that the numbers were too small to find meaningful relationships. Larger numbers were needed and were obtained in the Seven Countries Study.

The results of the Seven Countries Study presented in this book should be viewed in this broader context of the role of diet, lifestyle and risk factors in relation to all-causes deaths and to longevity. This should be the ultimate goal of epidemiologic research.

Minneapolis   Ancel Keys
January 2002

Foreword

In the second half of the last century, epidemiological and experimental evidence was presented that the development of coronary heart disease is related to cigarette smoking, the blood cholesterol, and blood pressure level, a family history of the disease and other factors. This type of evidence was later supported by that of intervention trials, which demonstrated a reduction in incidence of coronary heart disease by smoking cessation, lowering blood cholesterol and lowering blood pressure.

The epidemiological evidence was collected in a series of observational studies within specific populations, and by studies across different populations and cultures. The Seven Countries Study, initiated by Ancel Keys from Minneapolis, Minnesota, U.S.A., compared population characteristics and the presence and development of coronary heart disease across seven countries in North America, Europe and Japan. These studies were continued by his collaborators and successors, following the original populations over four decades.

The Seven Countries Study showed that major differences in personal characteristics, lifestyle and diet across the study populations were associated with large differences in prevalence and incidence of coronary heart disease. During follow up it was established that the levels of major risk factors were associated with the population and the individual risk for future coronary heart disease events. While initial epidemiological studies focused on single risk factors, the Seven Countries Study and other studies demonstrated the concept that such risk is multifactorial.

In the last decades we have observed a reduction in the deaths and incidence of early coronary heart disease in Western European and North American populations. This reduction is most likely related to improved coronary care and to reduction of several risk factors in the population, albeit that one of the strongest risk factors, smoking, has not been abolished. This reduction in population risk is certainly related to the impact of the Seven Countries Study together with other epidemiological studies, preventive practice, and public policy. More recently, clinical trials have shown a reduction in risk of development of coronary heart disease through reduction of blood pressure and blood cholesterol levels.

In this book, an overview is given of the results of the Seven Countries Study, with detailed descriptions of the populations which were studied, the prevalence and incidence of coronary heart disease in the seven countries, and the impact of specific risk factors as smoking, diet, physical activity, overweight, cholesterol and blood pressure levels, as well as diabetes. As such, this book contains important reference material for epidemiologists, physicians, and health care authorities interested in coronary heart disease, which remains the number one cause of death in Western Europe and North America, and which will shortly be the most prominent cause of death and disability in all continents.

The European Society of Cardiology, the American Heart Association, the European Atherosclerosis Society, the European Society for Hypertension, the Heart Foundations and many other organizations share a mission to improve the quality of life and life expectancy through reduction of cardiovascular diseases. The measures proposed by these organizations to reduce cardiovascular risk in the population, and to improve prognosis of individuals including patients with established coronary heart disease, have been derived from observations such as the Seven Countries Study. Accordingly, I strongly recommend this book to all who are interested in fighting heart disease and stroke.

Maarten L.Simoons, M.D.
Professor of Cardiology
Thoraxcenter
Erasmus Medical Center
Rotterdam, The Netherlands
President European Society of Cardiology

Acknowledgements

More than 40 years of research in the Seven Countries Study has depended on many people. In the first phase of the study, 12,763 men aged 40-59 were examined at baseline from 1958 to 1964. Repeat examinations took place after 5 and 10 years and mortality data were collected up to 25 years. Thereafter, repeat examinations in elderly men were carried out in Finland, The Netherlands, rural Italy, Serbia and Crete and mortality follow-up was continued in 13 of the 16 cohorts. To all participants we are most grateful. They were examined repeatedly, in some cases up to 20 visits. Without their interest and patience this study would not have succeeded.

The 40-year research period started with the "classic period," 1958-1985, carried out under the leadership of Ancel Keys from the Laboratory of Physiological Hygiene, University of Minnesota, Minneapolis, Minnesota. The surveys at baseline, 5 and 10 years follow-up were carried out by local teams of clinical and diet investigators in close collaboration with Minneapolis. Ancel Keys, Henry Blackburn and Alessandro Menotti did the central coordination in this critical phase.

The principal investigators in the different countries were:
U.S.A.: Ancel Keys, Henry Taylor, Henry Blackburn (direction and medical examinations)
Ancel Keys, Joseph Anderson, David Jacobs (dietary surveys),
Rose Hilk, John Vilandre, David Jacobs (data processing and statistical analyses)
Finland; Martti Karvonen, Sven Punsar (direction and medical examinations),
Paavo Roine, Maija Pekkarinen (dietary surveys).
Netherlands: Frans van Buchem, Louise Dalderup, Edward Bosschieter (direction and medical examinations),
Cees den Hartog, Theodora van Schaik (dietary surveys)
Italy: Flaminio Fidanza, Alessandro Menotti, Vittorio Puddu (direction and medical examinations),
Flaminio Fidanza (dietary surveys)
Greece: Christ Aravanis, Andy Dontas (direction and medical examinations),
Christ Aravanis, Helen Sdrin (dietary surveys)
Croatia: Ratko Buzina, Ivan Mohacek (direction and medical examinations),
Ratko Buzina, Anna Brodarec (dietary surveys)
Serbia: Bozidar Djordjevic, Srecko Nedeljkovic (direction and medical examinations),
Bozidar Simic, Srecko Nedeljkovic (dietary surveys)
Japan: Noburu Kimura, Hironori Toshima (direction and medical examinations),
Noburu Kimura (dietary surveys)

Fieldworkers for the baseline, 5 and 10 year follow-up survey were acknowledged in the 1967, 1970 and 1980 monographs as were the sources of financial support from both the USA and local funds.

In the second phase of the Seven Countries Study, about 1985 to the present, repeated field surveys in the elderly were carried out in Finland, The Netherlands, and rural Italy, and formed the Finland, Italy, Netherlands, Elderly (FINE) Study. Similar surveys in the elderly were carried out in Serbia and Crete. Mortality follow-up was continued in the USA, Corfu, and Japan. The fieldwork activities were coordinated by Daan Kromhout, The Netherlands and the mortality follow-up by Alessandro Menotti.

The responsible investigators of the FINE Study are:

Finland: Aulikki Nissinen (direction), Juha Pekkanen, Paula Kivinen (medical examinations).

Leena Räsänen (dietary surveys).

The Netherlands: Daan Kromhout, Bennie Bloemberg, Edith Feskens, Sandra Kalmijn (fieldwork coordinators),

Edward Bosschieter, Ans Thomassen-Gijsbers, Janny Willemsen-ten Arve (medical examinations),

Marianne Bouterse-Van Haaren, Hester Goddijn, Annemarie Jansen, Lucie Viet (coordinators dietary surveys),

Bennie Bloemberg (coordinator data processing)

Italy: Simona Giampaoli (fieldwork coordinator)

Alessandro Menotti (medical examinations),

Flaminio Fidanza (dietary surveys)

The responsible investigators of the surveys in the elderly in Serbia and Crete are:

Serbia: Srecko Nedeljkovic (direction), Miodrag Ostojic, Miodrag Grujic, Nikola Vojvodic, Slobodan Imshiragic (medical examinations),

Crete: Anthony Kafatos, Andy Dontas (medical examinations)

Anthony Kafatos (dietary surveys).

The 40-year mortality follow-up of baseline cohorts not receiving repeated examinations was carried out by:

U.S.A.: Henry Blackburn, Alessandro Menotti, Rose Hilk

Corfu: Andy Dontas, Cleo Dontas

Japan: Hironori Toshima, Yoshinori Koga, Tsutomu Imaizumi, Hisashi Adachi

Data analyses were carried out by investigators in several countries. Ph.D. students used data from each national study and from the Seven Countries Study for their theses.

This overview of collaborators during 40 years indicates that an enormous network was built over the years to carry out these population-based, multidisciplinary, cross-cultural studies. It was a pleasure and stimulus to work with so many fine colleagues from the different countries.

This book provides an overview of the main results from the Seven Countries Study, published earlier in different monographs and peer-reviewed journals. The editors took the initiative and take responsibility for this book and its conclusions. Chapters were prepared by one or two of the editors, sometimes in collaboration with a colleague, and were critically reviewed by all editors and other colleagues from The Netherlands and Belgium. We are particularly grateful to Prof. Hugo Kesteloot, Prof. Wim Saris, Prof. Evert Schouten, Prof. Jaap Seidell, Dr. Edith Feskens, Dr. Volkert Manger Cats, Dr. Jantine Schuit, Dr. Tommy Visscher, and Dr. Peter Zock for their critical comments and thoughtful remarks.

Coordination of the editing process was skillfully done by Anke Roccuzzo. Without her patience and endurance this book would never have been published. Bennie Bloemberg, who was a co-author of three chapters, was responsible for preparing the tables and graphs. The board of directors of RIVM provided Daan Kromhout the possibility to do most of his writing during the beautiful summer of 2001. We gratefully acknowledge their contributions.

PART I: BACKGROUND AND THE BURDEN OF CARDIOVASCULAR DISEASES

CHAPTER 1.1

OBJECTIVES AND HISTORY OF
THE SEVEN COUNTRIES STUDY

Henry Blackburn

The Seven Countries Study was the first to examine systematically the relation among diet, lifestyle, risk factors and the rates of coronary heart disease and stroke in contrasting populations (1-6). The idea of the study arose in various forms in the minds of individuals capable of integrating clinical, laboratory, and population evidence and curious about the origins and possible prevention of these diseases. Ancel Keys, the leader of the study, gave the concept its scope, design, impetus, and direction. He coordinated the program in seven countries, the United States, Finland, The Netherlands, Italy, Yugoslavia, Greece and Japan working from the Laboratory of Physiological Hygiene, School of Public Health, University of Minnesota, Minneapolis, U.S.A.

In the mid-1950s, when the Seven Countries Study was mounted, there was no "big science" and nothing like a Program Project existed in the agenda of the new National Institutes of Health of the U.S.A.. So there was neither precedent nor support for an optimally organised, rigorously and centrally directed, adequately funded, multi-center epidemiological undertaking. The Seven Countries Study was, nevertheless, pioneering and forward-looking for its day. It developed methods and tested major hypotheses of diet, lifestyle, and disease. It measured risk characteristics, prevalence, incidence, and mortality rates of major cardiovascular diseases, both for individuals and among contrasting populations.

HYPOTHESIS

Keys and colleagues posed the hypothesis that differences among populations in the frequency of coronary disease and stroke would occur in some orderly relation to physical characteristics and lifestyle, particularly composition of the diet, and especially of fatty acids in the diet, and to levels of serum cholesterol.

BACKGROUND AND PILOT STUDIES

The background of the study lies in Keys's application to health of physiological principles and knowledge in a quantitative human biology that he called physiological hygiene. The wartime observations and experiments of Keys and colleagues at Minnesota profoundly changed their thinking about the modifiability, by diet composition, calorie restriction, exercise, and bed rest, of such presumably immutable attributes as body build and type, circulatory responses, and blood pressure and cholesterol levels. Moreover, Keys facility with computation, including regression equations, extended their thinking to correlations among individual levels, and then among population levels, of risk attributes, diet, behaviour, and disease rates. Keys was also particularly impressed at the time with news reports of an apparent "epidemic" of heart attacks among executives in the U.S. and with reports in the medical literature of a dramatic fall and subsequent rise of cardiac deaths, especially in northern Europe, during and after World War II. He set about to study the characteristics of healthy executives with the intention to follow them for the risk of later disease. Inadequate in numbers and ranges of variables, the Minnesota Business and Professional Men's Study became, nevertheless, a pioneer longitudinal epidemiological study of cardiovascular diseases and a crucial predecessor to the Seven Countries Study.

But it was Keys's Sabbatical year at Oxford and related world travels in 1951-1952, which opened the larger issues of cultural differences in diet, behaviour, cholesterol levels and disease risk. It led to discussions with nutritional and clinical scientists such as Hugh Sinclair, Flaminio Fidanza, John Brock and others already beginning to ponder such population differences. The contrasts they explored together in the course of a few years of the early 1950s, in eating patterns, nutrient intake, blood cholesterol levels (and vital statistics on heart attack rates) by social or occupational class, in Italy, Spain, Yugoslavia, South Africa, and Japan, set off Keys's wider questioning. This led, in turn, to his conceptual formulations about the relation of mass cultural phenomena to the population burden of major heart diseases.

This rich preparation and experience led Keys and colleagues in the mid 1950s to a broad view of human biology and health. At the same historical moment, opportunities for research grew from expansion in the U.S.A. of the review and support role of the National Institutes of Health and its new National Heart Institute. At this time also, Keys's match-up with great clinicians completed the picture: he sought out, or they sought him, such leaders as Paul Dudley White of Boston (then the first Executive Director of the new National Heart Institute), Christ Aravanis of Athens, John Brock of Capetown, Martti Karvonen of Helsinki, Noboru Kimura of Japan, and Vittorio Puddu of Rome. All these remarkable physicians saw beyond the clinic and beyond the individual patient to the origins of common heart attacks in the population, its environment and culture. Distinguished nutritionists were soon brought into the picture: Paavo Roine in Finland, Cees den Hartog in the Netherlands, Flaminio Fidanza in Italy, and Ratko Buzina in Yugoslavia. Keys formulated all the ideas into grant proposals, and over the years of the study, into syntheses of the study's major monographs. But first, there were field methods to develop and pilot studies to carry out to provide evidence sufficient to back the assumptions of the central proposal and grant application to NIH. Keys, Anderson, and Grande in Minnesota pioneered modifications of chemical measurement of blood lipids and diet analyses, including measured serum samples dried on filter paper. Taylor developed sampling and recruitment and scheduling strategies for the field surveys; Brozek established standard anthropometric measures related to body mass, body configuration, and body fat distribution, while Blackburn, Rautaharju, Rose and colleagues developed protocols for medical history and physical examinations, blood pressure, electrocardiography and stress testing, and diagnosis-related classifications including the Minnesota Code (7).

Keys then enlisted the collaboration of enthusiastic colleagues in Finland (Karvonen), the Netherlands (Dalderup), Italy (Fidanza and Puddu), Yugoslavia (Buzina and Djordjevic), Greece (Aravanis and Dontas), Japan (Kimura), and the U.S.A. (Taylor and Blackburn), and launched pilot surveys in Finland in the fall of 1956 and in Italy and Crete in 1957. There the feasibility of recruitment and survey examinations was tested among total samples of rural populations of men in the target ages, 40-59. This pilot experience was conveyed in a formal application to NIH for central coordination of the study at Minnesota and for conduct of field surveys in selected regions. Henry Taylor's NIH-funded study among U.S. railworkers was treated at the outset as a non-comparable industrial U.S. population; its counterpart in Italy, the Rome Railroad Study, was added in 1962. Ancel Keys recruited the core of investigator teams and coordinated the study from the Laboratory of Physiological Hygiene located in offices under Memorial Stadium, Gate 27, at the University of Minnesota. Henry Blackburn served as Project Officer in the early years and in 1972, central coordination of follow-up and field clinical data was shifted to Alessandro Menotti at the Center for Cardiovascular Diseases, S. Camillo Hospital, Rome and the

Laboratory of Epidemiology and Biostatistics, Istituto Superiore di Sanitá (National Institute of Public Health), Rome. All field studies were carried out under the aegis of a National Heart Institute grant (#HE04697). Local support was substantial throughout. Both public and private sources, as well as the American Heart Association and World Health Organization, provided either direct or logistic support. Since 1985 the Dutch and Italian centers supported central data processing and data analysis.

SEVEN COUNTRIES STUDY SURVEYS

The baseline round of Seven Countries surveys was carried out from 1958 to 1964 in total populations of men ages 40-59, in 16 areas of the seven countries. The second and third rounds were carried out in the same season of the year, 5 and 10 years later. Follow-up for deaths in the cohorts continues to the present day. Most of the areas were stable and rural and had large and obvious contrasts in habitual diet. Central chemical analysis of foods consumed among randomly selected families in each area, plus diet recall measures in some areas, allowed an effective test of the dietary hypothesis. Little more than hearsay and crude vital statistics were then available about comparative coronary or stroke death rates in those regions. At the time, women were not considered for study because of the apparent great rarity of cardiac events among them and the invasiveness of the field examinations.

The Seven Countries Study has been extended since this early history to consider elderly cohorts in the FINE Study (Finland, Italy, the Netherlands) and in Serbia, and Crete; it has been enhanced by new dietary surveys and by new probing analyses from the younger collaborators among the investigative teams. The Seven Countries Study has in these ways periodically renewed itself and continued to seek new insights from the ongoing data.

PUBLICATIONS OF THE SEVEN COUNTRIES STUDY

The methods, baseline findings, and the first 5 and 10-years' observations of the Seven Countries Study were published in major monographs referenced below in 1967, 1968, 1970, and 1980 (1-4). Since then, emphasis has shifted to individual presentations in the world literature.

The 10 most cited publications according to the Science Citation Index till November 30, 2001 are listed in Table 1. They represent the whole spectrum of the Seven Countries Study such as the three monographs from 1967, 1970 and 1980, and papers about the Minnesota Code, serum cholesterol, obesity and different aspects of diet.

The current monograph integrates all previously published information from the Seven Countries Study on diet, lifestyle, risk factors, and coronary heart disease. It brings up to date the results, elaborates on the analyses, and summarises the long-term implications of the study, both for preventive medical practice and public health policy.

Table 1. Ten most-cited papers in the Seven Countries Study

Article	citations
Blackburn H, Keys A, Simonson E, Rautaharju PM, Punsar S. The electrocardiogram in population studies. A classification system. Circulation 1960;21:1160-1175.	309
Keys A, Aravanis C, Blackburn HW, Van Buchem FSP, Buzina R, Djordjevic BS. Dontas AS, Fidanza F, Karvonen MJ, Kimura N, Lekos D, Monti M, Puddu V, Taylor HL. Epidemiological studies related to coronary heart disease. Characteristics of men aged 40-59 in Seven Countries. Acta Med Scand 1967;460, Suppl 180:1-392	179
Keys A (Ed). Coronary heart disease in seven countries. Circulation 1970;41, Suppl 1:1-211.	707
Keys A, Fidanza F, Karvonen MJ, Kimura N, Taylor HL. Indices of relative weight and obesity. J Chron Dis 1972;25:329-343.	421
Keys A, Aravanis C, Blackburn H, Buzina R, Djordjevic BS, Dontas AS, Fidanza F, Karvonen MJ, Kimura N, Menotti A, Mohacek I, Nedeljkovic S, Puddu V, Punsar S, Taylor HL, Van Buchem FSP. Seven countries. A multivariate analysis of death and coronary heart disease. Cambridge, MA; Harvard University Press, ISBN: 0-674-80237-3, 1980:1-381.	825
Keys A, Menotti A, Karvonen MJ, Aravanis C, Blackburn H, Buzina R, Djordjevic BS, Dontas AS, Fidanza F, Keys M, Kromhout D, Nedeljkovic S, Punsar S, Seccareccia F, Toshima H. The diet and 15-year death rate in the Seven Countries Study. Am J Epidemiol 1986;124:903-915.	310
Kromhout D, Bosschieter EB, De Lezenne Coulander C. The inverse relation between fish consumption and 20-year mortality from coronary heart disease. N Engl J Med 1985;312:1205-1209.	1020
Hertog MGL, Feskens EJM, Hollman PCH, Katan MB, Kromhout D. Dietary flavonoids and the risk of coronary heart disease. (The Zutphen Elderly Study). Lancet 1993;342;1007-1011.	780
Hertog MGL, Kromhout D, Aravanis C, Blackburn H, Buzina R, Fidanza F, Giampaoli S, Jansen A, Menotti A, Nedeljkovic S, Pekkarinen M, Simic BS, Toshima H, Feskens EJM, Hollman PCH, Katan MB. Flavonoid intake and long-term risk of coronary heart disease and cancer in the Seven Countries Study. Arch Intern Med 1995;155:381-386.	322
Verschuren WMM, Jacobs DR, Bloemberg BPM, Kromhout D, Menotti A, Aravanis C, Blackburn HW, Buzina R, Dontas AS, Fidanza F, Karvonen MJ, Nedeljkovic S, Nissinen A, Toshima H. Serum total cholesterol and long-term coronary heart disease mortality in different cultures. Twenty-five year follow-up of the Seven Countries Study. JAMA 1995;274:131-136.	151

SUMMARY

The Seven Countries Study is a prototypical comparison of populations made across a wide range of diet, lifestyle, risk, and disease experience. It was the first to explore associations among diet, lifestyle, risk, and disease in contrasting populations (ecological correlations). There were, of course, limitations: the relatively small number of units for ecological correlations; the selection of the samples in the different geographic areas in part for reasons of convenience; and the technical challenges of conducting surveys across cultures by national teams, often working under difficult field conditions. However, the study was unique for its time in standardization of measurements for diet, risk factors, and disease; in training its survey teams; for its high response rates, and for the central, blindfold coding and analysis of the data. The Seven Countries Study has produced, in the end, powerful evidence for the causes of cardiovascular diseases for individuals and among different cultures, and thus provided a sound base for preventive practice and public policy.

BOOKS AND MONOGRAPHS

1. Keys A, Aravanis C, Blackburn HW, Van Buchem FSP, Buzina R, Djordjevic BS. Dontas AS, Fidanza F, Karvonen MJ, Kimura N, Lekos D, Monti M, Puddu V, Taylor HL. Epidemiological studies related to coronary heart disease. Characteristics of men aged 40-59 in Seven Countries. Acta Med Scand 1967;460, Suppl 180:1-392.
2. Den Hartog C, Buzina R, Fidanza F, Keys A, Roine P. Dietary studies and epidemiology of heart diseases. Stichting tot wetenschappelijke voorlichting op voedingsgebied, The Hague, The Netherlands 1968: 1-157.
3. Keys A (Ed). Coronary heart disease in seven countries. Circulation 1970;41, Suppl 1:1-211.
4. Keys A, Aravanis C, Blackburn H, Buzina R, Djordjevic BS, Dontas AS, Fidanza F, Karvonen MJ, Kimura N, Menotti A, Mohacek I, Nedeljkovic S, Puddu V, Punsar S, Taylor HL, Van Buchem FSP. Seven countries. A multivariate analysis of death and coronary heart disease. Cambridge, MA; Harvard University Press, ISBN: 0-674-80237-3, 1980:1-381.
5. Kromhout D, Menotti A, Blackburn H (Eds). The Seven Countries Study: A scientific adventure in cardiovascular disease epidemiology. Brouwer Offset b.v., Utrecht, ISBN 90-6960-048-x, 1994:1-219.
6. Toshima H, Koga Y, Blackburn H, Keys A (Eds). Lessons for science from the Seven Countries Study. Springer Verlag, Berlin, Heidelberg, New York, Tokyo. ISBN 3-540-70140-0, 1994:1-243.
7. Rose G, Blackburn H. Cardiovascular Survey Methods. World Health Organization, Geneva. 1968:1-188.

CHAPTER 1.2

POPULATIONS AND ORGANIZATION OF THE SURVEYS IN THE SEVEN COUNTRIES STUDY

Alessandro Menotti

The Seven Countries Study required a multi-centered population study to satisfy the aim. Feasibility studies were carried out in Finland, Italy, and Greece. Field operations were preceded by intense efforts to standardize procedures and measurements suitable to different cultures and remote areas. The first pilot field survey was conducted in Nicotera, a village in Calabria in southern Italy in the fall of 1957.

THE 16 COHORTS

The cohorts in the Seven Countries were chosen to represent cultures with apparent contrasts in lifestyle, eating habits, risk factor levels, and, presumably, incidence of and mortality from coronary heart disease (CHD), though the latter was unknown. They were not representative of the corresponding countries and their choice was partly made from convenience. However, the object was to recruit *all* men of a civic department aged 40 to 59 years at the time of their first examination.

The U.S. railroad cohort consisted of men working in the railroad industry in the midwest and northwest of the U.S., selected on the basis of their occupation involving more or less physical activity.

The East Finland cohort was a "chunk sample" of all men in the rural village of Ilomantsi and its surroundings in the region of North Karelia, Finland. The choice was linked to the allegedly high incidence of and mortality due to CHD in that area and their unusual high-fat diet.

The West Finland cohort was recruited in the southwest part of the country as a "chunk sample" of all men in the rural villages of Pöytyä and Mellilä. This was an area where incidence of CHD was thought to be lower than in the eastern part of the country on the basis of vital statistics.

The Zutphen cohort represented a 4/9 statistical sample of all men resident in the commercial town of Zutphen in the eastern part of the Netherlands.

The Crevalcore cohort was a "chunk sample" of all men living in the rural village of Crevalcore, located in northern Italy in a plains area where the traditional diet was apparently rich in animal fat.

The Montegiorgio cohort was a "chunk sample" of all men living in the rural village of Montegiorgio, located in central Italy, in a hilly area about 30 km inland from the Adriatic Sea. They apparently followed a more "Mediterranean diet" than in Crevalcore.

The Rome railroad cohort represented the Italian counterpart of the U.S. railroad group. Men working in four occupations and at different levels of physical activity were recruited in Rome and surroundings.

The Dalmatia cohort was from a number of villages along the Adriatic Sea coast, south of the town of Split in Dalmatia, Republic of Croatia within former Yugoslavia, and characterized by a Mediterranean, high vegetable diet.

The Slavonia cohort was recruited from a number of scattered villages centered around the village of Dalj in the Slavonia plain, Republic of Croatia within former Yugoslavia; the diet was presumably high in animal products.

The Zrenjanin cohort was made up of men working in an agro-industrial cooperative located in the town of Zrenjanin, north of Belgrade in the Republic of Serbia, former Yugoslavia.

The Belgrade cohort was formed by the faculty members of the University of Belgrade, located in the capital of the Republic of Serbia within former Yugoslavia.

The Velika Krsna cohort was a "chunk sample" of all men in the rural village of Velika Krsna located not far south of Belgrade, Republic of Serbia within former Yugoslavia.

The Corfu cohort, made up of men residents of rural villages located in the northern part of the island of Corfu, Greece; it was also characterized as one of the highest olive oil consuming regions.

The Crete cohort, made up of men residents of rural villages centered at Kastelli, located inland from the northern coast, and east of the capital of Heraklion on Crete, Greece. It was characterized by a high olive oil intake.

The Tanushimaru cohort was a "chunk sample" of all men resident in the rural village and farming community of Tanushimaru on the island of Kyushu, Japan.

The Ushibuka cohort was a "chunk sample" of all men resident in the village of Ushibuka, on the island of Kyushu, Japan, who were predominantly fishermen, with a high fish intake.

The cohort of Nicotera in Italy as well as another rural cohort enrolled in southern Hungary, did not become part of the study because full standardisation was not accomplished.

FIELD OPERATIONS

The field operations were carried out during periods of several weeks or months (two years for the U.S. railroad), depending on size of the cohort and logistic difficulties, which were particularly severe in remote rural areas. An international team of physicians, other professionals, technicians and nurses participated in the survey, most of the professionals having been trained at the Laboratory of Physiological Hygiene, University of Minnesota, Minneapolis. Further formal training was given to all before the start of each survey operation. Local people were assigned tasks requiring knowledge of the language and customs, while international visitors ran operations mainly involving machines and procedures. Members of the central staff of the study participated in all field examinations.

The examination of each participant included completing a questionnaire for general information, lifestyle, dietary habits and family history, anthropometric measurements, blood collection for biochemical tests, urine collection and analysis, a medical history questionnaire, and a physical examination. Blood pressure was also measured, and a resting and a post-exercise electrocardiogram were recorded; in most cohorts spirometry was done. There was a regular sequence in the various measurements.

For subsamples of men, information on habitual diet was repeatedly collected using several dietary survey methods. In some cohorts, dietary recall information was obtained from all participants. Other ancillary measurements, not belonging to the basic protocol, were taken for special purposes, including a pulse-wave recording, and work intensity questionnaires. All measurements and procedures followed standardized protocols. Several measurements and coding were made centrally, including serum cholesterol determination, ECGs, and evaluation and coding of clinical diagnoses and causes of death.

Table 1. The 16 cohorts examined in the Seven Countries Study

Area	Year(s) of entry examination	Number of subjects enrolled	Participation rate (%)
U.S. railroad, U.S.A.	1957-1959	2,571	75.0
East Finland, Finland	1959	817	99.3
West Finland, Finland	1959	860	97.0
Zutphen, The Netherlands	1960	878	84.3
Crevalcore , Italy	1960	993	98.5
Montegiorgio, Italy	1960	719	99.0
Rome railroad, Italy	1962	768	80.6
Dalmatia, Croatia, YU	1958	671	98.0
Slavonia, Croatia, YU	1958	696	91.0
Zrenjanin, Serbia, YU	1963	516	98.0
Belgrade, Serbia, YU	1964	538	80.0
Velika Krsna, Serbia, YU	1962	511	96.7
Corfu, Greece	1961	529	95.3
Crete, Greece	1960	686	97.6
Tanushimaru, Japan	1958	508	100.0
Ushibuka, Japan	1960	502	99.6
Total		12,763	90.4

PARTICIPATION RATES AT BASELINE AND FOLLOW-UP OPERATIONS

Table 1 reports, for each cohort, the year(s) of baseline examination, the number of men enrolled and the participation rate against the basic rosters; seven years were needed to complete enrollment in all areas. The participation rate averaged more than 90%, with very high rates achieved especially in rural areas.

Follow-up operations were characterized by two types of activities:
- re-examination of survivors after 5 and 10 years, following the same procedures as in the baseline examination;
- periodic collection of mortality data and causes of death;

The re-examinations after 5 and 10 years, part of the basic protocol, were performed in all cohorts, except for the 5-year anniversary in Japan and the 10-year anniversary for the U.S. railroad. Collection of data on mortality and causes of death continued in all cohorts for a minimum of 25 years, and much longer – up to 35 years – for 13 of the16 cohorts. A systematic monitoring of non-fatal cardiovascular events was possible in some areas.

After the 10-year anniversary re-examination, central funding stopped. Additional field examinations were performed with local funding and organization outside the central coordination of the international study. The list of field examinations following the baseline is given in Table 2.

Table 2. Re-examination, incidence and mortality data in the 16 cohorts of the Seven Countries Study, including the contribution of the FINE study

Area	Years of re-examinations	Follow-up period for incidence (y)	Follow-up period for mortality (y)
U.S. railroad	5	5	35
East Finland	5, 10, 15, 25*, 30*, 35*	10	35
West Finland	5, 10, 15, 25*, 30*, 35*	10	35
Zutphen	5, 10, 25*, 30*, 35*	25	35
Crevalcore	5, 10, 20, 25*, 31*, 35*	25	35
Montegiorgio	5, 10, 20, 25*, 31*, 35*	25	35
Rome railroad	5, 10	10	25
Dalmatia	5, 10	10	25
Slavonia	5, 10	10	25
Zrenjanin	5, 10, 25, 35	10	35
Belgrade	5, 10, 25, 35	10	35
Velika Krsna	5, 10, 25, 35	10	35
Corfu	5, 10	10	35
Crete	5, 10, 31	10	35
Tanushimaru	10	10	35
Ushibuka	10	10	35

* Formally part of the FINE Study

THE FINE STUDY

In the 1980s, investigators from Finland, The Netherlands and Italy organized a 25-year field re-examination in their areas according to the standard rules. A new "epigon" study was organized among the elderly – the men aged 65-84 – taking as baseline the 25-year anniversary examination. The Dutch cohort, Zutphen, was supplemented at that examination with another subgroup of men, then aged 65-84, who had not been included at the launch of the study in 1960. The new study, called FINE (Finland, Italy, The Netherlands, Elderly), had a total of 2284 men (716 in Finland, 886 in the Netherlands and 682 in Italy), with participation rates of 92%, 74%, and 76% respectively. A grant obtained from the National Institute of Aging in the United States, with Aulikki Nissinen from Finland as principal investigator, was instrumental in the development of the FINE Study.

On the occasion of the new FINE entry examination, and in subsequent examinations, some changes in the procedures were introduced to better characterize the health status of elderly men. Data were collected on physical activity, physical skill and performance, mental depression, cognitive function, and daily living habits. Re-examination took place after 5, 10, and 15 years, corresponding to years 30, 35 and 40 of the follow-up of the Seven Countries Study. A continuous monitoring of mortality and causes of death was also made.

Long-term follow-up studies on elderly men were also carried out by colleagues in Serbia and Crete, who used the Seven Countries Study protocol. In Serbia, re-examination took place after 25 and 35 years and on Crete after 31, 37 and 40 years.

The surveys to promote standardization of data collection in Serbia and Crete were supervised by Daan Kromhout and members of his team. Databases comparable to the FINE database were prepared for the Serbian and Cretan cohorts.

COORDINATION AND DATA ANALYSIS

The coordination of the Seven Countries Study was done by the Laboratory of Physiological Hygiene, University of Minnesota, under the guidance of Ancel Keys. Henry Blackburn coordinated the fieldwork during the first 10 years of follow-up. Centralized data analyses using all the study material were carried out under the leadership of Ancel Keys. After his retirement in 1972, and until 1993, the majority of the centralized analyses were done at the Istituto Superiore di Sanità (National Institute of Public Health) in Rome under the coordination of Alessandro Menotti. In 1990, Alessandro Menotti and Daan Kromhout, with the help of Bennie Bloemberg and Simona Giampaoli, prepared a new database containing risk factor data of the first three rounds, along with 25-year mortality data. This database was used for all subsequent data analyses.

Centralized analyses after 1993 were carried out jointly between the Division of Epidemiology, University of Minnesota (the successor of the Laboratory of Physiological Hygiene) and the National Institute of Public Health and Environment in Bilthoven in the Netherlands.

Daan Kromhout and Bennie Bloemberg, in cooperation with Alessandro Menotti, Aulikki Nissinen, Simona Giampaoli, Edith Feskens and co-workers, created a database containing common data in the FINE Study, with data collected in the baseline, 5- and 10- year follow-up survey and the 10-year mortality data.

The database created in 1990 for the first 25 years of follow-up, is currently being expanded for 13 of the 16 cohorts, including mortality data of at least up to 35 years. A new database was created as well; it contained not only 35-year mortality data but also risk factor data collected at baseline in the Finnish, Dutch, rural Italian, Serbian, and Cretan cohorts, with 5, 10, 25, 30 and 35 years of follow-up, respectively.

CHAPTER 1.3

PREVALENCE AND INCIDENCE OF CARDIOVASCULAR DISEASES IN THE SEVEN COUNTRIES STUDY

Alessandro Menotti

Prevalence and incidence are the two major measures of disease frequency. Prevalence is a static measurement, counting individuals with a disease at a given time. Incidence is a dynamic measurement, the occurrence of new events or cases of a disease during a defined time period. For cardiovascular diseases prevalence is a numerical indicator of the burden of disease for the society and its medical services. Incidence, on the other hand, is the prerequisite measure to estimate risk in the population through the associations between baseline characteristics (risk factors) and subsequent occurrence of the disease. The association is, of course, not necessarily causal. Moreover, incidence of cardiovascular manifestations, such as myocardial infarction or stroke, is relevant to needs for health services, since these acute and severe conditions require immediate assistance and intervention.

In the Seven Countries Study, prevalence of coronary heart disease (CHD) and other cardiovascular diseases was ascertained at entry examination and thereafter at the 5th and 10th anniversary examination. This prevalence measurement was used mainly to exclude subjects for subsequent computation of incidence rates, secondarily for a first look at comparative disease rates. After 25 years of follow-up, information on the prevalence of cardiovascular diseases was collected in the FINE Study and in the Serbian cohorts.

Ascertainment of incident cases of CHD in different cohorts and cultures was one of the primary purposes of the Seven Countries Study, and this was possible through the first 10 years of follow-up in all cohorts except the U.S. railroad where it was confined to the first 5 years. Following the 10th anniversary, collection of data on incidence was limited to the Dutch, and rural Italian cohorts. This measurement was mainly used for prediction.

This chapter provides an overview of the prevalence and incidence during the first 10 years of follow-up. In addition, the cumulative prevalence of myocardial infarction and stroke during 35 years of follow-up is described.

DEFINITIONS OF PREVALENCE AND INCIDENCE RATES OF
CARDIOVASCULAR DISEASES

Information on prevalence and incidence of different manifestations of cardiovascular diseases was collected during the first 10 years of follow-up. Diseases were angina pectoris, myocardial infarction, chronic heart disease of possible coronary origin, hypertensive heart disease, and cerebrovascular disease or stroke. Long-term information on the cumulative prevalence of cardiovascular diseases up to 35 years' follow-up is available only for myocardial infarction and stroke.

Diagnostic criteria were outlined *a priori* and can be summarized as follows:
Angina pectoris was based on the Rose questionnaire (1) and criteria applied at entry to a survey examination.
Myocardial infarction was based on a combination of clinical judgment from the Rose questionnaire (2) and on medical history of myocardial infarction, plus ECG findings from records taken at field examination. Details are reported elsewhere (2,3). Myocardial infarction was classified as definite or possible.
Chronic heart disease of possible coronary origin was based only on clinical data and corresponded to rare cases of definite or possible heart failure, or chronic arrhythmia of possible coronary origin.
Hypertensive heart disease also needed the presence of definite hypertension (160 or 95 or more mmHg), or a history of hypertension.

16

Other etiologically defined heart disease was based on clinical judgement of the examining physician.

Stroke was based on history and objective evidence of stroke with permanent paralysis, paresis or aphasia, or a history of cerebral insufficiency of short duration and objective evidence of carotid pulse deficit. It could also be based on a bruit, or evidence of paralysis or paresis only, after excluding other causes. Definite and possible diagnoses were made on the basis of slight differences. The possible diagnosis also included cases of TIA.

During the first 10 years of follow-up, both prevalence and incidence criteria were applied in a hierarchical fashion. Prevalence of CHD was defined as the prevalence of angina pectoris, myocardial infarction, or chronic heart disease of possible coronary origin. The prevalence of other heart diseases is represented by the combination of hypertensive heart disease and other etiologically defined heart disease.

CHD incidence was computed by choosing the most severe manifestation occurring in a given period among those classed as CHD deaths (see chapter 1.4) and/or incidence, after excluding prevalent cases at baseline examination. The following subgroups were used in different analyses:

- CHD deaths only
- CHD death + definite myocardial infarction = Hard CHD
- Possible myocardial infarction + angina pectoris + chronic heart disease of possible coronary origin = Soft CHD
- CHD death + definite myocardial infarction + possible myocardial infarction + angina pectoris + chronic heart disease of possible coronary origin = Any CHD

Collection of data on prevalence of cardiovascular diseases after 25 years of follow-up within the FINE Study and the independent Serbian cohorts followed the same pattern. However, the coding followed different rules:

- the diagnosis of myocardial infarction did not include the contribution of the ECG recorded at field examination and the diagnosis of possible myocardial infarction was not considered;
- the diagnosis of chronic heart disease of possible coronary origin was not considered;
- a specific diagnosis of heart failure, based on clinical history in the judgment of the examining physician (resting dyspnea at minimal effort, leg edema, etc.), and the use of specific drugs;
- the diagnosis of stroke followed the same criteria used during the first 10 years of follow-up; however, the physical examination made no contribution, and the diagnosis of a possible stroke was not considered;
- coding and analyses allowed a single individual to be treated as having several manifestations, whereas the coding and analysis system of the first 10 years' follow-up was based on a hierarchical, mutually exclusive procedure.

PREVALENCE OF CARDIOVASCULAR DISEASES

A summary of the prevalence of heart diseases at entry examination is given in Table 1. Three diagnostic categories are considered here:

- a diagnosis of CHD (any manifestation),
- diagnoses of other heart diseases due to different etiology,
- the presence of major ECG findings.

Table 1. Age-adjusted prevalence rates of heart diseases per 1,000 at entry examination in the 16 cohorts. Rates are mutually exclusive. Reconstructed and modified from reference 2.

Cohort	Any CHD	Other heart diseases	Major ECG findings
U.S. railroad	45	23	39
East Finland	55	30	21
West Finland	17	25	32
Zutphen	16	18	60
Crevalcore	11	21	50
Montegiorgio	8	35	26
Rome Railroad	14	29	37
Dalmatia	1	8	38
Slavonia	6	17	32
Zrenjanin	17	15	19
Belgrade	14	14	30
Velika Krsna	15	27	27
Corfu	5	2	62
Crete	6	24	22
Tanushimaru	6	-	61
Ushibuka	4	-	38

The ECG findings class corresponds to particular Minnesota Codes (MC, see chapter 3.5) in the absence of clinically defined heart disease: intermediate and small Q waves (MC 1.2-3), deeply negative T waves (MC 5.1-2), atrio-ventricular blocks of first and second degree (MC 6.1-2), complete left, right, and intraventricular bundle branch blocks (MC 7.1-2 and 7.4), and atrial fibrillation (MC 8.3). The criteria were applied in a hierarchical way, making figures exclusive one from the other (2).

Although large differences exist among cohorts for the three categories, they are definitely larger for CHD manifestations than for other heart diseases and ECG findings. This is partly due to some of the ECG findings being incorporated into the diagnoses of CHD. This applied especially to cohorts where CHD prevalence is high. In general, higher prevalence rates for CHD were observed in North America and northern Europe than in the other areas. This is not necessarily true for other heart diseases or ECG findings. Among other heart diseases the majority were rheumatic heart diseases.

More detailed analyses on prevalence of CHD were reported using 10 year follow-up data (3), but the numbers in each cohort were relatively small and a subdivision of data into more detailed categories proved of little use. However, it is clear that prevalence data cannot be used to detect disease associations with risk factors or possible causes due to their nature. The main use of this information has always been to exclude one or more categories from the denominators when estimating incidence, or when searching for associations between baseline characteristics and incident events.

After 25 years of follow-up, large increases in prevalence were observed in elderly men aged 65-84 (4). Table 2 shows prevalence rates for different cardiovascular manifestations in the cohorts of three European countries. These findings suggest that angina pectoris and myocardial infarction are common conditions in Finland and in

Table 2. Prevalence of cardiovascular diseases per 1,000 in elderly men aged 65-84. Rates are not mutually exclusive. Reconstructed and modified from reference 4.

Cardiovascular disease	Finland	Netherlands	Italy
Angina pectoris	19.7[b]	10.3	9.5[c]
Myocardial infarction	13.6	12.2	4.8[c, d]
Coronary heart disease[a]	24.8[b]	16.0	13.2[c]
Heart failure	4.0	4.3	4.6
Stroke	9.3[b]	3.6	5.0[c]

a = Angina pectoris + myocardial infarction   c = Finland vs Italy, p< 0.05
b = Finland vs Netherlands, p < 0.05   d = Netherlands vs Italy, p < 0.05

the Netherlands. Prevalence rates of heart failure were similar in the three countries. Stroke was most common in Finland followed by Italy. The lowest stroke rates were observed in the Netherlands.

TRENDS IN CUMULATIVE PREVALENCE OF MYOCARDIAL INFARCTION AND STROKE DURING 35 YEARS

Long-term trend analysis could only be made after re-coding the diagnoses of the first 10 years of the Seven Countries Study follow-up, so as to render them comparable to those of the FINE Study and the independent Serbian cohorts. For this analysis the contributions of the physical examination and the ECG taken at field examination during the first 10 years of follow-up were excluded and the hierarchical coding system was abandoned. The cumulative prevalence was calculated by dividing the number of prevalent cases accumulated over time by the number of men examined in each survey.

During the first 25 years of follow-up, the highest cumulative prevalence rate of definite myocardial infarction was observed in East Finland (Table 3). At 35 years of follow-up similar rates were noted in the three northern European cohorts. Substantial increases in the cumulative prevalence of definite myocardial infarction during 35 years of follow-up were observed in the Italian cohorts Crevalcore and Montegiorgio and during the first 25 years in the three Serbian cohorts. At year 35, slightly lower rates were seen in East Finland, Zrenjanin and Belgrade, compared to year 25. This could be attributed to natural selection among severely ill patients.

Similar data on the prevalence of definite stroke were only available starting in 1970 due to a stricter application of the diagnostic criteria (Table 4). Between 1970 and 1985 a substantial increase in the prevalence of stroke was observed in all eight European cohorts. During the next 10 years the prevalence of stroke stayed stable or increased in six of the eight cohorts but was more than 50% lower in the Serbian cohorts Zrenjanin and Velika Krsna. This was due to the high death rates in these cohorts (see chapter 1.4)

Table 3. Trends in age-adjusted cumulative prevalence of definite myocardial infarction cases (%) during 35 years of follow-up.

| Year | 1960 | | 1970 | | 1985 | | 1995 | |
| Age | 40-59 | | 50-69 | | 65-84 | | 75-94 | |
Cohort	N	%	N	%	N	%	N	%
East Finland	817	5.5	656	11.5	313	18.1	119	16.1
West Finland	860	1.2	720	4.5	380	10.1	149	15.7
Zutphen	878	0.8	627	5.8	361	14.3	146	17.8
Crevalcore	997	0.2	799	3.1	373	7.0	147	9.0
Montegiorgio	719	0.1	606	2.4	309	3.0	124	7.3
Zrenjanin	517	0.9	436	1.4	177	7.3	55	5.9
Belgrade	538	0.6	436	2.2	288	8.0	142	6.9
Velika Krsna	511	0.2	437	0.6	227	2.0	74	3.5

Table 4. Trends in age-adjusted cumulative prevalence of definite stroke cases (%) during 25 years of follow-up

| Year | 1970 | | 1985 | | 1995 | |
| Age | 50-69 | | 65-84 | | 75-94 | |
Cohort	N	%	N	%	N	%
East Finland	656	4.0	318	13.1	120	15.9
West Finland	720	2.7	386	10.5	148	13.9
Zutphen	627	0.8	360	4.3	146	8.2
Crevalcore	799	2.2	373	6.0	146	7.8
Montegiorgio	606	4.8	304	9.6	122	9.3
Zrenjanin	436	2.5	180	10.6	52	4.1
Belgrade	436	1.5	286	9.6	139	10.3
Velika Krsna	437	0.7	227	8.7	74	3.1

INCIDENCE OF CORONARY HEART DISEASE

The 5-year Seven Countries Study monograph published in 1970 reported incidence data for all cohorts (2). Large differences were observed, but rates were based on small numbers of events. In any case it was the first time that a systematic study conclusively demonstrated large differences in CHD incidence among different cultures and populations.

Numbers derived from the 10-year follow-up gave more solid rates, with a summary reported in Table 5 and Figure 1. Manifestations were computed on the basis of a hierarchical system, while a subject with more than one event during the period is classified only for the most severe event, based on an empirical classification (death, major, non-fatal, soft). Due to the data collection procedure and diagnostic criteria, the most reliable figures are considered to be those for CHD deaths and hard CHD events. "Hard criteria" CHD practically corresponds to definite fatal and non-fatal myocardial infarction, including sudden death of coronary origin and other fatal coronary conditions. Large differences were seen among cohorts for all of the endpoints considered. High incidence rates in North America and northern

Table 5. Age-adjusted CHD incidence rates per 1,000 during 10 years of follow-up, with rates mutually exclusive. Reconstructed and modified from reference (3)

Cohort	CHD deaths	Hard non-fatal CHD	Hard[a] CHD	Soft CHD	Any[b] CHD
U.S. railroad	42	39	81[c]	153[c]	234[c]
East Finland	68	39	107	180	287
West Finland	25	29	54	104	158
Zutphen	32	19	51	56	107
Crevalcore	23	22	45	63	108
Montegiorgio	12	23	35	62	97
Rome railroad	25	11	36	43	79
Dalmatia	7	11	18	45	63
Slavonia	17	8	25	31	56
Zrenjanin	15	9	24	47	71
Belgrade	25	7	32	47	79
Velika Krsna	7	6	13	32	45
Corfu	15	19	34	35	69
Crete	0	3	3	18	21
Tanushimaru	7	8	15	20	35
Ushibuka	5	15	20	26	46

a = Hard CHD = CHD deaths + hard non-fatal CHD;

b = Any CHD = hard CHD + soft CHD

c = Estimation based on average ratios between coronary death and other events derived from other areas.

Figure 1. CHD incidence rates in eight countries. Age-standardized rates per 1,000 in 10 years.

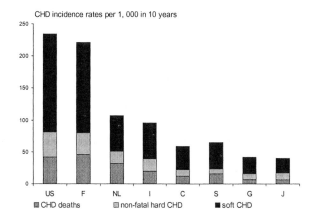

US = U.S.A.; F = Finland; NL = The Netherlands; I = Italy; C = Croatia; S = Serbia; G = Greece; J = Japan

Europe contrasted with low rates in southern Europe and Japan. The highest rates were those in East Finland, the lowest in Crete and the Japanese areas.

The ratios between pairs of CHD manifestations were quite uniform. On average, out of 100 hard CHD cases there were 50 CHD deaths; out of 100 any CHD cases there were 38 hard events and 20 coronary deaths. The most interesting ratio is CHD death to hard CHD events; this was 0.50, suggesting that persons free of CHD at baseline who experience a major CHD event in the course of 10 years' follow-up have a 50% risk of dying in 10 years. This figure, although approximate, represents the fatality rate for major CHD events in the Seven Countries Study.

A correlation matrix was constructed to evaluate the relationship among different components of CHD events, although some are composite and contain part of the information of other components (data not reported here in detail). All the correlation coefficients found were about 0.90 and some were close to 1, except for that of CHD deaths with hard non-fatal events (0.78). This suggests that beyond possible bias and uncertainties in classification of the several CHD manifestations, there is substantial coherence in the incidence of CHD manifestations in the different cohorts.

Figure 2. Correlation between 10-year hard CHD incidence and 25-year CHD death rates.

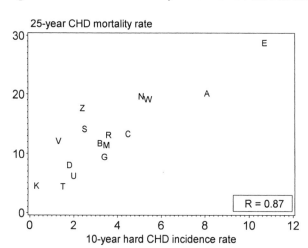

For legend see appendix

In the same matrix we considered the correlation between 25-year mortality from CHD and all possible components of incidence after 10 years of follow-up. The original values of 25-year CHD death rates can be found in chapter 1.4. In this case, the correlation of 10-year incidence of hard CHD with 25-year CHD mortality is high (0.87), although it is known that during the 10- to 25-year period cohorts were characterized by different increments in the rates of CHD deaths (Fig. 2). The associations of the other 10-year CHD incidence manifestations with the 25-year CHD death rates were high but lower than the previous ones.

These results suggest that CHD death rates are a good approximation of incidence, at least for relatively short periods. With increasing follow-up periods the association among different CHD death rates may wane due to changes in the occurrence of events in different cohorts.

COMMENTS

During the early phase of cardiovascular epidemiology, the Seven Countries Study was the only study specifically designed to detect differences in CHD rates among different populations. It is not possible to directly compare prevalence and incidence findings of the Seven Countries Study with those of other longitudinal investigations because detailed information on diagnostic criteria used in the different studies is lacking. Thus any comment on the literature can only refer to the capability of other studies in showing cross-cultural differences in the burden posed by CHD.

The Seven Countries Study showed a high CHD prevalence in U.S.A. and northern Europe and a low prevalence in southern Europe and Japan. Other comparisons were attempted among a few populations (e.g. the Ni-Hon-San Study (5), and among the Framingham, Honolulu and Puerto Rico Studies (6), as well as between the Framingham and Yugoslavia Heart Studies (7)). The Ni-Hon-San Study had the opportunity to compare men of the same ethnic background living in fairly different environments; it found higher rates of the disease in California, lower in Japan, and intermediate in Hawaii. The CHD burden was systematically higher in Framingham than in the other areas.

The CHD incidence data of the Seven Countries Study during the first 10 years of follow-up formed the first reliable indication that different populations and cultures suffer different proportions of disease measured by standardized criteria. The highest 10-year CHD incidence rates were observed in Finland and The Netherlands. The lowest rates were observed in southern Europe and Japan.

The procedure used for measuring incidence was the same in all cohorts; it was based on information collected during baseline, and 5- and 10-year surveys. To calculate incidence, information on both fatal and non-fatal cases is needed. The actual number of new events during 10 years of follow-up has been underestimated for the following reasons:

- incidence data were not obtained from people not present at 5- and 10-year examinations;
- subjects who died from a non-coronary disease before a given survey could have had a major non-fatal coronary event during the interval between the last examination and death; this event could not be classified as an incident event.

Information on this type of bias was obtained from Italian rural areas, where a systematic monitoring system was organized. It was shown that during 25 years of follow-up, the number of hard CHD events observed by the standard procedure underestimated the total number of actual events by 17% (8), the difference being major non-fatal coronary events. This underestimate would likely have been smaller during the first 10 years of follow-up because of lower incidence rates during this period. The influence of this type of bias has probably been small due to the high participation rates in the follow-up surveys of all cohorts.

Recently a large study, the WHO-MONICA Project (9), based on a different methodological approach, confirmed the existence of large differences in major CHD events among populations. Direct comparisons cannot be made since the MONICA registration system has produced, so far, the average of 10-year incidence data in population groups geographically defined but no data for cohorts followed longitudinally. The age range was comparable (35 to 64 years), but each year one new age group came in and one went out from the denominator. Therefore there was no aging effect in the estimate of incidence. Moreover, the diagnostic criteria were not entirely comparable. Despite the large changes in CHD mortality rates (and probably CHD incidence rates) observed during the years before and during the observation period (about 1985 to 1995), the highest CHD incidence rates were still present in Finnish areas. Incidence rates in the U.S. were lower than in Finland, but higher than the two Italian areas. The Yugoslavian areas (located in Serbia) had higher rates than the Italian ones. The ranking of the population rates was practically the same for the MONICA Project as for the 25-year CHD mortality ranking in the Seven Countries Study, but data from the Netherlands, Croatia, Greece and Japan were not available from the MONICA Project.

Incidence rates beyond the 10th anniversary were collected only in a few areas and following different procedures and criteria. As an example, incidence of a first major coronary event was 177 per 1,000 in 25 years in the pool of the two rural Italian areas (8). Taking the 10-year incidence of major CHD events reported in Table 5 as a reference (an average of 40 per 1,000 in 10 years), this means that between year 10 and year 25 the cumulative incidence has increased fourfold.

SUMMARY AND CONCLUSIONS

The Seven Countries Study was the first to show true differences in prevalence, incidence and mortality for CHD among populations with different geographical, ethnic, and cultural characteristics. The possible existence of such differences could be hypothesized on the basis of official mortality data and anecdotal findings, but only this study was able to show them on the basis of a uniform and standardized approach.

At baseline, high prevalence rates of CHD were observed in the U.S.A. and East Finland and low rates in the southern European and Japanese cohorts. Data from eight European areas showed that during 25 years of follow-up the cumulative prevalence of myocardial infarction was highest in East Finland and increased in Crevalcore (northern Italy), and in the Serbian cohorts Zrenjanin and Belgrade. Till 1985, the cumulative prevalence of stroke increased substantially in all European cohorts. When these populations reached the gerontological age of 65 to 94 years the prevalence of myocardial infarction and stroke remained high. In northern Europe the prevalence for both myocardial infarction and stroke varied between 10 and 18% and in southern Europe between 2 and 10%.

The large differences in 10-year incidence of and mortality from CHD (strongly correlated) showed high rates in northern European and North American cohorts, with exceedingly high levels in East Finland, lower rates in southern Europe and the lowest in some Mediterranean areas, as well as in Japan. The differences in 10-year hard CHD, substantially representing the incidence of myocardial infarction, were on the order of fivefold or greater between the extremes. The fatality rate, based on hard incidence data, although somewhat variable, was on average about 50%.

REFERENCES

1. Rose G, Blackburn H. Cardiovascular Survey Methods. Geneva. World Health Organization. 1968: 1-188.
2. Keys A (Ed). Coronary heart disease in seven countries. Circulation 1970, 41, Suppl 1: 1-211.

3. Keys A, Aravanis C, Blackburn H, Buzina R, Djordjevic BS, Dontas AS, Fidanza F, Karvonen MJ, Kimura N, Menotti A, Mohacek I, Nedeljkovic S, Puddu V, Punsar S, Taylor HL, Van Buchem FSP. Seven countries. A multivariate analysis of death and coronary heart disease. Cambridge MA; Harvard University Press, ISBN:0-674-80237-3, 1980:1-381.

4. Menotti A, Mulder I, Nissinen A, Giampaoli S, Feskens EJ, Kromhout D. Prevalence of morbidity and multimorbidity in elderly male population and their impact on 10-year all cause mortality: The FINE study (Finland, Italy, The Netherlands, Elderly). J Clin Epidemiol 2001; 54: 680-686.

5. Robertson TL, Kato H, Gordon T, Kagan A, Rhoads GC, Land CE, Worth RM, Belsky JL, Dock DS, Miyanishi M, Kawamoto S. Epidemiological studies of coronary heart disease and stroke in Japanese men living in Japan, Hawaii and California. Am J Cardiol 1977; 39: 244-249.

6. Gordon T, Garcia-Palmieri MR, Kagan A, Kannel WB, Schiffman J. Differences in coronary heart disease in Framingham, Honolulu and Puerto Rico. J Chron Dis 1974; 27: 329-344.

7. Kozarevic D, Pirc B, Racic Z, Dawber TR, Gordon T, Zukel WJ. The Yugoslavia Cardiovascular Disease Study. 2. Factors in the incidence of coronary heart disease. Am J Epidemiol 1976; 104: 133-140.

8. Menotti A, Verdecchia A, Dima F. The estimate of coronary incidence following different case finding procedures. Eur Heart J 1989;10:562-572.

9. Tunstall-Pedoe H, Kuulasmaa K, Mahonen M, Tolonen H, Ruokokoski E, Amouyel P, for the WHO MONICA Project. Contribution of trends in survival and coronary event rates to changes in coronary heart disease mortality: 10-year results from 37 WHO MONICA Project populations. Lancet 1999; 353: 1547-1557.

CHAPTER 1.4

CARDIOVASCULAR AND ALL-CAUSES MORTALITY PATTERNS IN THE SEVEN COUNTRIES STUDY

Alessandro Menotti, Mariapaola Lanti

In prospective population studies, mortality data are relatively easy to collect. Their diagnostic accuracy is usually acceptable, and the fact and date of death are certain. They allow us to use mathematical models based on life tables. Moreover, mortality data for a population sample can be compared with those of other studies and with official national mortality statistics. Finally, in the absence or incompleteness of non-fatal event ascertainment, mortality data represent a good approximation to incidence, especially if adjustment can be made relating fatal to non-fatal events.

Mortality data are important indicators of the health status of a population. This justifies the considerable attention paid to secular trends in death rates, which, during the last few decades, have characterized coronary heart disease (CHD), cardiovascular diseases, and all-causes mortality. Downward trends for CHD, stroke, and cardiovascular deaths were seen in most Western countries. This started in the late 1960s in the U.S.A. and spread to Europe, Australia, New Zealand, and Japan in the 1970s and 1980s. These trends mark new phenomena in the history of public health (1,2). Before the 1970s there had been a definite up-turn in these diseases in the Western world, from a predominance of infectious diseases to chronic non-communicable diseases, primarily cardiovascular diseases and cancer, as leading causes of death. This trend is seen now in the developing countries. Projections made to the year 2020 (3) estimate that worldwide there will be a predominance of non-communicable diseases as the major causes of death, led by CHD and stroke. This will lead to a change in health status in developing and developed countries and a further increase in life expectancy.

In the Seven Countries Study, mortality data were collected during the 1960-1985 period. These data are used to describe trends in mortality from cardiovascular and all-causes mortality for a period of 25 years. Also mortality data for elderly men collected between 1985 and 1995 are reported.

CODING MORTALITY DATA

Data on mortality and causes of death were collected systematically in all cohorts for 25 years of follow-up. Altogether only 56 men (0.4 %) were lost to follow-up, all of whom were members of cohorts in former Yugoslavia. In addition elderly men from Finland, The Netherlands and Italy were followed for 10 years. Only 7 men (0.3%) were lost to follow-up.

Methodology for collection of data was similar in the cohorts. Deaths occurring in a given sample were periodically reported at the local registry offices, or in special files if the sample was occupational, for the 25 years of follow-up. Usually the underlying causes of death reported on the official certificate were used as a preliminary indication by the research team, and other sources were considered for assigning the final cause of death. The search was made by collecting and reviewing data from previous clinical records completed by the research group, from hospital and necropsy records, family and hospital doctors. Information was also gained from relatives, friends and other witnesses, from the police in cases of violent causes or death suddenly in public places or without witnesses, and medical records made available by the family. This procedure was used in all cohorts except the U.S. railroad, for which only subsamples of cases were validated by hospital records, and for the Finnish samples, where after 15 years of follow-up only death certificates were available. This information was evaluated by two investigators (H. Blackburn and A. Menotti for the first 10 years and subsequently A. Menotti only), who assigned the

28

final diagnosis, exploiting all possible data and following defined diagnostic criteria reported elsewhere (4).

The 8th revision of the WHO-ICD was used for coding causes of death (5). A special code was added (A795) for the identification of sudden coronary death (within 2 hours of onset of the symptoms) when other causes could be reasonably excluded. Systematic priorities were adopted in the assignment of first and subsequent causes of death in the case of apparent multiple causes. The following hierarchy was used:

- violent causes;
- cancer in advanced stage;
- coronary heart disease in its typical manifestations (angina, infarction, sudden death);
- stroke;
- "atherosclerotic or ischemic heart disease" in the absence of angina and infarction;
- others.

Priorities in the choice of secondary causes of death (up to three) were also defined and followed. Mortality codes, and especially coronary mortality, were further compacted according to the so-called LPH (Laboratory of Physiological Hygiene) codes, as related to the first cause of death assigned by the research group (4,6).

After 25 years of follow-up, new surveys were carried out among elderly men for eight cohorts (East Finland, West Finland, Zutphen in the Netherlands, Crevalcore and Montegiorgio in Italy, Zrenjanin, Belgrade, and Velika Krsna in Serbia). These men were then followed for another 10 years. Although the general rules for mortality collection and coding procedures for these elderly men were similar, the following differences were noted:

- death certificates were made available to only a single reviewer (AM);
- the WHO-ICD-9 (7) instead of the WHO-ICD-8 (5) was used;
- no special code was adopted for sudden CHD death, which was included in the rubrics 410-414;
- cardiac fatal events manifested by heart failure or chronic arrhythmia, in the absence of typical CHD manifestations or mention, were coded as such and not as CHD.

In addition, a parallel coding was produced following the traditional rules in order to make comparable all codes from year 0 to year 35 of follow-up.

CARDIOVASCULAR AND ALL-CAUSES MORTALITY RATES DURING 25 YEARS

Death rates from all-causes and CHD were described in the 5- and 10-year monographs of the Seven Countries Study (4,6). However, no details were given on causes of death other than all-causes and coronary, nor on time trends in death rates. Only recently a partial review of 25-year mortality rates has been carried out (8).

Table 1 summarizes the 25-year experience in the 16 cohorts for all-causes and cardiovascular diseases mortality. For all-causes mortality there is not a clear-cut geographical trend; the highest rates are located in Slavonia, closely followed by East Finland and Zrenjanin. The highest rate, in Slavonia, is due to high rates from stroke, chronic bronchitis, infectious diseases (mainly pulmonary tuberculosis), and violent deaths. In East Finland the high death rate is due to CHD and lung cancer, and in Zrenjanin to stroke and cancers other than lung cancer. Beyond these three cohorts,

29

Table 1. Age-adjusted 25-year cardiovascular and all-causes death rates per 1,000 in the 16 cohorts. Partly derived from reference 8.

Cohort	Cause of death				
	AC	CHD	STR	CVD	CA
U.S. railroad	451	202	36	263	114
East Finland	597	288	49	370	127
West Finland	503	192	45	263	123
Zutphen	480	197	38	248	178
Crevalcore	498	134	52	210	169
Montegiorgio	462	115	77	198	123
Rome railroad	397	132	47	197	122
Dalmatia	433	81	83	180	100
Slavonia	610	142	109	263	108
Zrenjanin	579	177	120	306	131
Belgrade	295	119	45	177	84
Velika Krsna	500	122	93	227	103
Corfu	404	95	68	183	109
Crete	314	46	72	127	89
Tanushimaru	394	45	84	131	131
Ushibuka	515	63	108	175	181

AC= all causes; CHD = coronary heart disease; STR = stroke;
CVD = all cardiovascular diseases; CA = cancer

only three (West Finland, Velika Krsna, and Ushibuka) experienced a death rate of 50% or more in 25 years. Low death rates were recorded in the Rome railroad and the Belgrade cohorts (occupational), in Crete and in Tanushimaru. The 25-year life expectancy was obviously highly related to death rates (e.g. 18.7 years in Slavonia and 18.7 years in East Finland, against 21.8 in Belgrade and 22.4 in Crete).

The geographic distribution of CHD death rates reflects the typical trend already known from analyses on shorter follow-up periods. The highest levels are located in the U.S. cohort and in northern Europe (especially East Finland), while lower levels are found in southern Europe and Japan. Crete and Tanushimaru have very low rates, whereas in the Serbian cohorts (mainly Zrenjanin) and Slavonia, rates are similar to or higher than in Italy. Despite the large cross-cultural differences, CHD is the first cause of death in all cohorts except Dalmatia, Crete, and the two Japanese cohorts.

The geographic trend for stroke death rate is the inverse of the one for CHD, the highest rates in areas of southern Europe, mainly Serbia and Croatia, and Japan; the lowest in the Netherlands. The highest death rates from cancer were found in Zutphen, Crevalcore, Zrenjanin and the two rural Japanese cohorts.

A summary of death rates for a selected number of major causes, considering eight entities instead of 16 cohorts is given in Fig. 1. The levels of all-causes mortality rate are mainly determined by major cardiovascular diseases (CHD and stroke), but in some areas cancer (in the Netherlands, Italy, and Japan) or "other diseases" (in Croatia) are major contributors. The picture is complex; only for some causes of death can a clear geographic trend be detected. A ratio of 0.40 or greater of CHD to all-causes mortality is typical for areas with the highest death rates from CHD (i.e. the

30

Figure 1. Age-adjusted 25-year death rates per 1,000 from combined causes in the eight entities.

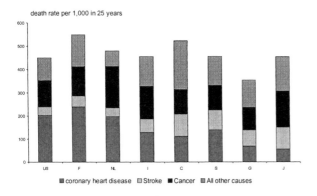

death rate per 1,000 in 25 years

■ coronary heart disease ☐ Stroke ■ Cancer ▨ All other causes

US = U.S.A.; F = Finland; NL = The Netherlands; I = Italy; C = Croatia; S = Serbia; G = Greece; J = Japan

Table 2. Correlation matrix among some pairs of death rates in the 16 cohorts.

Cause of death		Cause of death	Corr.coeff.
Coronary heart disease	vs	All-causes	0.58
Cardiovascular diseases	vs	All-causes	0.78
All cancers	vs	All-causes	0.42
Other causes	vs	All-causes	0.20
Coronary heart disease	vs	Stroke	-0.42
Cardiovascular diseases	vs	Coronary heart disease	0.94
Cardiovascular diseases	vs	All-cancers	0.15

U.S., northern Europe, and Belgrade). Four or five fatal CHD events occurred in North America and northern Europe for each stroke event, while the ratio in Dalmatia, Crete and Japan is less than 1.

Another way to look at the same problem is to inspect correlation coefficients between pairs of death causes, as given in Table 2. CHD and cancer are highly correlated with all-causes mortality, forming its major component, but they are not highly correlated with each other. On the other hand, CHD and stroke are inversely correlated (r = -0.42). The reasons for this finding have been explored in a separate paper (9).

MORTALITY RATES IN ELDERLY MEN

These data are derived from the five cohorts in three European countries, which participated in the FINE Study, with entry age of 65 to 84 years. A total of 716 men were enrolled in Finland (two rural cohorts: East and West Finland), 886 in the Netherlands (Zutphen, enhanced by a new subgroup of men of the same age, who were added to the 25-year survivors of the original study), and 682 in Italy (two rural cohorts from Crevalcore and Montegiorgio) (8).

Table 3. Age-adjusted 10-year death rates per 1,000 in the five cohorts of the FINE Study

Cohort	Cause of death					
	AC	CHD	STR	HF	CVD	CA
East Finland	600	226	99	3	328	145
West Finland	541	195	74	8	291	132
Zutphen	478	112	53	22	223	149
Crevalcore	426	93	62	14	243	110
Montegiorgio	451	44	102	46	210	134
Finland	567	209	86	7	309	137
Italy	438	72	79	28	224	123

AC = all-causes; CHD = coronary heart disease; STR = stroke; HF = heart failure; CVD = all cardiovascular diseases; CA = all cancers

The 10-year death rates in elderly men are summarized in Table 3. The grouping for different cardiovascular diseases and all-causes mortality was similar to that of the first 25 years of follow-up in the regular cohorts. In general, half the elderly men died during 10 years of follow-up. During the first 25 years of follow-up of younger men, also about 50% of the men died. The overall picture in elderly men is similar to that for the first 25 years of follow-up. Apart from the higher death rates, due to the effect of aging, the inter-cohort and inter-country differences are found along the same lines as in the previous period of follow-up. The Finnish cohorts show the highest rate for all-causes mortality, for CHD and cardiovascular diseases; the Dutch cohort shows an intermediate all-causes death rate, but has the highest rate of lung cancer and chronic bronchitis, and a low rate for stroke. The Italian cohorts show the lowest rates for all-causes and CHD mortality, and relatively high rates for stroke and cancer (mainly in Montegiorgio). The death rate for heart failure shows an increasing north-to-south trend, which may be due to death certificates recording. Overall, during these 10-years of follow-up among elderly men, mortality rates due to all cardiovascular

Figure 2. Age-adjusted 10-year death rates from combined causes per 1,000 in the three countries of the FINE Study.

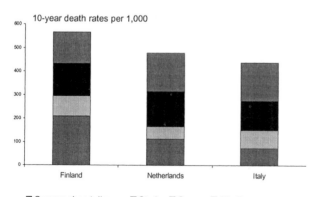

■ Coronary heart disease ☐ Stroke ■ Cancer ■ All other causes

diseases were similar in the Netherlands and Italy, due to higher rates as a result of CHD in the first country and from stroke in the latter.

A representation of death rates is given in Fig. 2; here, only CHD, stroke, cancer and other causes are considered in the three countries. The most striking differences are the high CHD rate in Finland and the low stroke rate in the Netherland.

TIME TRENDS IN CARDIOVASCULAR AND ALL-CAUSES MORTALITY RATES

The 16 cohorts were combined into eight regional entities to report trends in major causes of death and to obtain more stable rates. Former Yugoslavia was split in two parts (i.e. Croatia, the combination of Dalmatia and Slavonia, and Serbia, the combination of Zrenjanin, and Belgrade, and Velika Krsna).

Trends in mortality were modeled by a newer analytical approach, the accelerated failure time model, a log-linear model incorporating the Weibull distribution (10). Independent solutions were produced for each entity using only age as the co-variate. The back application of the coefficients (plus the constant and the scale factor) was applied to a man aged 50 (i.e. the mean or median age for all the cohorts at baseline), and the hazard was estimated for each year during a 25-year period. From these estimates, curves describing the time trend of the hazard were produced for CHD and stroke. For each cause, two curves were drawn:
- a curve describing the cumulative hazard in the 25 years,
- a curve describing the annual increment of hazard, year by year, during the 25 years.
- The first resembles any cumulative risk during a defined period; the second, changes in the risk of death year by year, independent of the cumulative risk of death reached. Curves for CHD and stroke are given in Figs. 3 to 6, where each curve is described.

Coronary heart disease, cumulative hazard (Fig.3). The increase in the cumulative hazard during the course of 25 years was universal, with three groups of countries being prominent: Finland, along with the Netherlands and the United States at the top; Greece and Japan at the bottom and the other three southern European entities (Italy, Croatia, and Serbia) in between. Large changes were observed. The cumulative hazard for the Netherlands reached that of the United States at year 24; the cumulative hazard for Serbia, among the lowest at the beginning of follow-up, overtook Greece and Japan during the first few years, Croatia at around year 17 and Italy at year 20.

Coronary heart disease, annual increment of the hazard (Fig. 4). The curves for Finland and the U.S. tended to flatten out (i.e. no increase in the annual hazard) around year 22, and that of the Netherlands towards the end of the follow-up period. The curve for Serbia rose higher than those for Greece and Japan at year 5, Croatia at year 11, Italy at year 13; the U.S. at year 18, the Netherlands at year 20 and Finland at year 23, showing a remarkable increase during the whole follow-up period. Although located at different levels, the curves for Italy and Croatia, and separately for Greece and Japan, increases at a regular rate along almost a straight line.

Figure 3. Cumulative hazard during 25 years of follow-up for CHD mortality in the eight entities derived from the accelerated failure time model.

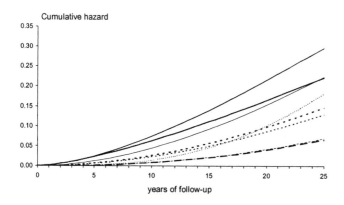

Figure 4. Annual increment of hazard during the 25-year follow-up for CHD mortality in the eight entities derived from the accelerated failure time model

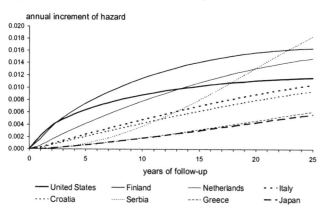

Stroke, cumulative hazard. (Fig. 5) The curves for all countries increased in an exponential fashion. The curve for Serbia rapidly overtook all others except that for Croatia, which remained the highest. Curves at the lowest levels are those of the U.S. and the Netherlands.

Stroke, annual increment of hazard.(Fig. 6) All curves tend to rise during the 25 years, except for a slight tendency to flattening for the U.S. and Italy. After the first few years, the curve of the annual increment for Serbia overtook all except that of Croatia, which was overtaken around year 17.

COMMENTS

Since it is uncommon to find detailed mortality data on causes of death in population studies, comparisons cannot be made. On the other hand, a comparison with official mortality statistics by country is not *a priori* a proper one, since the cohorts examined in the Seven Countries Study are not random or representative samples of each country. Despite this, coherent relationships were found for death rates from all-

Figure 5. Cumulative hazard during 25 years of follow-up for stroke mortality in the eight entities derived from the accelerated failure time model.

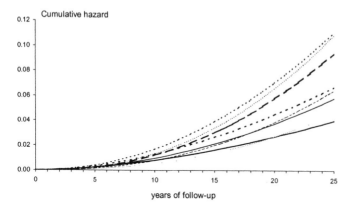

Figure 6. Annual increment of hazard during 25 years of follow-up for stroke mortality in eight entities, derived from the accelerated failure time model.

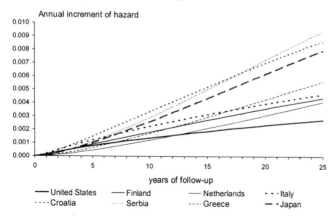

causes and CHD during the first 5 and 10 years of follow-up. The rank in mortality rates matched well the rank of official vital statistics of CHD mortality for those years (4,6).

Differences in all-causes, CHD, stroke and other conditions in the Seven Countries Study, were tentatively explained in papers dealing with inter-cohort (ecological) analyses, reported in different chapters in this book. These differences pointed to different cultural-geographic distributions of the several causes of death. These were characterized by high rates for CHD in northern Europe and the U.S., high rates for stroke in some areas of southern Europe and Japan, high rates for lung cancer in northern Europe, and high rates for other cancers in Japan. Although limited to five European cohorts, the picture given by the 10-year follow-up mortality rates among elderly men in the FINE Study is similar to the one observed during the previous 25 years of follow-up, which started from the age range of 40 to 59 years.

The findings indicate that the dynamics of CHD, stroke, cardiovascular diseases, and cancer mortality in the eight entities of the Seven Countries Study had different forms, characterized by different accelerations or decelerations of risk, during the 25 years of follow-up. Studying the first five years of follow-up in Figs. 3 to 6, we see that large changes in trends could not be expected, and the only conclusions from the early reports dealing with 5- and 10-year data are that large cross-cultural differences exist in several causes of death (3,4). What happened later was largely unexpected, mainly in relation to the Serbian cohorts, whose mortality from CHD and stroke, accelerated at a greater rate than in any other group. These included the Finnish group where the cumulative rates were and remained among the highest. During the first five years of follow-up even the Serbian death rates from CHD and stroke were very low and expected to remain low, like those from Greece and Japan. They were also partly accounted for by low levels of important risk factors such as serum cholesterol and blood pressure (4,6). The increases became evident after the first 10 years of follow-up and appeared even larger when risk factor measurements were taken at 25 years of follow-up (11-13).

Earlier ecological analysis of the Seven Countries Study data showed a direct relationship between change in average population serum cholesterol level and subsequent coronary deaths (14). Other analyses, carried out at the individual level, showed how increases of systolic blood pressure during the first 10 years of follow-up were associated with an excess of cardiovascular and stroke deaths in the late follow-up period (15). Although we remain cautious, because of the limited statistical units, rises in the mean population levels of major coronary risk factors, largely documented in Serbia, would seem to offer a reasonable explanation for the form of the annual hazard during the last part of the follow-up period, at least for CHD.

A relative decrease, or a lesser increase, in the instantaneous annual hazard for CHD was shown for cohorts belonging to three countries, that is, the U.S.A., Finland, and the Netherlands. These are the same countries where, in the same historical period – starting in the late 1960s or early 1970s – a marked decline in official CHD mortality (and perhaps incidence) rates was recorded. On the other hand, it is known that a decline in CHD mortality started at least 10 years later in Italy, was uncertain in Japan, and poorly documented in Greece and elsewhere. The situation of Serbia, instead, could be compared to that reported in national statistics of other Central and Eastern European countries, where an extraordinary increase in death rates from CHD was recorded for the same years. This has been reported by many studies using official mortality data (1,2,16), including a specific review of the issue made especially for the countries of the Seven Countries Study (17); here, it was clearly shown that extraordinary increases in CHD mortality occurred in Serbia in those years. On the other hand, the northern European and American cohorts, where the rate of increase of the hazard tended to flatten, showed smaller increases or even a decline in mean population levels of major risk factors (8).

Caution should be taken, however, in interpreting these data and in making comparisons with official mortality statistics. In fact, trends described in this analysis could reflect only in part those of official CHD and cardiovascular diseases mortality in the corresponding countries. This is because the changing hazards described here refer to aging populations during a 25-year period, while the official decline or increase in CHD mortality rates are usually reported for specific age-adjusted death rates, and for defined age ranges (different in the various reports).

These observational changes anticipated the final results of the WHO-MONICA Project, where spontaneous risk factor changes in either direction were correlated to increases or declines in coronary incidence and mortality (18,19). However, these findings from the MONICA Project are seen only when there is a four-year gap between risk factor change and coronary events. This means that a lag time must be taken into account before observing the possible effects of risk factor changes. In this regard, the MONICA Project suffers from a relatively short observation period.

Overall, a long-term observational study, such as the Seven Countries Study, provides findings that larger, more recent, and shorter duration studies are now starting to reveal. Long-term trends in population risk factor levels are found to anticipate and predict changes in CHD and cardiovascular diseases mortality.

SUMMARY AND CONCLUSIONS

Data on mortality and causes of death were systematically collected in the Seven Countries Study cohorts for 25 years. The major causes of death in most of the cohorts were cardiovascular diseases, although in different proportions and with different composition. CHD was the most common cardiovascular disease in all cohorts except in Crete, Dalmatia, and the Japanese areas, where stroke was the predominant condition. The highest death rates from CHD were located in Finland, the U.S., and the Netherlands, while the lowest rates were seen in Mediterranean areas and Japan, and intermediate rates in inland southern Europe. Despite the major role of cardiovascular diseases in determining all-causes mortality, overall death rates were highest in Slavonia, and due to other causes of death such as infectious diseases, chronic bronchitis and violence, and in East Finland in relation to CHD and in Zrenjanin due to stroke. Among the lowest all-causes death rates, were those seen in Mediterranean southern Europe and in the occupational cohorts of Belgrade professors and Rome railroad men.

The mortality experience of elderly men in five cohorts from Finland, The Netherlands and Italy, was not basically different from that during the previous 25 years. The highest all-causes and CHD mortality rates were found in Finland, with the Netherlands at an intermediate position and Italy at a lower level. The highest stroke mortality rate was located in one of the Italian areas (Montegiorgio); the same cohort had shown fairly high death rates from this cause of death in the past. Overall, the 10-year mortality experience for these men, aged 65 to 84 years, was of the same magnitude as for those enrolled at the age of 40 to 59 years and followed for 25 years. Secular trends in these aging cohorts differed among countries. Any cause of death increased in a roughly exponential fashion in all countries. However, the annual increment of death rates showed different pictures. In particular, the annual increment of rates for CHD declined until almost stable rates were reached in the U.S., Finland and The Netherlands; it was relatively stable in other areas except in Serbia, where the annual increment increased markedly until it overtook that of all other countries. The trend of death rates in Serbia has been largely explained by changes occurring in population risk factor levels and was similar to trends found in other countries of Central and Eastern Europe. Trends in stroke mortality were less diverse, but again, a larger increase in rates in Serbia and Dalmatia characterized the changing epidemic of cardiovascular diseases during those years.

Summing up, the mortality findings in the 16 cohorts and 8 entities of the Seven Countries Study mirrored well the mortality trends occurring in the second part of the

20th century in several parts of the world. Despite the large changes in mortality during this period the overwhelming contribution of cardiovascular diseases to total deaths remained basically unchanged.

REFERENCES

1. Uemura K, Pisa Z. Trends in cardiovascular diseases mortality in industrialized countries since 1950. Wld Hlth Statist Quart 1988; 41: 155-178.
2. National Heart Lung and Blood Institute. Report of the Task Force on Research in Epidemiology of Cardiovascular Diseases. Bethesha MD, US DHHS, 1994.
3. Murray CJ, Lopez AD. Alternative projections of mortality and disability by cause 1990-2020: Global Burden of Disease Study. Lancet 1997; 349: 1498-1504.
4. Keys A (Ed). Coronary heart disease in seven countries. Circulation 1970;41, Suppl 1: 1-211.
5. World Health Organization. International classification of diseases and causes of death. 8th Revision. Geneva, World Health Organization, 1965:1-616.
6. Keys A (ed), Aravanis C, Blackburn H, Buzina R, Djordjevic BS, Dontas AS, Fidanza F, Karvonen MJ, Kimura N, Menotti A, Mohacek I, Nedeljkovic S, Puddu V, Punsar S, Taylor HL, Van Buchem FSP. Seven countries. A multivariate analysis of death and coronary heart disease. Cambridge MA; Harvard University Press 1980:1-381.
7. World Health Organization. International classification of diseases and causes of death. 9th Revision. Geneva, World Health Organization, 1975:1-773.
8. Menotti A, Blackburn H, Kromhout D, Nissinen A, Adachi H, Lanti M, for the Seven Countries Study Research Group. Cardiovascular risk factors as determinants of 25-year all-causes mortality in the Seven Countries Study. Eur J Epidemiol 2001;17:337-346.
9. Menotti A, Blackburn H, Kromhout D, Nissinen A, Karvonen M, Aravanis C, Dontas A, Fidanza F, Giampaoli S. The inverse relation of average population blood pressure and stroke mortality rates in the Seven Countries Study: a paradox. Eur J Epidemiol 1997;13: 379-386.
10. Afifi AA, Clark V. Computer aided multivariate analysis. Van Nostrand Reinhold Co. New York 1990:1-505.
11. Nedeljkovic S, Menotti A, Keys A, Ostojic MC, Grujic MZ, Kromhout D, Stojanovic G. Coronary heart disease in three cohorts of men in Serbia followed-up for 25 years as a part of the Seven Countires Study. Kardiologija 1992, 1-2: 35-44.
12. Nedeljkovic S, Ostojic MC, Grujic MZ, Josipovic V, Keys A, Menotti A, Seccareccia F, Lanti M, Kromhout D. Coronary heart disease in 25 years. The experience in the three Serbian cohorts of the Seven Countries Study. Acta Cardiol 1993; 48: 11-24.
13. Kromhout D, Nedeljkovic S, Grujic MZ, Ostojic MC, Keys A, Menotti A, Katan MB, Van Oostrom MA, Bloemberg BPM. Changes in major risk factors for cardiovascular diseases over 25 years in the Serbian cohorts of the Seven Countries Study. Int J Epidemiol 1994; 23: 5-11.
14. Menotti A, Blackburn H, Kromhout D, Nissinen A, Fidanza F, Giampaoli S, Buzina R, Mohacek I, Nedeljkovic S, Aravanis C, Toshima H. Changes in population cholesterol levels and coronary heart disease deaths in seven countries. Eur Heart J 1997; 18: 566-571.
15. Menotti A, Keys A, Blackburn H, Karvonen M, Punsar S, Nissinen A, Pekkanen J, Kromhout D, Giampaoli S, Seccareccia F, Fidanza F, Nedeljkovic S, Aravanis C, Dontas A, Toshima H. Blood pressure changes as predictors of future mortality in the Seven Countries Study. J Hum Hypertension 1991, 5: 137-144.
16. Thom T, Epstein FH, Feldman JJ, Leaverton PE, Wolz M. Total mortality and mortality from heart disease, cancer and stroke from 1950 to 1987 in 27 countries. NIH, NHLBI, NIH Publication No.92-3088, Bethesda, MD 1992.

17. Toshima H, Koga Y, Blackburn H, Keys A (Eds). Lessons for science from the Seven Countries Study. A 35-year collaborative experience in cardiovascular diseases epidemiology. Tokio, Springer, 1994;1-243

18. Tunstall-Pedoe H, Kuulasmaa K, Mahonen M, Tolonen H, Ruokokoski E, Amouyel P. Contribution of trends in survival and coronary-event rates to changes in coronary heart disease mortality: 10-year results from 37 WHO MONICA Project populations. Monitoring trends and determinants in cardiovascular disease. Lancet 1999; 353: 1547-1557.

19. Kuulasmaa K, Tunstall-Pedoe H, Dobson A, Fortmann S, Sans S, Tolonen H, Evans A, Ferrario M, Tuomilehto J. Estimation of contribution of changes in classic risk factors to trends in coronary-event rates across the WHO MONICA Project populations. Lancet 2000; 355: 675-687.

PART II: DIET, LIFESTYLE AND CORONARY HEART DISEASE

CHAPTER 2.1

DIET AND CORONARY HEART DISEASE
IN THE SEVEN COUNTRIES STUDY

Daan Kromhout, Bennie Bloemberg

During the first part of the past century, research on diet and coronary heart disease focused on cholesterol. The original diet–heart hypothesis related cholesterol in the diet to cholesterol in blood and cholesterol in the atherosclerotic plaque. This hypothesis was based on dietary experiments in rabbits, carried out at the beginning of the 20th century by Ignatowski and Anitskow in Leningrad, and by cross-cultural comparisons made by the Dutch physician, De Langen (1). He compared the diet, plasma cholesterol concentrations, and the frequency of coronary heart disease among the natives of the island of Java and Dutch immigrants (2). Compared with the largely vegetarian and rice-eating Javanese, the Dutch consumed a Western diet. The blood cholesterol concentrations were twice as high in the Dutch as in the Javanese. Western "metabolic diseases" such as diabetes, gallstones, nephritis, and CHD were almost non-existent among the Javanese.

In the original diet–heart hypothesis the emphasis was on the detrimental effect of dietary cholesterol and animal fat. In his book "Chinese lessons to Western Medicine," which appeared in 1941, Snapper was probably the first who pointed to a possible protective effect of polyunsaturated fat (3). Sinclair stressed the importance of different fatty acids in the etiology of CHD in a letter to the editor published in the Lancet in 1956 (4). He pointed to the detrimental effects of saturated fatty acids and unsaturated *trans* fatty acids produced by partial hydrogenation of polyunsaturated fatty acid-rich oils for margarine production. He hypothesized that a high intake of saturated fatty acids and of unnatural *trans* fatty acids in combination with a chronic relative deficiency of essential fatty acids would promote coronary atherosclerosis and thrombosis. Essential fatty acids are polyunsaturated fatty acids from the N-6 family (i.e. linoleic acid and arachidonic acid) present in vegetables oils and of the N-3 family (i.e. eicosapentaenoic acid and docosahexaenoic acid) present in seafood. These fatty acids may protect against coronary atherosclerosis and thrombosis.

Research in the second part of the 20th century was dominated by studies on the effects of different saturated, monounsaturated and polyunsaturated fatty acids on blood lipoproteins and coronary atherosclerosis, and thrombosis. Besides interest in the role of fatty acids, the interest in antioxidants also boomed, especially after experimental work suggested that not native LDL but modified LDL (oxidized LDL) plays a central role in the development of atherosclerosis (5). In this context it is not only nutritive antioxidants (e.g. carotenoids, tocopherols, and vitamin C) that may play a role, but also so-called non-nutritive antioxidants (e.g. polyphenols abundantly present in plant foods).

This chapter, then, summarizes the ecological relationships between diet and CHD in the Seven Countries Study. First, the dietary survey methods, and food and nutrient patterns of the cohorts around 1960 will be described, and trends in diet over a period of 30 years will be reported. Secondly, the role of diet in explaining population rates of CHD will be dealt with, special attention being paid to the Mediterranean dietary pattern.

DIETARY SURVEY METHODS

In the Seven Countries Study different dietary survey methods were used. The record method was used to determine the average food consumption of small subsamples of the 16 cohorts (6). The dietary history method was used in surveys in which the food consumption of all members of different cohorts was determined. In 1960 this method was introduced in the Zutphen cohort and later on in the Italian and Finnish cohorts (7-9).

In most cohorts the seven-day food record was used in combination with precise weighing (6). Generally 20 to 50 families were selected. The participant or the nutritionist recorded the type of foods and the amount eaten. The same amount as consumed by the participant was weighed and put into a container for chemical analysis. The food samples were analyzed for water, ash, protein, total fat, and fatty acids in central laboratories of the Universities of Minnesota and Naples. The nutrient intake was also determined using food tables and comparative studies were carried out. Seasonal variation in food consumption was substantial, but variation in macro nutrient intake (e.g. fatty acids) was small (10). It is possible that substantial variation in dietary antioxidants occurred but this was not investigated.

The fatty acid content of the diet was determined by both chemical analysis and food tables (10). The fatty acid content of fat-rich foods (e.g. meat, milk, lard, and olive oil) varies considerably. For instance, around 1960 the fat content of beef varied from 14% in lean beef to 39% in very fat beef (10). This means that a valid estimate of the fat intake can only be obtained from accurately collected food consumption data. It is therefore necessary to validate nutrient intake data obtained from calculations using food tables by data obtained from direct chemical analysis. Several of these comparative studies were carried out in the Seven Countries Study, and showed good agreement between the average intake of fatty acids obtained by both methods (6).

The record data were used to characterize groups and not individuals. For characterization of the food consumption pattern of individuals and for studying relationships between foods or nutrients, and the occurrence of coronary heart disease, information on *habitual* food consumption is needed. The cross-check dietary history provides this type of information. The interview is generally carried out by a nutritionist or dietician and consists of three steps. First, information is collected about the usual food consumption pattern during weekdays and weekends. This is checked by collecting information on the average consumption of food for the duration of a day or a week. The second check consists of either keeping a 3-day record or estimating the quantities of food bought for the whole family during a week (7,11). This test revealed yet undetected errors, such as incorrect estimates. On the basis of all information collected, the usual food consumption was calculated. The interview generally takes at least an hour and coding the data takes a couple of hours per participant. This method is therefore very time-consuming and was only carried out in the Dutch, Italian, and Finnish cohorts, where special funds for dietary surveys in individuals were available. These data were converted into nutrients using national food tables. Computerized versions of these food tables became available after 1975. It therefore took a long time before the data were coded in a comparable way - according to both food groups and nutrients - for analysis in the different countries (12).

The concept differs, depending on whether the record or the dietary history method is used. The record method provides information on the *current* food consumption, while the dietary history methods provide information about the *usual* food consumption. This leads, for instance, to a difference in energy intake between the two methods. The dietary history method overestimates the average energy intake, compared with the record method (13). This is due to the fact that participants in a study tend to overestimate the intake of infrequently consumed foods. Because of the different concepts behind the two dietary survey methods, and the different results obtained by the two methods, we will describe separately the results obtained by the record and the dietary history method.

FOOD AND NUTRIENT INTAKE AROUND 1960

Between 1959 and 1964, dietary surveys using the record method were carried out in 14 of the 16 cohorts (14). Two surveys were held around 1970. It took, however, till 1986 before all data collected were coded in a standardized way. All foods were coded as the edible part of raw products, and were combined in 15 homogeneous food groups and a heterogeneous group. The average consumption of these 16 food groups was calculated per person per day for each cohort.

In 1987 equivalent food composites representing the average food intake of each cohort *at baseline* were collected from local markets (15). These foods were transported in cooling boxes to the laboratory of the Department of Human Nutrition, Wageningen University in the Netherlands. The foods were cleaned and equivalent food composites prepared according to the average consumption pattern of each cohort. The foods were homogenized and frozen until chemical analyses of the different nutrients could take place. In this chapter the emphasis will be on fatty acids and antioxidants. The methods for determining these nutrients have been described in detail in several publications (16-18).

Characteristic food patterns were established in 1960. In the United States the consumption of fruit, meat, and pastries was high (14) (Tables 1-3). The northern European diet was characterized by a high consumption of milk, potatoes, butter or margarine, and sugar products. The continental diet of several Yugoslavian cohorts

Table 1. Average amount of vegetable foods consumed per person in g per day of the 16 cohorts in 1960 (14).

Cohort	Bread	Cereals	Potatoes	Legumes	Vegetables	Fruit
U.S. railroad	97	26	124	1	171	233
East Finland	380	71	273	1	108	40
West Finland	356	99	296	8	104	34
Zutphen	252	17	252	2	227	82
Crevalcore	349	149	30	5	140	191
Montegiorgio	358	171	56	21	194	28
Rome railroad	249	113	29	6	260	150
Dalmatia	435	64	214	7	200	6
Slavonia	440	120	129	40	198	1
Zrenjanin	425	83	136	15	245	185
Belgrade	244	50	86	12	179	145
Velika Krsna	794	29	28	22	115	1
Corfu	450	45	150	30	191	462
Crete	380	30	190	30	191	464
Tanushimaru	5	497	95	103	174	26
Ushibuka	10	449	34	79	222	42

Table 2. Average amount of animal foods consumed per person in g per day of the 16 cohorts in 1960 (14).

Cohort	Meat	Fish	Eggs	Cheese	Milk
U.S. railroad	273	3	40	18	231
East Finland	105	58	11	19	1192
West Finland	107	7	35	18	1090
Zutphen	138	12	27	31	447
Crevalcore	154	22	54	24	313
Montegiorgio	85	35	39	9	8
Rome railroad	226	30	25	33	77
Dalmatia	117	96	31	4	434
Slavonia	188	35	51	21	228
Zrenjanin	212	7	19	16	184
Belgrade	175	19	27	51	335
Velika Krsna	70	0	37	203	191
Corfu	35	60	5	14	70
Crete	35	18	25	13	235
Tanushimaru	8	93	19	0	28
Ushibuka	8	207	39	0	23

Table 3. Average amount of food remaining and consumed per person in g per day of the 16 cohorts in 1960 (14).

Cohort	Edible fats	Sugar products	Pastries	Alcohol 100%	Rest
U.S. railroad	33	24	95	6	91
East Finland	96	91	13	1	39
West Finland	72	101	12	2	28
Zutphen	79	72	29	3	29
Crevalcore	58	38	6	79	25
Montegiorgio	63	7	4	64	19
Rome railroad	51	19	12	65	56
Dalmatia	88	39	0	95	3
Slavonia	70	22	0	21	51
Zrenjanin	55	26	2	12	12
Belgrade	49	54	6	5	24
Velika Krsna	28	1	0	12	2
Corfu	75	13	0	31	109
Crete	95	20	0	15	107
Tanushimaru	3	13	0	18	23
Ushibuka	7	26	5	25	25

was generally high in bread and meat or cheese. The Italian cohorts had a high consumption of cereals and wine. The four Mediterranean cohorts two from Greece, one from Croatia, and one from Italy, had a high intake of olive oil in combination with a high intake of fruit in Greece, a high intake of fish and wine in Croatia, and a high intake of cereals in Italy. The Japanese cohorts were characterized by a high intake of fish, rice, and soy products.

Table 4. Type and average amount of visible fats consumed per person in gram per day of the 16 cohorts in 1960 (18).

Cohort	Butter	Margarine	Lard	Olive oil	Sunflower oil	Other
U.S. railroad	26	4				3[a]
East Finland	89	8				
West Finland	66	7				
Zutphen	21	56	2			
Crevalcore	13		7	32	4	3[b]
Montegiorgio			40	24		
Rome railroad	4		2	43		
Dalmatia			17	72		
Slavonia			62	8		
Zrenjanin			44		12	
Belgrade	18		9		28	
Velika Krsna			24		5	
Corfu				75		
Crete				95		
Tanushimaru						3[c]
Ushibuka						7[b]

a= soy bean oil   b = peanut oil   c = rapeseed oil

Detailed analysis of the type and amounts of visible fats consumed showed a very high average intake of butter in Finland (about 75 g per day) and intermediate amounts in the United States, The Netherlands and Belgrade (about 20 g per day; Table 4) (18). Margarine consumption was high in the Netherlands (about 55 g per day) and lard consumption in the Italian cohorts, Crevalcore and Montegiorgio, and in Slavonia (30-60 g per day). Olive oil consumption was highest in Crete (95 g per day) followed by Corfu and Dalmatia (about 75 g per day). Sunflower oil consumption was highest in Belgrade and Zrenjanin (12-28 g per day), and in the Japanese cohorts the most commonly consumed oil was rapeseed oil (3-7 g per day). This shows large variation in the type of fats consumed by the different cohorts.

The fatty acid analyses in duplicate portions of foods collected during the baseline survey were repeated 25 years later in food composites, representing the average food consumption of the 16 cohorts around 1960 (15). This was done because in 1960 it was not possible to determine the different *trans* fatty acids and the N-3 polyunsaturated fatty acids. At that time there was also no interest in the role of antioxidants in the etiology of CHD.

For 13 of the 16 cohorts information was available on fatty acid determinations carried out 25 years apart (15). The correlation between the two determinations of the average population intake was 0.92 ($p < 0.001$) for saturated fatty acids, 0.93 ($p < 0.001$) for monounsaturated fatty acids and 0.52 ($p = 0.07$) for polyunsaturated fatty acids. The relatively low correlation for polyunsaturated fatty acids was due to a mere twofold range in intake compared to a 6-or 7- fold range for saturated and monounsaturated fatty acids.

Figure 1. Average intake of different saturated fatty acids (SAFA) (g per day) of the 16 cohorts in 1960.

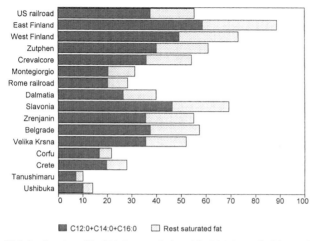

C12:0 = lauric acid, C14:0 = myristic acid, C16:0 = palmitic acid

Figure 2. Average intake of different monounsaturated fatty acids(MUFA) (g per day) of the 16 cohorts in 1960.

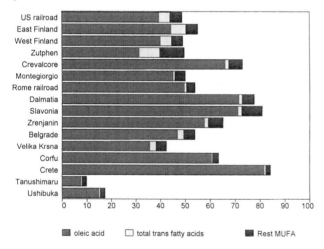

49

Figure 3. Average intake of different polyunsaturated fatty acids (PUFA) (g per day) of the 16 cohorts in 1960.

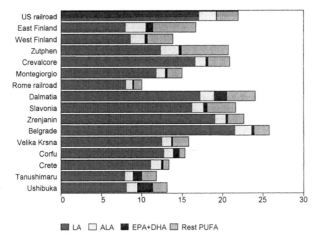

LA = linoleic acid   ALA= α-linolenic acid,
EPA = eicosapentaenoic acid   DHA = docosahexaenoic acid

Figure 4. Average population intake of different antioxidants (mg per day) of the 16 cohorts in 1960.

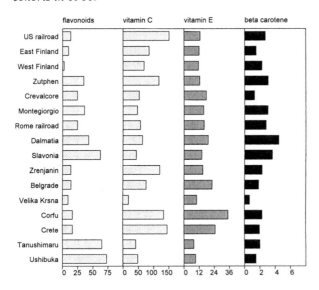

Chemical analysis of the fatty acids carried out in 1987 showed that the average intake of saturated fatty acids was highest in east and west Finland, and Slavonia (70-90 g per day), and the lowest in the Mediterranean and Japanese cohorts (10-30 g per day (Fig. 1) (15). The intake of *trans* fatty acids was highest in Zutphen (The Netherlands) (8 g per day) and the consumption was close to zero in the Mediterranean and Japanese cohorts (Fig. 2). The intake of monounsaturated fatty acids was highest in the Mediterranean cohorts (50-85 g per day) and lowest in Japan (10-20 g per day). The consumption of polyunsaturated fatty acids was divided into N-6 and N-3 polyunsaturated fatty acids (Fig. 3). The most important contributor to the N-6 polyunsaturated fatty acids is linoleic acid (C 18:2, N-6) and to the N-3 polyunsaturated fatty acids α-linolenic acid (ALA, C18:3, N-3) , eicosapentaenoic acid (EPA, C20:5, N-3) and docosahexaenoic acid (DHA, C 22:6, N-3). The highest intake of linoleic acid was found in Belgrade and Zrenjanin (Serbia) (about 20 g per day) and the lowest in Finland and Japan (about 8 g per day). The highest intake of ALA was present in the Finnish diet (2 – 2.5 g per day) and the lowest in the Italian, Greek, and Japanese diet (0.8 – 1.3 g per day). The cohorts characterized by a high fish intake, the Japanese cohorts and Dalmatia, had the highest intake of EPA and DHA (1 – 2 g per day). The lowest intake was found in Velika Krsna (0.2 g per day).

Large differences were also observed in the average population intake of antioxidants. The intake of beta-carotene (Fig. 4) was the highest in the Croatian cohorts, Dalmatia and Slavonia (3 – 4 mg per day), and the lowest in Velika Krsna (Serbia) (0.6 mg per day) (17). Vitamin E intake was highest in the Greek cohorts (about 30 mg per day) and lowest in the Japanese cohorts (about 8 mg per day). The United States and the Greek cohorts had the highest intake of vitamin C (about 135 mg per day), and Velika Krsna (Serbia) had the lowest intake (17 mg per day). The intake of flavonoids was highest in Japan (about 65 mg per day) and lowest in Finland (about 5 mg per day) (16).

Characteristic food and nutrient patterns were concluded to be present in 1960. The consumption of dairy food (e.g. milk and butter) was high in Finland, The Netherlands, and the United States. Also the consumption of meat was very high in the United States. The cohorts from the United States, Finland and the Netherlands, were also characterized by a high intake of saturated fatty acids (>20% of energy). The continental diet, as observed in Serbia, was characterized by a high consumption of bread, meat or cheese. The saturated fat intake of these cohorts was intermediate and varied between 15 and 20% of energy. The Italian cohorts Crevalcore and Rome had a relatively high consumption of meat (150-225 g per day) and eggs (40-55 g per day) and their intake of saturated fat varied between 10 and 15% of energy. The Mediterranean diet characterized by a high consumption of olive oil, either in combination with cereals (Montegiorgio), fish (Dalmatia) or fruit (Crete and Corfu) was low in saturated fat (7 – 10% of energy) and high in monounsaturated fat and vitamin E. The Japanese cohorts had a high intake of fish, rice, and tea, a very low (≤ 5% of energy) intake of saturated fat, and a high intake of flavonoids (> 60 mg/d).

TRENDS IN FOOD AND NUTRIENT INTAKE IN THE COURSE OF 30 YEARS

Dietary data were, with some exceptions, not collected repeatedly in the cohorts of the seven countries. In Finland and The Netherlands food consumption data were collected using the record method in middle-aged men studied outside the context of the Seven Countries Study around 1985 (19,20). In Finland cross-sectional dietary surveys were carried out in the context of the FIN MONICA Project in east and west Finland in 1982. For the purpose of this overview the data from east and west Finland were averaged. The data of the Dutch men in Zutphen in 1960 could be compared with those of a representative sample of Dutch men of the same age surveyed in 1987-1988. For Italy only repeatedly collected dietary data with the dietary history are available. In 1965 all men in the cohorts of Crevalcore and Montegiorgio were surveyed using this method. The total number of men was 1541 and their average age was 55 years. In 1991 small samples of men with an average age of 41 years with 23 men from Crevalcore and 18 men from Montegeorgio were surveyed (21). These men were the sons and nephews of the men who participated in the Seven Countries Study since 1960. The data of these men were averaged.

Repeat dietary survey data in men of the same age were also collected in Dalmatia and Japan (22,23). These data were less detailed than those collected in Finland, The Netherlands, and Italy and will therefore be shortly summarized. In Dalmatia sons of the men who participated in the Seven Countries Study were surveyed. This provided the possibility to compare dietary data of men aged 40-49 in 1960 and 1989 (22). In Japan repeat dietary surveys using the 24-hour recall method were carried out in men age 40-64 between 1958 and 1989 (23).

Between 1959 and 1982 a decrease in the consumption of cereal products, potatoes, milk, fats and oils, and sugar was found in middle-aged men from Finland (Table 5). A substantial increase was noted in the consumption of meat and fruit. Generally, although less pronounced, similar changes were observed in the Netherlands between 1960 and 1988. The most remarkable increase in the Netherlands in that period was in the consumption of alcohol. In Italy large increases were observed in the consumption of vegetables, cheese, and pastries between 1965 and 1991. The consumption of legumes, potatoes, fruit, meat, and milk increased also. Substantial decreases were observed in the consumption of bread, eggs, fats and oils, and wine. These differences are partly confounded by the 14 year average difference in age between the men surveyed in 1965 and 1991. However especially the large decreases and increases in the consumption of different food groups cannot be explained by this age difference.

In Dalmatia middle-aged men showed large increases in the consumption of vegetables, fruit, meat, eggs, and milk products, and decreases in the consumption of fish, oils, and wine (22). In Japan the consumption of meat increased from 13 g per day to 75 g per day, and of milk from 13 g per day to 74 g per day (23). The fish consumption increased from 56 g per day in 1958 to 97 g per day in 1968, and varied thereafter around 100 g per day . The rice consumption decreased from 593 g per day to 232 g per day.

The consequences of these changes in the diet were a decrease in total and saturated fat in Finland and the Netherlands, and more polyunsaturated fat in Finland (Table 6). In Italy small changes were observed in the intake of total fat and different fatty acids but the intake of dietary fiber decreased substantially. The largest changes were found in the contribution of alcohol to energy intake. This increased from less than 1% of energy to 2% of energy in Finland, and about 6% of energy in the Netherlands. In Italy a decrease from about 20% to about 14% of energy was observed. The changes in the diet in Dalmatia suggest that the intake of saturated fat probably increased and the intake of unsaturated fat decreased (22). As in Italy, a decrease of more than 50% occurred in the contribution of alcohol intake to total energy. In Japan the total fat intake increased from 5% to 22% of energy; a concomitant decrease in carbohydrate was observed from 78 to 61% of energy (23).

Individual dietary data using the dietary history method were collected in1960 in Zutphen, 1965 in Montegiorgio and Crevalcore, and 1969 in east and west Finland (7-9). These surveys were repeated in these cohorts at regular intervals. The changes in

Table 5. Trends in average food groups (g per day) in middle-aged men from Finland, The Netherlands and Italy from 1959 to 1991. Derived from references 14, 19, 20, 21, 26.

Year	1959	1982	1960	1987/88	1965	1991
Number	60	441	45	661	1541	41
Age (y)	40-59		40-59		45-64	28-53
Method	Record		Record		Diet hist	
Food group	Finland		Netherlands		Italy	
Cereal products	443	270	269	218	460	366
Legumes	5	-	2	8	9	20
Potatoes	285	167	252	157	24	40
Vegetables	106	89	227	162	55	246
Fruit	37	279	82	117	175	248
Meat	106	175	138	143	112	175
Fish	33	41	12	11	22	27
Eggs	23	29	27	19	17	8
Cheese	19	24	31	36	13	32
Milk	1141	770	447	334	97	131
Fats and oils	84	64	79	59	60	38
Sugar	96	46	72	58	13	14
Pastries	13	-	29	38	12	71
Alcohol (100%)	2	3	3	22	82	59

Table 6. Trends in average energy and nutrient intake in men from Finland, The Netherlands, and Italy from 1959 to 1991. Derived from references 15, 19, 20, 26, and personal communication Fidanza.

Year	1959	1982	1960	1987/88	1965	1991
Number	60	441	45	661	1541	41
Age (y)	40-59		40-59		45-64	28-53
Method	Record		Record		Diet hist	
Energy/nutrient	Finland		Netherlands		Italy	
Energy (kcal)	3467	2909	2702	2696	2897	3023
Energy (MJ)	14.5	12.2	11.3	11.3	12.2	12.6
Protein (%E)	12.9	14.7	13.2	13.4	10.5	13.7
Fat (%E)	40.0	38.5	45.5	40.3	26.6	28.1
Carbohydrate (%E)	46.8	44.5	40.7	40.7	43.0	44.7
Alcohol (%E)	0.4	2.3	0.7	5.7	20.0	13.5
Saturated fat (%E)	21.0	19.6	20.3	16.5	7.8	7.0
Monounsaturated fat (%E)	13.5	13.1	16.5	15.5	16.3	18.6
Polyunsaturated fat (%E)	4.0	4.9	6.9	6.9	2.5	2.5
Cholesterol (mg)	515	514	476	359	238	255
Fiber (g)	47	-	25	27	39	25

Table 7. Trends in average food groups (g per day) in aging men from Finland from 1969 to 1989. Derived from references 12, 24.

	East Finland			West Finland		
Year	1969	1969	1989	1969	1969	1989
Age (y)	50-69	50-69	70-89	50-69	50-69	70-89
Food group	N=612	N=96[a]	N=96[a]	N=694	N=127[a]	N=127[a]
Cereal products	321	339	234	350	355	216
Legumes	7	7	3	7	7	3
Potatoes	262	271	152	306	304	160
Vegetables	87	98	142	71	70	104
Fruit	76	80	242	91	88	212
Meat	145	159	116	148	145	102
Fish	59	56	68	22	17	42
Eggs	23	22	20	34	36	30
Cheese	9	11	16	13	16	24
Milk	1094	1177	952	1101	1074	887
Fats and oils	81	85	58	73	71	58
Sugar	102	119	41	70	77	41
Alcoholic drinks	17	18	21	23	23	46

Table 8. Trends in average energy and nutrient intake in aging men from Finland from 1969 to 1989. Derived from references 12, 24.

	East Finland			West Finland		
Year	1969	1969	1989	1969	1969	1989
Age (y)	50-69	50-69	70-89	50-69	50-69	70-89
Energy/nutrient	N=612	N=96[a]	N=96[a]	N=694	N=127[a]	N=127[a]
Energy (kcal)	3664	3986	2719	3731	3746	2672
Energy (MJ)	15.4	16.7	11.4	15.7	15.7	11.2
Protein (%E)	13.1	12.9	15.9	12.9	12.8	14.4
Fat (%E)	37.9	38.1	36.5	38.1	37.4	39.1
Carbohydrate (%E)	50.9	50.7	46.9	50.4	51.2	44.9
Alcohol (%E)	0.9	1.0	0.7	1.3	1.3	1.6
Saturated fat (%E)	22.2	22.3	19.3	22.1	21.7	20.6
Monounsaturated fat (%E)	11.8	11.8	11.7	11.8	11.6	12.7
Polyunsaturated fat (%E)	2.9	2.9	4.4	3.0	3.0	5.2
Cholesterol (mg)	662	704	465	696	694	497
Fiber (g)	41	43	30	38	38	26

a = Same individuals surveyed 20 years apart

Table 9. Trends in average food groups (g per day) in aging men from Zutphen from 1960 to 1985 (25).

| Year | 1960 | 1960 | 1970 | 1985 |
| Age (y) | 40-59 | 40-59 | 50-69 | 65-84 |
Food group	N=1049	N=315 [a]	N=315 [a]	N=315 [a]
Bread	261	263	183	133
Cereals	17	20	16	17
Legumes	12	12	4	8
Potatoes	341	329	187	173
Vegetables	200	201	180	168
Fruit	112	120	170	201
Meat	111	104	138	111
Fish	20	19	17	17
Eggs	34	30	31	19
Cheese	30	33	31	33
Milk	533	548	423	390
Fats and oils	89	87	61	48
Sugar	81	84	78	56
Pastries	22	24	33	39
Alcoholic drinks	64	43	95	101

Table 10. Trends in average energy and nutrient intake in aging men from Zutphen from 1960 to 1985 (25).

| Year | 1960 | 1960 | 1970 | 1985 |
| Age (y) | 40-59 | 40-59 | 50-69 | 65-84 |
Energy/nutrient	N=1049	N=315 [a]	N=315 [a]	N=315 [a]
Energy (kcal)	3070	3056	2622	2237
Energy (MJ)	12.8	12.8	11.0	9.4
Protein (%E)	11.8	11.8	12.4	14.6
Fat (%E)	41.9	41.5	41.4	39.9
Carbohydrate (%E)	44.8	45.5	43.2	41.4
Alcohol (%E)	1.0	0.6	2.5	4.1
Saturated fat (%E)	17.5	17.4	17.0	17.2
Monounsaturated fat (%E)	18.0	17.7	17.4	14.9
Polyunsaturated fat (%E)	5.8	5.8	6.7	6.3
Cholesterol (mg)	442	416	412	344
Fiber (g)	33	33	25	25

a = Same individuals surveyed during 25 years

Table 11. Trends in average food groups (g per day) in aging men from Italy from 1965 to 1991 (26).

	Crevalcore			Montegiorgio		
Year	1965	1965	1991	1965	1965	1991
Age (y)	45-64	45-64	71-90	45-64	45-64	71-90
Food group	N=879	N=171[a]	N=171[a]	N=662	N=82[a]	N=82[a]
Bread	321	357	190	368	398	251
Cereals	114	116	74	118	115	91
Legumes	10	10	14	8	9	14
Potatoes	20	21	36	27	26	29
Vegetables	39	42	153	70	71	215
Fruit	265	281	279	85	79	220
Meat	143	156	121	81	77	115
Fish	17	16	16	26	26	29
Eggs	17	19	7	17	17	8
Cheese	16	16	33	10	7	20
Milk	175	173	222	20	15	64
Fats and oils	58	57	37	61	61	42
Sugar	18	20	14	7	7	13
Pastries	20	26	35	5	4	22
Alcoholic drinks	815	778	336	764	748	443

Table 12. Trends in average energy and nutrient intake in aging men from Italy from 1965 to 1991 (26).

	Crevalcore			Montegiorgio		
Year	1965	1965	1991	1965	1965	1991
Age (y)	45-64	45-64	71-90	45-64	45-64	71-90
Energy/ nutrient	N=879	N=171[a]	N=171[a]	N=662	N=82[a]	N=82[a]
Energy (kcal)	3003	3111	2279	2790	2806	2361
Energy (MJ)	12.6	13.0	9.5	11.7	11.7	9.9
Protein (%E)	11.1	11.4	13.8	9.8	9.7	12.3
Fat (%E)	26.7	26.4	31.3	26.2	25.9	27.5
Carbohydrate (%E)	42.1	43.7	44.5	43.8	45.1	46.7
Alcohol (%E)	19.8	18.2	10.9	20.0	19.2	13.5
Saturated fat (%E)	8.6	8.2	8.9	6.8	6.6	6.6
Monounsaturated fat (%E)	15.6	15.7	18.7	16.9	17.0	18.4
Polyunsaturated fat (%E)	2.5	2.5	3.5	2.5	2.3	2.5
Cholesterol (mg)	290	309	187	187	182	162
Fiber (g)	38	41	21	39	41	20

a = Same individuals surveyed 20 years apart

food and nutrient intake patterns of these aging cohorts in the course of about 25 years are reported here (12). The structure of the tables 7-12 is the same. The first columns of each cohort represent the total number of men examined at the baseline survey. The next columns provide the results for the same men examined in the different rounds. In this way information is obtained about the possible differences in the average intake of food groups and nutrients between all men examined at baseline and the same men surveyed repeatedly during the follow-up period.

The most remarkable changes in the dietary pattern of aging men in Finland were the large decreases in consumption of cereal products, potatoes, meat, milk, and fats and oils, and sugar (8,24) (Table 7). Increases were noted in the consumption of vegetables, fruit, fish (West Finland), cheese, and alcoholic beverages (West Finland). These changes lead to a decrease in the intake of energy, saturated fat, dietary cholesterol, and dietary fiber and an increase in polyunsaturated fat (Table 8).

Similar changes were also observed in the aging men from Zutphen, The Netherlands, although there were also differences compared with the Finnish situation (25). The consumption of bread, potatoes, vegetables, eggs, milk, fats and oils, and sugar decreased in the 25 years (Table 9). In contrast, an increase was found in the consumption of fruit, pastries and alcoholic beverages. This was associated with a decrease in the intake of energy, total and monounsaturated fat, dietary cholesterol, and dietary fiber. The alcohol intake increased from less than 1 to more than 4% of energy.

In the Italian cohorts a large decrease in the consumption of bread and cereals was in aging men observed (26) (Table 11). The consumption of eggs, fats and oils, and wine also decreased substantially. Large increases were observed in the consumption of vegetables, fruit (Montegiorgio), cheese, milk, and pastries. This leads to an increase in total fat (Crevalcore), and monounsaturated and polyunsaturated fat (Crevalcore) (Table 12). Large decreases were observed in the intake of energy, alcohol, cholesterol (Crevalcore), and dietary fiber.

We conclude that characteristic patterns of food consumption could be identified in the different cohorts around 1960. After 30 years these differences were still present, although less pronounced. The most impressive changes in Europe were the decreases in the consumption of bread, and fats and oils, and the increase in fruit consumption. In northern Europe there were also substantial reductions in the consumption of potatoes, milk, and sugar and in Italy a large increase in he consumption of vegetables, cheese and pastries was noted. Large changes were observed in alcohol consumption. In countries with a traditional very low level of alcohol consumption (e.g. The Netherlands), a substantial increase was found between 1960 and 1985. In cohorts with a very high wine consumption (Italy and Croatia) a 50% reduction was noted. In Japan a large increase in animal foods (meat and milk) occurred, and the intake of rice fell by more than 50%.

In spite of these changes the characteristic fatty acid patterns are still present. The intake of saturated fatty acids is still highest in northern Europe. The Mediterranean cohorts are characterized by a high olive oil and monounsaturated fatty acid intake; wine and alcohol intake are still higher than in northern Europe in spite of a 50% decrease in wine consumption. Despite the increase in animal food consumption in Japan, the intake of total and saturated fat is still low compared with northern Europe, and N-3 polyunsaturated fatty acid intake is still high because of the high intake of fish and shellfish.

DIET, NUTRIENTS, AND CORONARY HEART DISEASE FROM A CROSS-CULTURAL PERSPECTIVE

The food and nutrient intake data of the 16 cohorts collected for the baseline survey, were also used to study the relationships with long-term CHD mortality rates. The average population consumption of 18 homogeneous food groups was related to 25-year CHD mortality rates (27). Animal food groups, with the exception of fish, were positively associated with CHD mortality and plant food groups, except for potatoes, were inversely associated. Multivariate analysis showed that the average population consumption of butter, margarine and lard, and meat were the strongest correlates of 25-year CHD mortality rates. These three food groups together explained 92% of the variance in population CHD mortality rates.

Figure 5. The relationship of factor score derived from factor analysis on 18 food groups with age-adjusted 25-year coronary heart disease death rates (27).

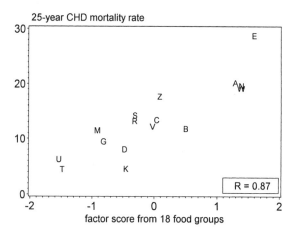

The factor score represents the dietary pattern of each cohort.
For legend see appendix

Factor analyses were carried out using the 18 food groups. Among the factor loadings, those corresponding to foods typical of the Mediterranean and Japanese cohorts had negative signs: cereals, vegetables, oils, legumes, fish, and alcohol. The ones for bread, fruit, and eggs were close to zero and all the others were positive. The summary factor score was positive for a dietary pattern rich in animal foods and negative for a pattern rich in plant foods. The population factor scores were strongly correlated with 25-year population CHD mortality rates (r= 0.87, p< 0.001) (Fig. 5).

For studying relationships between the population intake of nutrients and population CHD mortality rates at the beginning of the Seven Countries Study most emphasis was put on the intake of chemically analyzed fatty acids. After five years of follow-up a strong association had been observed between the average population intake of saturated fat and 5-year CHD mortality rates (28). This association was confirmed using 10-year mortality follow-up data (29). An analysis using the 15-year mortality data suggested a relationship between the ratio of monounsaturated to saturated fatty acids in the diet and CHD mortality rates (30). An additional analysis showed that the population intake of saturated fatty acids and 15-year CHD mortality rates were strongly positively associated (31). The inverse relationship between the intake of monounsaturated fatty acids and CHD mortality did not reach statistical significance. We conclude from these results that the average population intake of saturated fatty acids in contrast to monounsaturated fatty acids, is strongly related to long-term population CHD mortality rates.

The effect of the average intake of different fatty acids and antioxidants in relation to population CHD mortality rates could only be investigated using the results of the chemical analyses carried out in 1987 (15-17). Of the different fatty acids, the

Figure 6. Average intake of saturated fatty acids (%E) in 1960 and 25-year age-adjusted mortality rates from coronary heart disease (15).

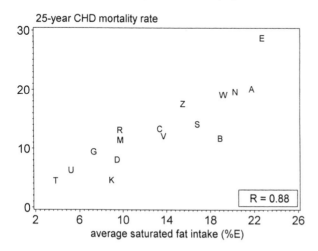

Figure 7. Average intake of trans fatty acids (%E) in 1960 and 25-year age-adjusted mortality rates from coronary heart disease (15).

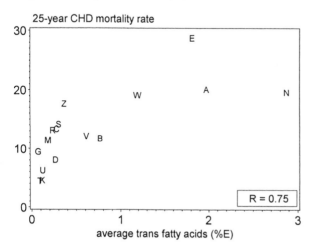

For legend see appendix

population's average intake of saturated fatty acids was the most related to 25-year CHD mortality rates (15) (Fig. 6). The intake of *trans* fatty acids was also strongly related to 25-year CHD mortality rates (Fig. 7). This association was slightly weaker than that for saturated fatty acids (r = 0.75 vs. r = 0.88). Because of the strong correlation between these two classes of fatty acids (r = 0.84) only saturated fatty acids were used in multivariate modeling. The relationships among the total, mono-, and polyunsaturated fatty acids and CHD mortality were not statistically significant.

The polyunsaturated fatty acids can be divided into the N-6 and N-3 fatty acids. The most important N-6 fatty acid in the diet is linoleic acid. The average population intake of linoleic acid was not related to 25-year CHD mortality rates. The most important N-3 fatty acids are α-linolenic acid (ALA), eicosapentaenoic acid (EPA) and docosahexaenoic acid (DHA). Contrary to expectations the average population intake of ALA was positively associated with 25-year CHD mortality rates (r = 0.70, p< 0.01). However, the population average intake of ALA was also strongly related to saturated fatty acids (r = 0.65, p< 0.01). After multivariate analyses, ALA was not associated with CHD mortality. The logarithm of average population intake of EPA and DHA was inversely (r = -0.36), but not significantly, associated with 25-year CHD mortality rates. The logarithm of average population fish consumption was inversely related to 25-year population CHD mortality rates (r = -0.50, p <0.05) (Fig. 8) (21). However, this association did not survive after multivariate analysis (17).

The relationships among the average population intake of different antioxidants and CHD mortality rates were investigated for β-carotene, vitamin E, vitamin C, and flavonoids (16, 17). The average population intake of the different vitamins with antioxidant properties was not related to long-term CHD mortality rates in the population (17). However, population average intake of flavonoids was inversely (r = 0.50, p< 0.05) related to 25-year CHD mortality rates (16) (Fig. 9).

Figure 8. Logarithm of average fish consumption (g per day) in 1960 and 25-year age-adjusted mortality rates from coronary heart disease (17).

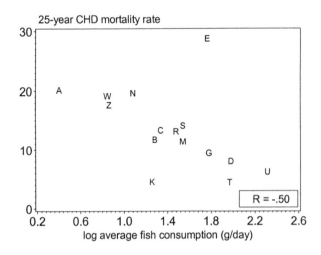

For legend see appendix

Figure 9. Average intake of flavonoids (mg per day) in 1960 and 25-year age-adjusted mortality rates from coronary heart disease (16).

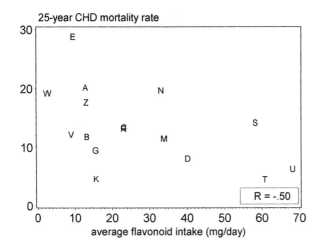

For legend see appendix

CHD is a multifactorial disease. Therefore multivariate models are needed to explain the occurrence of CHD mortality. Based on what is known about the etiology of CHD, a multivariate model for ecological correlations should include fatty acids, antioxidants, and cigarette smoking. Multivariate modeling showed that dietary saturated fatty acids and the prevalence of cigarette smokers were positively associated with 25-year CHD mortality rates, while population average flavonoid intake was inversely related (Table 13). The population mortality rates from CHD could be 90% explained by differences in the average population intake of saturated fatty acids, flavonoids, and the prevalence of cigarette smokers.

Table 13. Multivariate model for population average intake of different exposures and 25-year age-adjusted population coronary heart disease mortality rates (16).

Factor	β	SE	P-value
Saturated fat (%E)	0.905	0.117	<0.001
Flavonoids (mg)	-0.091	0.040	0.041
Cigarette smokers (%)	0.323	0.081	0.002

β = multivariate regression coefficient   SE = Standard error

The multivariate model provides the possibility to estimate the possible population protective effect of dietary interventions (Table 13). If the population average intake of saturated fatty acids decreases from 15 to 10% of energy this would reduce the estimated CHD mortality rate by 4.5%. If the population average flavonoid intake is increased from 30 to 60 mg per day the population rate of CHD mortality should decrease by 2.7%. At an average 25-year CHD mortality rate of 15% this means that about 50% of the long-term mortality from CHD might be prevented by optimizing the diet.

That this is not only theory but also reality can be shown by the results of an ecological study from Poland (32). After two decades of rising rates of CHD mortality, a sudden decline occurred. For ages 45 to 64, a decrease of about 25% in mortality from CHD and atherosclerosis was noted between 1991 and 1994. This change could be attributed to a marked shift from animal fats (-23%) to vegetable fats (+48%) and increased imports of fruit (100%). No major changes occurred in smoking, drinking, stress, or medical care.

We conclude that population differences in long-term mortality due to CHD can, to a large extent, be "explained" by population differences in the intake of saturated fatty acids and flavonoids in combination with cigarette smoking. We calculated that a decrease in population average for saturated fatty acid intake from 15 to 10% of energy, and an increase in intake of flavonoids from 30 to 60 mg per day, reduces the population CHD mortality rate by 50% (Table 13). If, in addition, the prevalence of smokers could be reduced from 60% (the average at the beginning of the Seven Countries Study) to about 35% CHD mortality could be eliminated from the population. This shows the large potential of intervention on diet and smoking in relation to a public health strategy for prevention of CHD.

THE MEDITERRANEAN DIET

The Mediterranean Sea borders on 18 countries that differ markedly in geography, economic status, health, lifestyle, and diet. This rules out the existence of *"the* Mediterranean diet." In general terms, however, the Mediterranean diet is defined by Fidanza as the diet "which is usual for people from countries whose coasts are washed by this sea, and is moderate in cereal products, fish, legumes, olive oil, fruit and vegetables in combination with little meat and wine. This type of diet, with variants characteristic for each Mediterranean population, results from an amalgamation over a period of time of local and foreign cooking cultures (first, the Greek-Latin, and then the Arabian)"(33). The main characteristics of this diet are that it is plant-food based, with olive oil as the principal source of fat. Many variants are present. The Italian Mediterranean diet is moderate in olive oil and high in cereals. The olive oil content of the Greek, Spanish, and Dalmatian Mediterranean diet is much higher than in the Italian one. The Greek Mediterranean diet is also characterized by a high intake of fruits, and the Spanish and Dalmatian diet by a high intake of fish.

The "reference" Mediterranean diet seems to differ according to country. Italian researchers favor the southern Italian diet (i.e. the diet in Nicotera during the baseline survey of the Seven Countries Study) as the reference diet (33,34). Greek researchers view the Cretan diet as the reference diet (35,36). These diets are called reference diets because they are associated with good health and a long life expectancy (37). For Crete the association between diet and health could be studied in the Cretan cohort of the Seven Countries Study. For Italy this could not be studied in the men from Nicotera, because that study was abandoned after the baseline survey due to lack of funds, but it was studied in Montegiorgio a farming village in the center of Italy close to Ancona. Dalmatia, on the coast of the Adriatic Sea in Croatia, is taken as a third Mediterranean cohort of the Seven Countries Study, because, besides a high intake of olive oil, this cohort also had a high consumption of fish in contrast to Crete and Montegiorgio.

62

In quantitative terms the Cretan diet was first described in 1948 on the basis of an extensive nutritional epidemiological study supported by the Rockefeller Foundation (37). The report of that study concluded that "olives, cereal grains, pulses, wild greens and herbs, and fruits, together with limited quantities of goat meat and milk, game and fish have remained the basic Cretan foods for 40 centuries......., no meal was complete without bread ..... Olives and olive oil contributed heavily to the energy intake ... food seemed to be "swimming" in oil." A similar conclusion was drawn on the basis of the dietary surveys carried out in Crete 15 years later in the context of the Seven Countries Study (38). The composition of the diet of Cretan men is described in the Tables 1-3. However, the original dietary records of the surveys carried out around 1960 were lost. Therefore the diet had to be reconstructed on the basis of a general description of that diet and food balance sheet data of Greece (14, 38). This means that we only know the general characteristics of the Cretan diet because details were lost.

With respect to fatty acids we have a fair estimate of the average intake of saturated, monounsaturated fatty acids and N-6 polyunsaturated fatty acids by middle-aged Cretan men in 1960. The estimate of N-3 polyunsaturated fatty acids and especially of α-linolenic acid (ALA) can be questioned. The average intake of ALA was 1.2 g per day in 1960, compared with 2.2 g per day in the Zutphen cohort of the Seven Countries Study (18). In a comparative study in elderly men from Zutphen and Crete carried out in the 1980s, we found that the average concentration of ALA in the cholesteryl esters was three times higher in Crete compared with Zutphen (0.9 vs. 0.3%) (39). The other characteristic difference in the fatty acid composition of the Cretan and Zutphen diet, as a high intake of oleic acid in Crete and a high intake of linoleic acid in Zutphen were reflected in the fatty acid composition of the cholesteryl esters. It is therefore likely that the intake of ALA in the Cretan diet of 1960 was underestimated because information about the consumption of wild greens like purslane, commonly present in Cretan salads and an important source of ALA, was not available.

Wild greens are also important sources of antioxidants, especially flavonoids. In 1997 the flavonoid content of six major flavonoids, including quercetin, were analyzed in seven different wild greens (40). The quercetin content varied per 100 g wild greens from 1.1 to 86.2 mg, and was very high in fennel (46.8 mg) and Queen Anne's lace (86.2 mg.). These concentrations are higher than in onions (34.4 mg), a vegetable known for its high flavonoid content. These results show that wild greens are rich sources of flavonoids. In 1960 no information was available about the consumption of wild greens. It is therefore likely that the average flavonoid intake of the middle-aged Cretan men in 1960 (15.7 mg per day) was underestimated.

Crete has a very rich flora and more than 2,170 plant species have been identified. That is higher than the number of species identified in England. Wild greens, commonly used in the Cretan diet, may be important sources of ALA and antioxidants. A quantitative estimate of the wild greens in the Cretan diet is therefore needed. Currently, we are collecting information on this important issue in collaboration with our Cretan colleague, Prof. Kafatos and our French colleague Prof. Renaud.

Another commonly mentioned reference diet is the diet of middle-aged men in the southern Italian village, Nicotera. Dietary surveys carried out around 1960 in the context of the Seven Countries Study showed that this diet is largely plant- food based (33, 34). Compared to the Cretan diet it is lower in olive oil, fruit, and potatoes, and contains more cereals and wine. No follow-up of the Nicotera cohort took place. Therefore the cohort of Montegiorgio was chosen for comparison with the Cretan cohort. The diet of the middle-aged men from Montegiorgio, compared with that of their counterparts in Nicotera, contained more cereals, wine, meat, and eggs, and less fruit.

The third Mediterranean cohort of the Seven Countries Study is Dalmatia, Croatia. Like the Cretan cohort, this cohort also had a high intake of olive oil. The consumption of fish, meat, and wine was much higher, and the consumption of fruit much lower in Dalmatia compared with Crete. The fatty acid and antioxidant composition of Mediterranean diets from Crete, Montegiorgio, and Dalmatia are compared with that of the northern European cohort of Zutphen. Also the 25-year mortality rates are compared.

The average total fat content of the Cretan diet in 1960 was 40% energy (Table 14). In spite of the high fat content the intake of saturated fatty acids was the lowest of the three Mediterranean cohorts. The average total fat intake was lower in Dalmatia and Montegiorgio (30-34%E), but the average intake of saturated fatty acids was in all three cohorts about 10% of energy. The highest average total and saturated fatty acid intake was found in Zutphen (44 and 20% E, respectively). In the Mediterranean diets *trans* fatty acids were almost non-existent, but the diet of the Zutphen men contained about 8 g per day. A very high intake of monounsaturated fatty acids was

Table 14. Population average dietary fatty acid and antioxidant intake and 25-year mortality rates in the Mediterranean cohorts and in Zutphen (15-17).

Cohort	Fatty acids				
	Total (%E)	SFA (g)	TFA (g)	MUFA (g)	PUFA (g)
Crete	40.1	28.0	0.4	84.1	13.4
Dalmatia	33.7	39.9	1.1	77.6	24.0
Montegiorgio	30.1	31.4	0.5	49.9	15.0
Zutphen	43.7	60.9	8.1	49.5	20.7
	Antioxidants (mg)			
	β-carotene	Vitamin E	Vitamin C	Flavonoids
Crete	1.8	23.3	136	15.7
Dalmatia	4.2	17.8	60	40.2
Montegiorgio	2.9	14.5	44	33.9
Zutphen	2.9	11.6	110	33.1
	25-year mortality rate (%)		
	CHD	Cancer	All-causes
Crete	4.6	8.8	31.4
Dalmatia	8.1	10.0	43.3
Montegiorgio	11.5	12.2	46.2
Zutphen	19.7	17.8	48.0

SFA = Saturated Fatty Acids   MUFA = Mono Unsaturated Fatty Acids
TFA = *Trans* Fatty Acids   PUFA = Poly Unsaturated Fatty Acids

observed in Crete and Dalmatia, about 80 g per day compared with about 50 g per day in Montegiorgio and Zutphen. The intake of polyunsaturated fatty acids varied between 15 and 25 g per day.

Also in the intake of antioxidants characteristic differences were observed. The Cretan cohort had the highest intake of vitamin E and C (Table 14). The Dalmatian

Table 15. Trends in average food groups (g per day) in men from Crete from 1960 to 1991 (14, 41, 42).

Year	1960	1991	1988
Age (y)	40-59	70-89	40-59
Food group	N=31[a]	N=21[a]	N=181[b]
Bread	380	185	115
Cereals	30	140	28
Legumes	30	116	40
Potatoes	190	76	88
Vegetables	191	278	238
Fruit	464	228	322
Meat	35	43	91
Fish	18	62	34
Eggs	25	10	13
Cheese	13	26	60
Milk	235	183	57
Fats and oils	95	75	50
Sugar	20	17	21
Pastries	0		65
Alcohol (100%)	15	8	10

Table 16. Trends in average energy and nutrient intake in men from Crete from 1960 to 1991. Derived from references 15, 41, 42.

Year	1960	1991	1988
Age (y)	40-59	70-89	40-59
Energy/nutrient	N=31[a]	N=21[a]	N=181[b]
Energy (kcal)	2820	2454	2488
Energy (MJ)	11.8	10.3	10.4
Protein (%E)	12.5	12.4	
Fat (%E)	41.9	44.4	35.8
Carbohydrate (%E)	43.0	42.4	
Alcohol (%E)	2.7	1.8	
Saturated fat (%E)	8.9	10.2	9.5
Monounsaturated fat (%E)	26.8	24.2	16.7
Polyunsaturated fat (%E)	4.4	5.1	3.0
Cholesterol (mg)	211	216	274
Fiber (g)	43	25	

a = aging cohort from the Seven Countries Study   b= independent sample of middle-aged men cohort had the highest intake of beta-carotene, and flavonoids. The intake of in Montegiorgio and Zutphen was intermediate for beta-carotene, low for vitamin E, low for vitamin C (Montegiorgio only), and intermediate for flavonoids.

For the three Mediterranean cohorts the lowest 25-year mortality rates for CHD, cancer and all-causes were found in Crete and the highest in Montegiorgio. All-causes mortality was almost 50% higher in Montegiorgio compared with Crete. The all-causes mortality rate of Montegiorgio was close to that of Zutphen. Compared with Crete, the mortality rate for CHD was four times higher, for cancer twice as high, and for all-causes, 50%.

An intriguing question is why the all-causes mortality rate in Crete is so much lower than in the other Mediterranean cohorts, Dalmatia and Montegiorgio. This cannot be due to differences in cigarette smoking, because the prevalence of smokers varied only between 57 and 59% in 1960. The largest difference was observed in wine consumption. Expressed in pure alcohol, the average daily amount was 15 g per day in Crete, 95 g per day in Dalmatia and 64 g per day in Montegiorgio. Detailed analyses of the food and alcohol consumption patterns of the rural Italian cohorts of the Seven Countries Study showed that men with a high alcohol intake, averaged at about 1/3 total energy intake, had a 6-10% higher 20-year mortality rate from all-causes compared with the other men (9). This was due to higher mortality rates for cardiovascular diseases, cancer, and liver cirrhosis. These results suggest that the superiority in survival of the Cretan men was due to the combination of a healthy diet and moderate alcohol consumption.

The Cretan diet of middle-aged men in 1960 no longer exists. A follow-up survey of a small sample of 21 men from the Cretan cohort aged 70-89 in 1991 showed the current Cretan diet of elderly men to contain less bread, potatoes, fruit, eggs, fats and oils, and wine and more cereals, legumes, vegetables, fish, and cheese than the diet of middle-aged men 30 years earlier (41) (Table 15). This led to small changes in the fatty acid composition of the diet (Table 16). A substantial decrease was observed in the intake of dietary fiber.

The comparison of the diet of middle-aged and elderly men in an aging cohort is confounded by age. Confounding by age is excluded when men of the same age are compared. This was done by examining middle-aged men of the Agricultural Bank of Greece, Crete in 1988 (42). They were all Cretans by birth and had been residents of Crete for at least the previous 10 years. The average food and nutrient intake of these men was compared with those of the Cretan farmers in 1960.

Comparison between Cretan men aged 40-59 examined almost 30 years apart showed that middle-aged men in 1988 consumed less bread, potatoes, fruit, eggs, fats and oils, and wine and more vegetables, fish, and cheese (Table 15). These changes were similar to those observed for the aging cohort. In addition, the middle-aged men had in 1988 a higher consumption of meat and pastries, and a lower consumption of milk. The total fat and monounsaturated fatty acids intake was lower in 1988 compared with 1960 (Table 16). However, the intake of saturated fatty acids was below 10% of energy.

We conclude that of the Mediterranean diets investigated the Cretan diet was associated with the lowest mortality rates. This was due to the balanced food and nutrient content of this diet in combination with a moderate consumption of wine. The results of the Seven Countries Study suggest that the Mediterranean diet as consumed in Crete in 1960 is associated with a very low risk of coronary and all-causes mortality. Whether this association is causal might be tested in future interventions, but the observations provide sound evidence for food policy.

The positive health effects of the Mediterranean diet on CHD risk factors has been tested in intervention studies carried out in East Finland and Southern Italy. Middle-aged men and women changed their usual Finnish diet for six weeks to a Mediterranean type of diet (43). This change in diet was associated with a more than 20% decrease in total and LDL cholesterol and apoprotein B. A similar study showed a significant blood pressure lowering effect of such a change in diet (44). At about the same time a study was carried out in southern Italy investigating the effect of a change from a traditional Mediterranean diet to a diet higher in saturated fatty acids, and cholesterol (45). These dietary changes were associated with an increase of 15% in total cholesterol and 19% in LDL cholesterol. These results show convincingly that a Mediterranean type of diet improves the levels of major CHD risk factors, such as LDL cholesterol, and blood pressure.

The effect of a Cretan Mediterranean diet on coronary and all-causes mortality was tested in cardiac patients. For this trial 605 patients were randomized and followed for 27 months (46,47). The effect of a Cretan Mediterranean diet was compared with a usual prescribed diet. Both diets had a moderate amount of total fat (31-33% of energy) and saturated fatty acids (8.3% of energy in the experimental group and 11.8% of energy in the control group). The largest difference was in α-linolenic acid (1.8 g per day in the experimental group and 0.79 g per day in the control group). The experimental group also had a higher consumption of fruits and vegetables, as reflected in the higher intake of vitamin C. These differences in diet were associated with a 70% lower cardiac and all-causes mortality in the experimental compared with the control group. Because of the great preventive potential of the Cretan Mediterranean diet there is an urgent need to replicate this trial (48).

The results of the Seven Countries Study, and those of intervention studies on cardiovascular risk factors and endpoints, provide evidence for a protective effect of the Mediterranean diet. A diet as consumed on Crete in 1960 in combination with moderate alcohol consumption is associated with a low risk for CHD and all-causes mortality. Although the main characteristics of the original Cretan diet, a high consumption of olive oil and fruit, are still present, the diet is changing rapidly and shows large increases in meat and pastries consumption. From a public health point of view the original Cretan diet should be kept to preserve health.

SUMMARY AND CONCLUSIONS

At the beginning of the Seven Countries Study distinct food patterns were present in different regions. The food pattern in the U.S. was characterized by a high intake of fruit, meat, and pastries. The northern European food pattern, as observed in Finland and the Netherlands, was high in potatoes, milk, butter, or margarine, and sugar products. The continental diet of the Serbian men was high in bread, meat, or cheese. The Italians had a high intake of cereals and wine. The Mediterranean cohorts Italy, Dalmatia, and Greece were characterized by a moderate to high consumption of olive oil and wine in combination with either a high consumption of fruit, fish, or cereals. The Japanese cohorts had a high consumption of fish, rice, and soy products.

Repeated food consumption surveys were carried out in Finland, the Netherlands and Italy between 1959 and 1991. The most impressive changes in all three countries were the decreases in the consumption of bread, and fats and oils, and the increase in fruit consumption. In northern Europe there were also substantial reductions in the consumption of potatoes, milk and sugar and increases in alcohol consumption. In Italy a large increase in the consumption of vegetables, cheese and pastries and a substantial decrease in wine consumption were noted. We concluded that the differences in food consumption patterns between northern and southern Europe became smaller, but characteristic differences still exist (e.g. a moderate consumption of olive oil and a high consumption of wine in Italy).

As early as the end of five years of follow-up, it was shown that differences in mortality from CHD rates between populations were strongly associated with population differences in the intake of saturated fatty acids. The 25-year CHD mortality rates could, to a large extent, be explained by population differences in the intake of saturated fatty acids and flavonoids in combination with the prevalence of cigarette smokers. A Mediterranean diet, as consumed on the island of Crete around 1960, was characterized by a high intake of olive oil, and fruit in combination with a moderate consumption of alcohol, and associated with a very low risk for coronary and all-causes mortality. Although the main characteristics of the original Cretan diet are still present, the diet is changing rapidly and those changes will likely have negative effects on future health.

REFERENCES

1. Connor WE. Diet-heart research in the first part of the 20th century. Acta Cardiol 1999;54:135-139.
2. Langen CD de. Cholesterol metabolism and racial pathology. Geneesk Tijdschr Nederl Indië 1916;56:1-34 (in Dutch)
3. Snapper I. Chinese lessons for Western medicine. NY Interscience Publ Inc, 1941.
4. Sinclair HM. Deficiency of essential fatty acids and atherosclerosis, etcetera. Lancet 1956;i:381-383.
5. Steinberg D, Parthasarathy S, Carew TE, Khoo JC, Witzum JL. Beyond cholesterol. Modifications of low-density lipoprotein that increase its atherogenicity. N Engl J Med 1989;320:915-924.
6. Den Hartog C, Buzina R, Fidanza F, Keys A, Roine P. Dietary studies and epidemiology of heart diseases. Stichting tot wetenschappelijke voorlichting op voedingsgebied, The Hague, The Netherlands 1968:1-157.
7. Den Hartog C, Van Schaik TFSM, Dalderup LM, Drion EF, Mulder T. The diet of volunteers participating in a long-term epidemiological field survey of coronary heart disease in Zutphen, The Netherlands. Voeding 1965;26:184-201.
8. Pekkarinen M. Dietary surveys in connection with coronary heart disease studies in Finland. In: New trends in nutrition, lipid research and cardiovascular diseases. New York: AR Liss Inc, 1981;234-261.
9. Farchi G, Mariotti S, Menotti A, Seccareccia F, Torsello S, Fidanza F. Diet and 20-year mortality in two rural population groups of middle-aged men in Italy. Am J Clin Nutr 1989;50:1095-1103.
10. Keys A. Dietary survey methods in studies on cardiovascular epidemiology. In: Dietary studies and epidemiology of heart diseases. Stichting tot wetenschappelijke voorlichting op voedingsgebied, The Hague, 1968:9-28.
11. Burke BS. The dietary history as a tool in research. J Am Diet Assoc 1947;23:1041-1046.
12. Huijbregts PPCW, Feskens EJM, Räsänen L, Alberti-Fidanza A, Mutanen M, Fidanza F, Kromhout D. Dietary intake in five aging cohorts of men in Finland, Italy and the Netherlands. Eur J Clin Nutr 1995;49: 852-860.
13. Bingham S. The dietary assessment of individuals; methods, accuracy , new techniques and recommendations. Nutr Abst Rev Ser A 1987;57:705-742.

14. Kromhout D, Keys A, Aravanis C, Buzina R, Fidanza F, Giampaoli S, Jansen A, Menotti A, Nedeljkovic S, Pekkarinen M, Simic BS, Toshima H. Food consumption patterns in the nineteen sixties in Seven Countries. Am J Clin Nutr 1989;49:889-894.
15. Kromhout D, Menotti A, Bloemberg B, Aravanis C, Blackburn H, Buzina R, Dontas AS, Fidanza F, Giampaoli S, Jansen A, Karvonen M, Katan M, Nissinen A, Nedeljkovic S, Pekkanen J, Pekkarinen M, Punsar S, Räsänen L, Simic B, Toshima H. Dietary saturated and trans fatty acids, cholesterol and 25-year mortality from coronary heart disease. The Seven Countries Study. Prev Med 1995;24:308-315.
16. Hertog MGL, Kromhout D, Aravanis C, Blackburn H, Buzina R, Fidanza F, Giampaoli S, Jansen A, Menotti A, Nedeljkovic S, Pekkarinen M, Simic BS, Toshima H, Feskens EJM, Hollman PCH, Katan MB. Flavonoid intake and long-term risk of coronary heart disease and cancer in the Seven Countries Study. Arch Intern Med 1995;155:381-386.
17. Kromhout D, Bloemberg BPM, Feskens EJM, Hertog MGL, Menotti A, Blackburn H, for the Seven Countries Study Group. Alcohol, fish, fiber and antioxidant vitamins do not explain population differences in coronary heart disease mortality. Int J Epidemiol 1996;25(4):753-759.
18. Vries JHM de, Jansen A, Kromhout D, Bovenkamp P van de, Staveren WA van, Mensink RP, Katan MB for the Seven Countries Study Group. The fatty acid and sterol content of food composites of middle-aged men in seven countries. J Food Comp Anal 1997;10:115-141.
19. Pietinen P, Uusitalo U, Vartiainen E, Tuomilehto J. Dietary survey of the FINMONICA project in 1982. Acta Med Scand 1988;Suppl 728:169-177.
20. What eat the Netherlands. Results of a national food consumption survey 1987-1988. Rijswijk 1988. (in Dutch).
21. Alberti-Fidanza A, Paolacci CA, Chiuchiu MP, Coli R, Fruttini D, Verducci G, Fidanza F. Dietary studies on two rural Italian population groups of the Seven Countries Study. 1. Food and nutrient intake at the thirty-first year follow-up in 1991. Eur J Clin Nutr 1994;48:85-91.
22. Buzina R, Suboticanec K, Saric M. Diet patterns and health problems: Diet in Southern Europe. Ann Nutr Metab 1991;Suppl 1:32-40.
23. Koga Y, Hashimoto R, Adachi H, Tsuruta M, Tasiro H, Toshima H. Recent trends in cardiovascular disease and risk factors in the Seven Countries Study: Japan. In: Lessons for science from the Seven Countries Study. A 35-year collaborative experience in cardiovascular disease epidemiology. Toshima H, Koga Y, Blackburn H, Keys A (Eds). Springer-Verlag, Tokyo 1994:63-74.
24. Räsänen L, Mutanen M, Pekkanen J, Laitinen S, Koski K, Halonen S, Kivinen P, Stengard J, Nissinen A. Dietary intake of 70- to 89-year-old men in eastern and western Finland. J Intern Med 1992;232:305-312.
25. Kromhout D, De Lezenne Coulander C, Obermann-de Boer GL, Van Kampen-Donker M, Goddijn E, Bloemberg BPM. Changes in food and nutrient intake in middle-aged men during the period 1960-1985 (The Zutphen Study). Am J Clin Nutr 1990;51:123-129.
26. Alberti-Fidanza A, Fidanza F, Chiuchiu MP, Verducci G, Fruttini D. Dietary studies on two rural Italian population groups of the Seven Countries Study. 3. Trend of food and nutrient intake from 1960 to 1991. Eur J Clin Nutr. 1999;53:854-860.
27. Menotti A, Kromhout D, Blackburn H, Fidanza F, Buzina R, Nissinen A for the Seven Countries Study Group. Food intake patterns and 25-year mortality from coronary heart disease: Cross-cultural correlations in the Seven Countries Study. Eur J Epidemiol 1999;15:507-515.
28. Keys A (Ed). Coronary heart disease in seven countries. Circulation 1970;41 Suppl 1:1-211.
29. Keys A, Aravanis C, Blackburn H, Buzina R, Djordjevic BS, Dontas AS, Fidanza F, Karvonen MJ, Kimura N, Menotti A, Mohacek I, Nedeljkovic S, Puddu V, Punsar S, Taylor HL, Van Buchem FSP. Seven countries. A multivariate analysis of death and coronary heart disease. Cambridge, MA; Harvard University Press, ISBN: 0-674-80237-3, 1980:1-381.

30. Keys A, Menotti A, Karvonen MJ, Aravanis C, Blackburn H, Buzina R, Djordjevic BS, Dontas AS, Fidanza F, Keys MH, Kromhout D, Nedeljkovic S, Punsar S, Seccareccia F, Toshima H. The diet and 15-year death rate in the Seven Countries Study. Am J Epidemiol 1986;124:903-915.

31. Keys A, Karvonen MJ. The diet and 15-year death rate in the Seven Countries Study. The authors reply. Am J Epidemiol 1988;128:239-241.

32. Zatonski WA, McMichael AJ, Powles JW. Ecological study of reasons for sharp decline in mortality from ischaemic heart disease in Poland since 1991. BMJ 1998;316:1047-1051.

33. Fidanza F. The Mediterranean Italian diet: Keys to contemporary thinking. Proc Nutr Soc 1991;50:519-526.

34. Ferro-Luzzi A, Branca F. Mediterranean diet, Italian-style: prototype of a healthy diet. Am J Clin Nutr 1995;61 Suppl:1338S-1345S.

35. Kafatos A, Mamalakis G. Changing patterns of fat intake in Crete. Eur J Clin Nutr 1993;47 Suppl 1:S21-S24.

36. Trichopoulou A, Lagiou P. Healthy traditional Mediterranean diet: An expression of culture, history and lifestyle. Nutr Rev 1997;55:383-389.

37. Nestle M. Mediterranean diets: historical and research overview. Am J Clin Nutr 1995;61 Suppl:1313S-1320S.

38. Keys A, Aravanis C, Sdrin H. The diets of middle-aged men in two rural areas of Greece. Voeding 1966;27:575-586.

39. Sandker GW, Kromhout D, Aravanis C, Bloemberg BPM, Mensink RP, Karalias N, Katan MB. Serum cholesterol ester fatty acids and their relation with serum lipids in elderly men in Crete and The Netherlands. Eur J Clin Nutr 1993;47:201-208.

40. Trichoupoulou A, Vasilopoulou E, Hollman P, Chamalides Ch, Foufa E, Kaloudis Tr, Kromhout D, Miskaki Ph, Petrochilou I, Poulima E, Stafilakis K, Teophilou D. Nutritional composition and flavonoid content of edible wild greens and green pies: a potential rich source of antioxidant nutrients in the Mediterranean diet. Food Chem 2000;70:319-323.

41. Kafatos A, Diacatou A, Voukiklaris G, Nikolakakis N, Vlachonikolis J, Kounali D, Mamalakis G, Dontas AS. Heart disease risk-factor status and dietary changes in the Cretan population over the past 30 y: the Seven Countries Study. Am J Clin Nutr 1997;65:1882-1886.

42. Kafatos A, Kouroumalis I, Vlachonikolis I, Theodoron C, Labadarios D. Coronary heart disease risk factor status of the Cretan urban population in the 1980's. Am J Clin Nutr 1991;54:91-98.

43. Ehnholm C, Huttunen J, Pietinen P, Leino U, Mutanen M, Kostiainen E, Pikkarainen J, Dougherty R, Iacono J, Puska P. Effect of diet on serum lipoproteins in a population with a high risk of coronary heart disease. N Engl J Med 1982;307:850-855.

44. Puska P, Iacono JM, Nissinen A, Korhonen HJ, Vartiainen E, Pietinen P, Dougherty R, Leino U, Mutanen M, Moisio S, Huttunen J. Controlled, randomized trial of the effect of dietary fat on blood pressure. Lancet 1983;1:1-5.

45. Ferro-Luzzi A, Strazzullo P, Scaccini C, Siani A, Sette S, Mariani MA, Mastranzo P, Dougherty RM, Iacono JM, Mancini M. Changing the Mediterranean diet: effects on blood lipids. Am J Clin Nutr 1984;40:1027-1037.

46. Lorgeril M de, Renaud S, Mamelle N, Salen P, Martin JL, Monjaud I, Guidollet J, Touboul P, Delaye J. Mediterranean alpha-linolenic acid-rich diet in secondary prevention of coronary heart disease. Lancet 1994;343:1454-1459.

47. Renaud S, De Lorgeril M, Delaye J, Guidollet J, Jacquard F, Mamelle N, Martin JL, Monjaud I, Salen P, Toubol P. Cretan Mediterranean diet for prevention of coronary heart disease. Am J Clin Nutr 1995;61 Suppl:1360S-1367S.

48. Kris-Etherton P, Eckel RH, Howard BV, St Jeor S, Bazzarre TL. Nutrition Committee Population Science Committee and Clinical Science Committee of the American Heart Association. AHA Science Advisory: Lyon Diet Heart Study. Benefits of a Mediterranean-style, National Cholesterol Education Program/American Heart Association Step I Dietary Pattern on Cardiovascular Disease. Circulation 2001;103:1823-1825.

CHAPTER 2.2

DIET AND CORONARY HEART DISEASE IN THE ZUTPHEN STUDY

Daan Kromhout, Bennie Bloemberg

The Zutphen Study differed from the other cohorts by collection of dietary data in all cohort members at regular intervals. This provided the possibility to study the etiologic relationships between dietary variables and the occurrence of CHD in individuals. As in the ecologic studies described in the previous chapter emphasis was placed on investigating the relationships among dietary fatty acids, antioxidants and CHD. However, the analyses were not limited to those nutrients. Other nutrients also implicated in the etiology of CHD were studied.

Currently there is a great interest in the effect of dietary fiber, carbohydrates and glycemic load on CHD (1,2). Already in 1956 Sinclair pointed to the importance of whole grain products for the prevention of CHD (3). It took, however, a long time before this was seriously investigated. Also amino acids may be involved in the etiology of CHD. Evidence is accumulating that plasma homocysteine is an important risk factor for CHD, especially in cardiac patients (4). Plasma homocysteine levels are inversely associated with B vitamins, especially folic acid (5). The amino acid arginine plays a central role in nitric oxide formation, an important vasodilator (6)

The role of diet in the etiology of CHD can be viewed as a complex interplay among different dietary factors. Dietary factors, combined with lifestyle factors, superimposed – in turn – on genetic susceptibility, determine CHD risk of an individual. In this chapter the relationships among different dietary variables and CHD risk as observed in the Zutphen Study will be summarized. First considered are the relationships among dietary fatty acids, dietary cholesterol and CHD risk. Thereafter attention will be paid to studies on dietary antioxidants and other nutrients in relation to CHD risk.

DIETARY SURVEYS IN THE ZUTPHEN STUDY.

In the Zutphen Study data were collected on the diet of all cohort members since 1960. Information on food consumption was collected with the cross-check dietary history method described in chapter 2.1. Between 1960 and 1963 several comparative and seasonal variation studies were carried out (7) in subsamples of about 50 men. The cross-check dietary history method was compared with one-week recording of food consumption either by weighing or estimating food intake. Generally, the energy intake was about 200 kcal/day higher with the cross-check dietary history compared with the one-week record (7). Seasonal variation in the consumption of foods was small.

In 1985 the survivors of the Zutphen cohort formed together with a new random sample of men of the same age in Zutphen who had not been earlier examined, the Zutphen Elderly cohort. Again the dietary history method was used and data were collected in 1985, 1990, 1995, and 2000. The reproducibility of the food intake data was investigated in repeated dietary surveys carried out three (n = 115) and 12 (n = 145) months after the initial survey (8). The food groups bread, milk products, sugar products, and alcoholic beverages were well reproduced (correlation coefficients higher than 0.70). Correlation coefficients of 0.51 or less were found for meat and for vegetables. Information on the validity of the dietary history method was not collected.

For the conversion of food and drinks to energy and nutrients, different food tables were used. In 1980 a computerized version of the Netherlands food table was developed for the energy and nutrient content of foods in the period 1960-1970. These data were analyzed in relation to mortality and morbidity follow-up from 1960 to

1985 and related to the original Zutphen cohort of 871 men aged 40-59 in 1960. For the dietary data collected in 1985, 1990, 1995, and 2000 the computerized version of the Dutch food table for the corresponding year was used. For nutrients not available in these food tables (e.g. *trans* fatty acids and α-linolenic acid) primarily Dutch data from chemical analyses of relevant foods analyzed in those years were used. These data were related to mortality and morbidity data collected in the period 1985-1995. The Zutphen Elderly Study dealt with 805 men aged 65-84 in 1985.

DIETARY FATTY ACIDS, DIETARY CHOLESTEROL AND CORONARY HEART DISEASE

Studies on the associations between the intake of fatty acids and CHD have undergone quite some changes over the past 20 years. Initially, the intake of the major classes of fatty acids (e.g. saturated, monounsaturated and polyunsaturated fatty acids) were analyzed in relation to CHD incidence. Later on, more specific analyses took place on fish consumption as an indicator of the intake of the N-3 polyunsaturated fatty acids, eicosapentaenoic acid (EPA) and docosahexaenoic acid (DHA), and the intake of *trans* fatty acids in relation to CHD incidence.

In 1984 we reported on the results of analyses using the intake of major classes of fatty acids in relation to 10-year CHD mortality (9). This analysis was based on 30 fatal CHD cases. No association was observed between the intake of saturated, monounsaturated, and polyunsaturated fatty acids and the 10-year mortality from CHD. There are several reasons which may explain this finding. First, the number of CHD cases was small, giving the study little power. Second, the standard deviation of the intake of the different fatty acids classes was small (1.5-3.1% of energy), and the range in intake of the different fatty acid classes limited. Therefore the power of this study to detect statistically significant associations was limited. Third, analyzing only these broad classes of fatty acids will mask the effects of small amounts of metabolically potent fatty acids (e.g. N-3 polyunsaturated and *trans* fatty acids) on CHD occurrence.

In univariate analyses dietary cholesterol was positively associated with 10-year CHD mortality (9). However, this association disappeared after multivariate analyses. Using 20-year mortality follow-up data, dietary cholesterol was positively associated in a multivariate model, taking age and different dietary variables into account (10). After adjustment for other risk factors (serum cholesterol, blood pressure, and smoking) this risk ratio, amounting to 1.8 (95%CI 0.8-3.8) for an increase of 200 mg of dietary cholesterol per 1,000 kcal (equivalent to about two eggs per day), was no longer statistically significant. A pooled analysis of four cohort studies, including the Zutphen Study, found a risk ratio for CHD of 1.3 (95%CI 1.1-1.5), with an increase of 200 mg of dietary cholesterol per 1,000 kcal (11). These results provide evidence for a small independent effect of dietary cholesterol on the occurrence of CHD.

TRANS FATTY ACIDS INTAKE AND CORONARY HEART DISEASE

Monounsaturated fatty acids can be divided into *cis* and *trans* fatty acids. *Cis* monounsaturated fatty acids abundantly present in, for example, olive oil are neutral in relation to serum LDL cholesterol, and elevate serum HDL cholesterol levels compared with carbohydrates. *Trans* fatty acids elevate LDL cholesterol and decrease HDL cholesterol levels (12). This only recently became apparent in metabolic studies carried out in the early 1990s. Epidemiological investigations also showed a strong association between *trans* fatty acid intake and CHD risk (13).

Trans fatty acids are produced by partial hydrogenation of polyunsaturated fatty acid-rich oils. This is done to improve the shelf life of margarines and shortenings. *Trans* fatty acids are also produced in the rumen of cattle, resulting in low levels of isomers in dairy and beef fat. In the Netherlands the intake of *trans* fatty acids was high because of a high consumption of margarine. In 1960 the average intake of *trans* fatty acids of middle-aged men in Zutphen, at 8 g per day, was the highest of all cohorts of the Seven Countries Study. In margarine production in the Netherlands, fish oils were used alongside vegetable oils. This made it possible to study the effects of different isomers of *trans* fatty acids on CHD risk in the Zutphen Elderly Study (14).

Figure 1. Daily intake of trans fatty acids in the Zutphen Elderly Study in the period 1985-1995 (14).

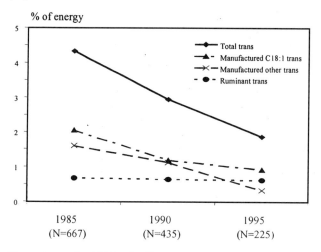

Since the early 1980s detailed information has been available in the Netherlands on the *trans* fatty acids content of different foods. This has made it possible to study the intake of manufactured C18:1 *trans* fatty acids and ruminant *trans* fatty acids, as well as the intake of total *trans* fatty acids. The average intake of total *trans* fatty acids decreased from 4.3% of energy in 1985 to 1.9% of energy in 1995 (Fig. 1). This decrease was seen for all manufactured *trans* fatty acids, but not for the low intake of ruminant *trans* fatty acids. The decrease in manufactured *trans* fatty acids was due to producers continuously reducing the content of *trans* fatty acids after publications on adverse health effects of these fatty acids (12,13)

Elderly men in Zutphen with a high intake of *trans* fatty acids (median: 6.4% of energy) in 1985 had an increased relative risk for 10-year CHD incidence (RR = 2.00, 95%CI 1.07-3.75) compared to those with a low intake (median: 2.4% of energy). A continuous analysis showed that the relative risk for a difference of 2% of energy amounted to 1.28 (95%CI 1.01-1.61). A pooled analysis, which also used the data of three other prospective studies, produced a relative risk of 1.25 (95%CI 1.11-1.40) (Fig. 2). We also analyzed the different isomers of *trans* fatty acids in relation to 10-

Figure 2. The fully adjusted relative risks (95 percent confidence interval) of CHD for an increase of 2% energy in trans fatty acid intake at baseline according to prospective population-based studies, and the pooled variance-weighted relative risk (14).

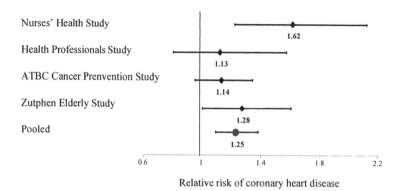

Relative risk of coronary heart disease

year CHD risk. These analyses showed all isomers to be positively associated with CHD risk.

The evidence of observational and dietary intervention studies suggests that a decrease in *trans* fatty acid intake will lower CHD mortality. We calculated that the decrease in *trans* fatty acid intake in the Netherlands of 2.4% of energy could have contributed to about 23% fewer coronary deaths (i.e. about 4,600 out of 20,000 coronary deaths). This suggests the large public health potential of optimizing the fatty acid composition of the diet.

FISH AND CORONARY HEART DISEASE

On May 9, 1985 the *New England Journal of Medicine* published three papers on the health effects of fish. The Zutphen Study reported a protective effect of a small amount of fish on 20-year mortality from CHD (10). Researchers from the United States showed that large quantities of fish oils (about 20 g of N-3 polyunsaturated fatty acids) reduced effectively trygliceride and VLDL lipoproteins in patients with hypertrygliceridemia (15). It was also shown that a daily dose of about 5 g N-3 polyunsaturated fatty acids had anti-flammatory effects by inhibiting the 5-lipoxygenase pathway in neutrophils and monocytes by inhibiting the leukotriene B4-mediated functions of neutrophils (16). These papers triggered interest in the role of fish and fish oils in the etiology of CHD.

Bang, Dyerberg, and Sinclair suggested that the low death rate from CHD among the Inuit of Greenland was due to their high consumption of seafood (17). The average consumption of seafood of an adult Inuit was estimated at 400 g per day. Kromann and Green showed that the incidence of acute myocardial infarction among the Inuit was 10 times lower than among Danes (18). This provided the basis for the hypothesis that the N-3 polyunsaturated fatty acids, EPA and DHA, present in seafood, protect against CHD.

Figure 3. Fish consumption in 1960 and 20-year mortality from coronary heart disease (10).

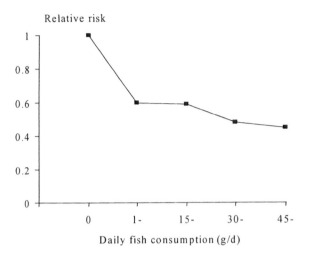

Daily fish consumption (g/d)

We were interested in the issue on whether a small amount of fish could also protect against CHD mortality. We investigated that issue in the Zutphen population, characterized by a low average fish consumption of 20 g per day, where 20% of the middle-aged men did not consume fish in 1960 (10). During 20 years of follow-up, 78 men died from CHD. An inverse dose-response relationship was observed between fish consumption in 1960 and death from CHD during 20 years of follow-up (Fig. 3). This relationship persisted after multivariate analyses. Mortality from CHD was more than 50% lower among those who consumed at least 30 g of fish per day than among those who did not eat fish. We concluded that the consumption of as little as 1 or 2 dishes of fish per week could be of preventive value in relation to CHD.

Ten years later we reported on this association using data collected in a small follow-up study from Rotterdam carried out in 272 elderly men in 1971 and followed for 17 years (19). During that period 58 persons died from CHD. In 1971 about 60% of the elderly ate fish and 40% did not eat fish. Multivariate analyses showed an inverse relation between fish consumption and 17-year mortality from CHD. The risk ratio for fish eaters compared with non-fish eaters differed significantly from unity (RR = 0.51, 95%CI 0.29-0.89)

In 2000 we reported on the relationship between the type of fish (fat or lean) in relation to 20-year mortality from CHD, using dietary data collected around 1970 in the Finnish, Dutch, and Italian cohorts (20). In total, more than 2,700 men aged 50-69 were interviewed on their dietary habits using the dietary history method. During 20 years of follow-up 463 men died from CHD. A differentiation was made between fatty (e.g. mackerel, herring) and lean (e.g. plaice, codfish) fish, because fatty fish is a rich source of the N-3 polyunsaturated fatty acids EPA and DHA. Fatty fish contains eight times more N-3 polyunsaturated fatty acids than lean fish (i.e. 400 mg N-3 polyunsaturated fatty acids vs. 50 mg per 15 g fish). Lean fish consumption was not associated with CHD mortality. Fatty fish consumption was inversely related to 20-year CHD mortality in all three cohorts. The pooled relative risk for fatty fish consumers was 0.66 (95%CI 0.49-0.90). These data suggest that fatty fish may protect against CHD mortality.

We also examined in the Zutphen Study the relationship between fish consumption and the 25-year incidence of stroke (21). Of the 552 men aged 50-69 in 1970, 42 developed a stroke. When men who consumed more than 20 grams of fish per day were compared with those who consumed less, the relative risk for stroke was significantly lower (RR = 0.49, 95%CI 0.24-0.99). These results suggest that consumption of at least one portion of fish per week may be associated with a reduced incidence of stroke.

The results of these observational studies suggest that a small amount of fish may protect against cardiovascular diseases. The most evidence is available for CHD. This evidence is, however, not entirely consistent (22). The inverse association between fish consumption and CHD is generally observed in high-risk cultures characterized by a low level of fish consumption. The association is also observed for the hardest endpoints (e.g. coronary mortality, cardiac arrest, or sudden death). However, results of experimental studies are needed to make a definite judgement on the causal nature of the association.

A randomized controlled trial, the so-called DART trial, on the effect of fatty fish consumption on mortality, was carried out in about 2000 cardiac patients from Wales (23). The experimental group was advised to take at least two portions of fatty fish weekly. The subjects who could not tolerate fish were asked to take daily three fish oil capsules. The difference in EPA content of the diet was about 250 mg per day. After two years of follow-up, CHD mortality was 33% and all-causes mortality was 29% lower in the experimental group. No significant difference was observed in the number of non-fatal myocardial infarctions. The authors suggest that the protective effect of fish may be due to prevention of ventricular fibrillation.

Several mechanisms such as effects on blood lipids and lipoproteins, hemostatic factors, and electrical stability of the heart have been hypothesized as being the explanation for the protective effect of fish. However, it should be realized that in most research on mechanisms large doses of fish oil were used. This is not compatible with the results of epidemiological studies showing a "protective effect" of a small amount of fish on CHD mortality. This should be taken into account when trying to explain the relationship of fish consumption to CHD.

Inuits are characterized by low triglyceride levels and long bleeding times. Intervention studies using large amounts of fish and fish oils showed a substantial decrease in serum triglycerides (12). We designed a study comparing habitual fish consumers of 26 years with controls. The habitual fish consumers ate on average about 33 g of fish per day and the controls 2 g per day. We studied the effect of a long-term difference of 30 g of fish per day on serum lipids and lipoproteins, and on platelet function (24, 25).

The average total triglyceride level of habitual fish consumers was 26% (p< 0.05) lower compared with controls (24). This is a similar difference to that obtained in short-term intervention studies in normolipidemic subjects consuming on average 5 g of N-3 polyunsaturated fatty acids per day. An even larger difference of 38% (p<0.05) was observed for the triglyceride content of the atherogenic Intermediate Density Lipoprotein (IDL) fraction. These results are suggestive for a role of N-3 polyunsaturated fatty acids in post-prandial metabolism of triglyceride-rich remnants.

Between habitual fish consumers and controls no differences were observed in cutaneous bleeding time, platelet number, collagen-induced platelet aggregation, and

ATP-release in whole blood (25). This also holds for the potential formation of thromboxane B2 in activated platelets, and for the activity of plasminogen activator inhibitor. The concentration of EPA in the phospholipids was twice as high in the habitual fish consumers as for the controls. A 30% higher content in the phospholipids of the habitual fish consumers was observed for DHA. These results suggest that platelet function did not contribute to the explanation of the protective effect of a small amount of fish. The higher content of EPA and DHA in the phospholipids of habitual fish consumers will increase cell membrane fluidity and may have a positive effect on electrical stability of the heart.

We conclude that there is substantial evidence that a small amount of fatty fish protects against CHD mortality. This effect is due to a higher intake of the N-3 polyunsaturated fatty acids EPA and DHA. There is some evidence that the atherogenic IDL lipoprotein fraction and membrane fluidity may be involved in the etiology of CHD. However, more research on the mechanisms behind the protective effect of a small amount of fatty fish is needed.

α-LINOLENIC ACID INTAKE AND CORONARY HEART DISEASE

Fish is an important source of the N-3 polyunsaturated fatty acids EPA and DHA. However, another major contributor to the intake of N-3 polyunsaturated fatty acids is the parent compound of this class of fatty acids, α-linolenic acid (ALA). Rich sources of α-linolenic acid are vegetable oils, salad dressing, mayonnaise, and nuts. Although the efficiency of conversion of ALA to EPA is low, there is evidence for beneficial effects of ALA on eicosanoid metabolism and platelet aggregation. These effects may be independent of the conversion of ALA to EPA.

We studied the relationship between the intake of ALA and 10-year incidence of CHD in the Zutphen Elderly Study (26). The intake of ALA was positively associated with CHD incidence. The relative risk between the highest and the lowest tertile of ALA intake was 1.68 (95%CI 0.86-3.29). The ALA intake was strongly correlated with the intake of *trans* fatty acids (r = 0.61). We therefore separated the total ALA intake into sources with and without *trans* fatty acids. The ALA intake from sources with *trans* fatty acids was non-significantly positively related to CHD risk. The ALA intake of foods without *trans* fatty acids was not associated with CHD risk (RR = 1.15, 95%CI 0.63-1.21).

The reason that we did not find a beneficial effect of ALA contrary to expectations may be due to the strong correlation between the intake of ALA and *trans* fatty acids. This association could also have complicated studying the association between ALA intake and CHD risk in other cultures where the intake of *trans* fatty acids is substantial (e.g. United States and northern Europe). In most of the prospective studies carried out in these cultures a protective effect of ALA was only found after multivariate analysis (27). Confounding by *trans* and other polyunsaturated fatty acids in ALA-rich oils hinders the interpretation of the results of these studies.

The Lyon Diet Heart Trial showed a strong protective effect on cardiovascular and all-causes mortality of a Mediterranean diet enriched with ALA (28, 29). The authors ascribe the success of their trial to the higher intake of ALA in the experimental group. This was however, not the only difference between the two groups. The experimental group had also a lower intake of saturated fat and a higher intake of vitamin C because of a high consumption of fruit and vegetables. It is therefore not possible to ascribe the protective effect of the Mediterranean diet only to differences in the intake of ALA.

We conclude that definite statements cannot be made about a possible beneficial effect of ALA, because of complexities in interpreting the results of observational and experimental studies.

DIETARY FLAVONOIDS AND CORONARY HEART DISEASE

Historically, research on antioxidants was focused on vitamins with antioxidant properties (e.g. carotenoids, tocopherols (vitamin E), and vitamin C). We became interested in so-called non-nutritive antioxidants after analyzing the effect of nutritive antioxidants on lung cancer in the Zutphen Study (30). We hypothesized that antioxidants could protect against lung cancer in smokers. We observed a protective effect of vitamin C but the protective effect of total fruits was stronger than that of citrus fruits and vitamin C. We therefore hypothesized that compounds other than vitamin C present in fruit could be of value in prevention of lung cancer in smokers. We started a research project on the health effects of flavonoids.

Flavonoids are secondary plant metabolites with strong antioxidant properties abundantly present in plant foods. More than 4,000 different types of flavonoids have been described. Six major classes of flavonoids can be distinguished: flavonols, flavones, catechins, flavanones, anthocyanidins, and isoflavones. We have studied the health effects of flavonoids, flavones, and catechins. When we started the program, analytical methods and quantitative data on the content of these flavonoids in foods were not available. We therefore had to develop and validate methods for the determination of flavonoids, flavones, and catechins. We also had to establish a food composition table on these flavonoids that could be used to determine the intake of flavonoids in humans. Thereafter the intake of different flavonoids could be related to the occurrence of CHD in the Zutphen Elderly Study.

For this program, expertise in nutrition, analytical chemistry, and epidemiology was needed. The program was carried out in close collaboration with Dr. Peter Hollman of the National Institute of Quality Control of Agricultural Products in Wageningen, The Netherlands. Multidisciplinary collaboration was a prerequisite for tackling the complex relationships between flavonoid intake and CHD risk.

First methods were developed and validated for measuring flavonoids in plant foods and drinks. For simplicity, we divided the flavonoids examined into flavonols and catechins. The concentration of flavones in foods is generally much lower than that of flavonols; for this reason, flavones, in the class of flavonols, are included. We determined the content of commonly consumed plant foods in the Netherlands in different seasons. The richest sources of flavonols are tea, apples, onions, and red wine, along with catechins in tea, apples, and chocolate. We were the first to discover that chocolate, and especially dark chocolate, is a rich source of catechins (31). We prepared a food table containing information on the content of different flavonoids in Dutch foods. This provided us the possibility to calculate the intake of different flavonoids of the elderly men in Zutphen.

The average intake of flavonols in elderly men in Zutphen in 1985 was 26 mg per day, with tea forming the major source (61%). The intake of flavonols was strongly inversely related to 5-year mortality from CHD. The relative risk for men who consumed more that 29.0 mg per day of flavonols, compared with those who

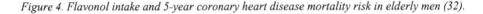

Figure 4. Flavonol intake and 5-year coronary heart disease mortality risk in elderly men (32).

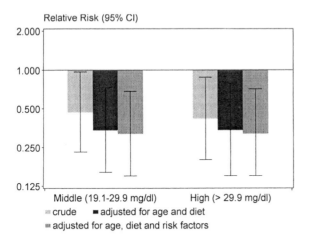

Relative Risk (95% CI)

Middle (19.1-29.9 mg/dl)   High (> 29.9 mg/dl)
▨ crude   ■ adjusted for age and diet
▨ adjusted for age, diet and risk factors

consumed less than 19.1 mg per day, was 0.32 (95%CI 0.15-0.71) (Fig.4) (32). These results were confirmed using 10-year mortality data from CHD (33). An inverse but not significant association was found between flavonol intake and the 5-year risk of fatal and non-fatal myocardial infarction (32). We analyzed also the relationship between the consumption of foods that contributed most to the flavonol intake and five-year mortality from CHD (32). Tea was significantly inversely associated with CHD mortality and the relative risk for the highest versus the lowest tertile of tea consumption was 0.45 (95%CI 0.22-0.95). For apples this risk ratio was 0.51 (95%CI 0.23-1.16), and for onions 0.85 (95%CI 0.46-1.61). These results show that tea and apple consumption contribute most to the protective power of flavonols.

Besides flavonols tea contains a lot of catechins; it contributes 87% to the total catechin intake (34). The average total intake of catechin was in the elderly men in Zutphen 72 mg per day in 1985. Catechin intake was inversely related to 10-year CHD mortality. Men with a catechin intake of more than 85.8 mg per day, compared with those with a catechin intake of less than 49.1 mg per day, had a relative risk of 0.49 (95%CI 0.27-0.88). Catechin intake was also inversely related with 10-year incidence of fatal and non-fatal myocardial infarction, however, this relationship was not statistically significant.

Catechin intake was highly correlated with both tea consumption ($r_s = 0.98$) and the intake of flavonols ($r_s = 0.85$). Therefore it was impossible to examine the effect of catechin intake on CHD mortality after adjusting for flavonol and tea intake. It is important, however, to examine whether flavonols or another component of tea is responsible for the observed effect of catechins. Therefore a model was developed with tea consumption, catechins from other foods than tea, and flavonols from other foods than tea as independent variables with 10-year CHD mortality as the dependent variable. The three independent variables were only weakly correlated with each other. Tea consumption and the catechins not from tea were inversely related with CHD mortality. These results suggest that catechins from tea and other sources may lower the risk of CHD mortality and that catechins are probably more important than flavonols.

Our results on the consumption of tea, the intake of different flavonoids and CHD risk were confirmed by some, but not all, epidemiological studies. It is therefore too early to make definite statements on the possible protective effect of tea consumption on CHD risk. More research is also needed on the health effects of different classes of flavonoids.

OTHER DIETARY FACTORS AND CORONARY HEART DISEASE RISK

Fatty acids and antioxidants have dominated research on the role of diet in the etiology of CHD. This does not mean that other nutrients or non-nutritive compounds are not important. Burkitt and Trowell suggested more than 20 years ago that dietary fiber could be an important determinant of chronic diseases, including CHD, in Western societies (1). B vitamins (e.g. folate, vitamin B6) are involved in homocysteine metabolism. Homocysteine is a risk factor for CHD. Dietary interventions trials provided evidence that supplements of B-vitamins lower homocysteine (35). The semi-essential amino acid L-arginine is the precursor of nitric oxide, a signaling molecule in the cardiovascular system that is involved in endothelial and platelet function (6). These dietary factors have been studied in relation to CHD risk in the Zutphen Study.

We studied the relationship between the intake of dietary fiber and 10-year mortality from CHD and all-causes (36). Mortality from CHD was about four times higher in men with a dietary fiber intake in the lowest quintile compared with those in the highest quintile. For all-causes mortality the ratio was about three. The inverse relationship between dietary fiber intake and mortality from CHD was of borderline significance in univariate analysis and disappeared after multivariate analysis. The inverse relation between dietary fiber intake and all-causes mortality remained after multivariate analysis. The number of fatal CHD cases was small (n = 27), therefore firm statements about a possible protective effect of dietary fiber intake on CHD cannot be made. On the other hand, it can be concluded that men with a dietary fiber intake of more than 37 grams per day had a significantly lower all-causes mortality.

Other epidemiological studies also found an inverse relation between dietary fiber intake and CHD risk (37-39). These studies suggest that especially cereal fiber is protective against CHD. This was in contrast to expectations because cereal fiber is a rich source of insoluble fiber. This type of fiber does not, however, lower serum total cholesterol levels in contrast to soluble fiber. Diets high in cereal fiber may have other beneficial effects such as an increased insulin sensitivity and lower serum triglyceride levels. We can conclude that evidence that dietary fiber may protect against CHD risk is accumulating. More research is needed on the effects of different types of fiber and their effect on lipoproteins, platelet function, and insulin sensitivity.

There is a great interest in homocysteine as a risk factor for cardiovascular diseases. However, it is still not clear whether serum homocysteine levels are independent predictors of cardiovascular risk. We found that serum homocysteine was a predictor for 10-year cardiovascular risk in the Zutphen Elderly Study (40). This association was stronger using a shorter (first five years) instead of longer follow-up period. As expected, we observed that the intake of folate and vitamin B6 was independently inversely associated with homocysteine level (41). We can conclude that many questions remain about the complex relationships between the intake of B vitamins, serum homocysteine levels, and CHD risk.

Basic research provides strong evidence for the involvement of nitric oxide in the athero-thrombotic process. We studied the relationship between the intake of the amino acid L-arginine, a precursor of nitric oxide, and CHD risk. The average intake of arginine in the Zutphen elderly men was 4.4 g per day (42). The major contributors to total arginine intake were: meat (37%), bread (13%), and milk products (12%). Arginine intake was not related to coronary risk. We also studied this association at the population level, using data of the 16 cohorts of the Seven Countries Study (43). The average population arginine intake was not related to 25-year population CHD mortality rates. We concluded that our analyses do not support a protective effect of arginine at intake levels observed in the Seven Countries Study.

Besides dietary factors studied in the Zutphen Study many more nutrients (e.g. minerals) and non-nutritive compounds (e.g. lignans) may play a role in the etiology of CHD. After decades of research the role of fatty acids in relation to coronary risk is becoming clear, although several important questions remain. For all other dietary factors much more observational and experimental research is needed before their role in the etiology of CHD is clarified.

SUMMARY AND CONCLUSIONS

Repeat dietary data of all members of the Zutphen cohort were collected at regular intervals. This made it possible to study the etiologic relationships between dietary variables and CHD occurrence in individuals. Emphasis was put on associations between the intake of fatty acids and antioxidants in relation to CHD mortality.

The intake of total saturated, mono and polyunsaturated fatty acids was not related to CHD mortality. The intake of *trans* fatty acids was positively associated with CHD risk. A small amount of fish was associated with lower CHD mortality risk. Fish is a rich source of the very long-chain N-3 polyunsaturated fatty acids EPA and DHA. However, a relationship between the intake of another N-3 polyunsaturated fatty acid, ALA and CHD risk could not be established.

The consumption of tea was inversely related to CHD risk. Tea is a rich source of different flavonoids; compounds present in plant foods with strong antioxidant properties. We found evidence for an inverse association of the flavonoids class, catechins. Finally we observed an inverse association of dietary fiber, especially with all-causes mortality.

We conclude that in the Zutphen Study the strongest effects of diet were found for fish consumption and the intake of *trans* fatty acids. Fish protects against fatal CHD and *trans* fatty acids increase CHD risk. Also evidence is accumulating that plant foods, more specifically dietary fiber and catechins in the diet, may be protective against CHD.

REFERENCES

1. Trowell HC, Burkett DP (Eds). Western diseases: their emergence and prevention. London: E Arnold Ltd , 1981.
2. Liu S, Willett WC, Stampfer MJ, Hu FB, Sampson L, Hennekens CH, Manson JE. A prospective study of dietary glycemic load, carbohydrate and risk of coronary heart disease in U.S. women. Am J Clin Nutr 2000;71:1455-1461.

3. Sinclair HM. Deficiency of essential fatty acids and atherosclerosis, etcetera. Lancet 1956;i:381-383.
4. Ueland PM, Refsum H, Beresford SA, Vollset SE. The controversy over homocysteine and cardiovascular risk. Am J Clin Nutr 2000;72:324-332.
5. De Bree A, Verschuren WMM, Blom HJ, Kromhout D. Association between B vitamin intake and plasma homocysteine concentration in the general Dutch population aged 20-65. Am J Clin Nutr 2001;73:1027-1033
6. Palmer RMJ, Ashton DS, Moncada S. Vascular endothelial cells synthesize nitric oxide from L-arginine. Nature 1988;333:664-666.
7. Den Hartog C, Van Schaik TFSM, Dalderup LM, Drion EF, Mulder T. The diet of volunteers participating in a long-term epidemiological field survey of coronary heart disease in Zutphen, The Netherlands. Voeding 1965;26:184-201.
8. Bloemberg BPM, Kromhout D, Obermann-de Boer GL, Van Kampen-Donker M. The reproducibility of dietary intake data assessed with the cross-check dietary history method. (The Zutphen Study). Am J Epidemiol 1989;130:1047-1056.
9. Kromhout D, De Lezenne Coulander C. Diet, prevalence and 10-year mortality from coronary heart disease in 871 middle-aged men (The Zutphen Study). Am J Epidemiol 1984;119:733-741.
10. Kromhout D, Bosschieter EB, De Lezenne Coulander C. The inverse relation between fish consumption and 20-year mortality from coronary heart disease. N Engl J Med 1985;312:1205-1209.
11. Stamler J, Shekelle R. Dietary cholesterol and human coronary heart disease. Arch Pathol Lab Med 1988;112:1032-1040.
12. Mensink RP, Katan MB. Effect of dietary *trans* fatty acids on high density and low-density lipoprotein cholesterol levels in healthy subjects. N Engl J Med 1990;323:439-445.
13. Willett WC, Stampfer MJ, Manson JE, Colditz GA, Speizer FE, Rosner BA, Sampson LA, Hennekens CH. Intake of *trans* fatty acids and risk of coronary heart disease among women. Lancet 1993;341:581-585.
14. Oomen CM, Ocke MC, Feskens EJ, Erp van-Baart MA, Kok FJ, Kromhout D. Association between *trans* fatty acid intake and 10-year risk of coronary heart disease in the Zutphen Elderly Study: a prospective population-based study. Lancet 2001;357:746-751
15. Phillipsen BE, Rothrock DW, Connor WE, Harris WS, Illingworth DR. Reduction of plasma lipids, lipoproteins, and apoproteins by dietary fish oils in patients with hypertriglyceridemia. N Engl J Med 1985;312:1210-1216.
16. Lee TH, Hoover RC, Williams JD, Sperling RI, Ravalese J 3rd, Spur BW, Robinson DR, Corey EJ, Lewis RA, Austen KF. Effect of dietary enrichment with eicosapentaenoic and docosahexaenoic acids on in vitro neutrophil and monocyte leukotriene generation and neutrophil function. N Engl J Med 1985;312:1417-1424.
17. Bang HO, Dyerberg J, Sinclair HM. The composition of the Eskimo food in north western Greenland. Am J Clin Nutr 1980;33:2657-2661.
18. Kromann N, Green A. Epidemiological studies in the Upernavik district, Greenland. Acta Med Scand 1980;208:401-406.
19. Kromhout D, Feskens EJM, Bowles CH. The protective effect of a small amount of fish on coronary heart disease mortality in an elderly population. Int J Epidemiol 1995;24:340-345.
20. Oomen CM, Feskens EJM, Räsänen L, Fidanza F, Nissinen AM, Menotti A, Kok FJ, Kromhout D. Fish consumption and coronary heart disease mortality in Finland, Italy and the Netherlands. Am J Epidemiol 2000;151:999-1006.
21. Keli SO, Feskens EJM, Kromhout D. Fish consumption and risk of stroke. The Zutphen Study. Stroke 1994;25:328-332.
22. Kromhout D. Fish consumption and sudden cardiac death. (editorial). JAMA 1998;279:65-66.
23. Burr ML, Fehily AM, Gilbert JF, Rogers S, Holliday RM, Sweetnam PM, Elwood PC, Deadman NM. Effects of changes in fat, fish and fibre intakes on death and myocardial re-infarction: diet and re-infarction trial (DART). Lancet 1989;ii:757-761.

24. Kromhout D, Katan MB, Havekes L, Groener A, Hornstra G, De Lezenne Coulander C. The effects of 26 years of habitual fish consumption on serum lipid and lipoprotein levels (The Zutphen Study). Nutr Metab Cardiov Dis 1996;6(2):65-73.
25. Van Houwelingen AC, Hornstra G, Kromhout D, De Lezenne Coulander C. Habitual fish consumption, fatty acids of serum phospholipids and platelet function. Atherosclerosis 1989; 75:157-165.
26. Oomen CM, Ocké MC, Feskens EJM, Kok FJ, Kromhout D. Alpha-linolenic acid intake is not beneficially associated with 10-year risk of coronary heart disease. Am J Clin Nutr 2001;74:457-463.
27. Ascherio A, Rimm EB, Giovannucci EL, Spiegelman D, Stampfer MJ, Willett WC. Dietary fat and risk of coronary heart disease in men: cohort follow-up study in the United States. BMJ 1996;313:84-90.
28. Lorgeril M de, Renaud S, Mamelle N, Salen P, Martin JL, Monjaud I, Guidollet J, Touboul P, Delaye J. Mediterranean alpha-linolenic acid-rich diet in secondary prevention of coronary heart disease. Lancet 1994;343:1454-1459.
29. Renaud S, De Lorgeril M, Delaye J, Guidollet J, Jacquard F, Mamelle N, Martin JL, Monjaud I, Salen P, Toubol P. Cretan Mediterranean diet for prevention of coronary heart disease. Am J Clin Nutr 1995;61 Suppl:1360S-1367S.
30. Kromhout D. Essential micronutrients in relation to carcinogenesis. Am J Clin Nutr 1987;45:1361-1367.
31. Arts IC, Hollman PC, Kromhout D. Chocolate as a source of tea flavonoids [letter]. Lancet 1999;354:488.
32. Hertog MGL, Feskens EJM, Hollman PCH, Katan MB, Kromhout D. Dietary antioxidant flavonoids and risk of coronary heart disease. The Zutphen Elderly Study. Lancet 1993;342:1007-12.
33. Hertog MGL, Feskens EJM, Kromhout D. Antioxidant flavonols and coronary heart disease risk [letter]. Lancet 1997; 349:699.
34. Arts IC, Hollman PC, Feskens EJ, Bueno de Mesquita HB, Kromhout D.Catechin intake might explain the inverse relation between tea consumption and ischemic heart disease: the Zutphen Elderly Study. Am J Clin Nutr 2001;74:227-232.
35. Clarke R, Collins R. Can dietary supplements with folic acid or vitamin B6 reduce cardiovascular risk? Design of clinical trials to test the homocysteine hypothesis of vascular disease. J Cardiovasc Risk 1998;5:249-255.
36. Kromhout D, Bosschieter EB, De Lezenne Coulander C. Dietary fibre and 10-year mortality from coronary heart disease, cancer and all-causes. The Zutphen Study. Lancet 1982;II:518-522.
37. Morris JN, Marr JW, Clayton DG. Diet and the heart: a postscript. BMJ 1977;ii:1307-1314.
38. Rimm EB, Ascherio A, Giovannucci E, Spiegelman D, Stampfer MJ, Willett WC. Vegetable, fruit, and cereal fiber intake and risk of coronary heart disease among men. JAMA 1996;275:447-451.
39. Wolk A, Manson JE, Stampfer MJ, Colditz GA, Hu FB, Speizer FE, Hennekens CH, Willett WC. Long-term intake of dietary fiber and decreased risk of coronary heart disease among women. JAMA 1999;281:1998-2004.
40. Stehouwer CDA, Weijenberg MP, Berg M van den, Jakobs C, Feskens EJM, Kromhout D. Serum homocysteine and risk of coronary heart disease and cerebrovascular disease in elderly men. Arterioscler Thromb Vasc Biol 1998;18:1895-1901.
41. Oomen CM, Verhoef P, Feskens EJM, Ocké M, Kromhout D. B vitamin intake, serum total homocysteine concentrations and 10-year risk of coronary heart disease in the Zutphen Elderly Study. Submitted.
42. Oomen CM, Erk MJ van, Feskens EJM, Kok FJ, Kromhout D. Arginine intake and risk of coronary heart disease mortality in elderly men. Arterioscler Thromb Vasc Biol 2000;20 2134-2139
43. Feskens EJ, Oomen CM, Hogendoorn E, Menotti A, Kromhout D. Arginine intake and 25-year CHD mortality: the Seven Countries Study. Eur Heart J 2001;22(7):611-612.

CHAPTER 2.3

CIGARETTE SMOKING, CORONARY HEART DISEASE
AND ALL-CAUSES MORTALITY IN THE SEVEN
COUNTRIES STUDY

Daan Kromhout

When the Seven Countries Study started in 1958 the relationship between cigarette smoking and lung cancer was already known (1,2). The 1962 data of the Framingham and Albany studies showed that cigarette smoking was also an important risk factor for CHD (3). At that time, high prevalence rates of cigarette smoking (75-90%) were observed in middle-aged men in Great Britain and the Netherlands (4,5). However, men who died from tobacco-related diseases in the 1950s had been exposed to the habit for a relatively short period. The full health consequences of long-term exposure to cigarette smoking have only recently become evident (6).

Of all lung cancer deaths in middle-aged men, more than 90% can be attributed to tobacco (7). A similar percentage is found for chronic obstructive pulmonary diseases. For vascular diseases (CHD and stroke) this percentage is about 35. However, the absolute number of vascular deaths attributed to smoking in the U.S. and northern European countries (Great Britain and the Netherlands) is higher than that for lung cancer. Of the 2.1 million deaths in 1985 in the U.S., 110,000 lung cancer deaths, 31,000 deaths from other cancers, and 143,000 vascular disease deaths were attributed to smoking. Tobacco causes as many deaths from vascular diseases as all types of cancer together. Vascular diseases are thus a major harmful health consequence of cigarette smoking.

This chapter summarizes trends in the prevalence of cigarette smoking in the Seven Countries Study for a 35-year period and the relationships between cigarette smoking and mortality from CHD and all-causes, both at the population and individual level.

TRENDS IN THE PREVALENCE OF CIGARETTE SMOKING IN A 35-YEAR PERIOD

Information on smoking was collected in the Seven Countries Study on the type of smoking (cigarette, cigar and pipe), past and current smoking and the amount smoked using a standardized questionnaire (8). With the exception of the Zutphen cohort, almost all men smoked cigarettes only. Because in Zutphen most pipe and cigar smokers also smoked cigarettes, only the results on cigarette smoking will be reported. The prevalence data are reported as the percentage of the population that smoked cigarettes.

In the Finnish cohorts of the Seven Countries Study the questionnaire data on smoking were validated by objective blood tests (9,10). In 1959 serum thiocyanate concentration was measured among 1,539 men aged 40-59, and in 1974, random measurements of the proportion of hemoglobin bound to carbon monoxide (COHb%) were carried out in 1,068 men, aged 55-74. Serum thiocyanate concentration effectively distinguished between men smoking at least 10 cigarettes per day from non-smokers (9). Light smokers with a daily consumption of 1-9 cigarettes per day had intermediate values of serum thiocyanate. Mean values for moderate and heavy smokers did not differ. COHb% was strongly related to cigarette smoking (10); concentrations above 2% were much more common in current smokers (70%) than in never-smokers (7%). Based on these validation studies, it can be concluded that current smokers identified with the Seven Countries Study questionnaire could be distinguished from never-smokers.

Figure 1. Prevalence of cigarette smokers in the 16 cohorts around 1960.

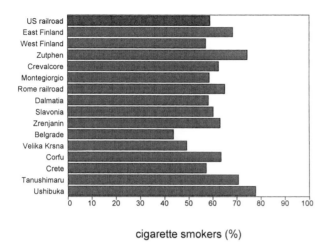

cigarette smokers (%)

In the baseline survey of the Seven Countries Study the prevalence of cigarette smokers in the 16 cohorts varied between 44% in Belgrade, and 78% in Ushibuka (Fig.1). Between 1960 and 1995, a substantial decrease in the prevalence of cigarette smokers was observed in eight European cohorts (Table 1). For example between 1960 and 1995 the prevalence of cigarette smokers fell from 75% to 27% in Zutphen and from 44% to 6% in Belgrade. The cohorts retained their relative position over time in the distribution of cigarette smokers. Also, the large variation in prevalence of cigarette smokers at age 75-94 is remarkable. A greater than fivefold range was observed between elderly men from Zutphen (27%) and West Finland (5%).

Trends in the prevalence of cigarette smokers presented in Table 1 are confounded by aging. In Table 2, trends are shown for men aged 40-59 examined in the Seven Countries Study in 1960, and in the WHO-MONICA Project in 1985 and 1995. During this 35-year period, the prevalence of cigarette smokers in middle-aged men in Finland decreased by about 50%, and absolute prevalence was less than 30% in 1995. In the Netherlands and Belgium a relative decrease of more than 40% was noted, and the prevalence of middle-aged cigarette smokers was 43% in 1995. In Italy a decrease in prevalence of middle-aged smokers of about 50% occurred between 1960 and 1995; in 1995 the prevalence was about 30%. The smallest relative decrease in the prevalence of cigarette smokers was observed in Serbia, and amounted to about 20%. Almost half of the middle-aged men in Serbia smoked cigarettes in 1995.

The prevalence of cigarette smokers among middle-aged men can be concluded to have decreased remarkably since 1960. Large absolute reductions (about 50%) were observed in Finland and Italy, and small ones (about 20%) in Serbia. Despite these decreases, cigarette smoking remains a major public health problem, with prevalence rates of cigarette smokers varying from 30 to 50% in middle-aged men, and 5 to 27% in elderly men.

Table 1. Trends in the prevalence of smokers in men aged 40-59 at baseline in several European cohorts of the Seven Countries Study in the period of 1960-1995.

| Year | 1960 | | 1970 | | 1985 | | 1995 | |
| Age(y) | 40-59 | | 50-69 | | 65-84 | | 75-94 | |
Cohort	N	%	N	%	N	%	N	%
East Finland	816	69	648	57	314	19	120	10
West Finland	857	57	715	42	383	17	150	5
Zutphen	878	75	701	54	361	34	123	27
Crevalcore	991	63	761	54	373	27	146	8
Montegiorgio	715	59	574	51	308	26	121	12
Zrenjanin	517	63	426	56	179	25	53	15
Belgrade	540	44	435	27	285	13	137	6
Velika Krsna	498	49	437	44	227	29	73	14

Table 2. Trends in the prevalence of cigarette smokers (%) in men aged 50 in the period of 1960-1995 in European populations.

Cohort	1960	1985	1995
North Karelia (FIN)	69	37	27
Turku/Looimaa (FIN)	59	39	29
Zutphen (NL)	76		
Ghent (B)		52	43
Crevalcore (I)	63		
Friuli (I)		38	29
Montegiorgio (I)	59		
Brianza (I)		47	34
Zrenjanin (SE)	63		
Novi Sad (SE)		52	49

The 1960 data represent the baseline data from the Seven Countries Study.
The 1985 and 1995 data are from the WHO-MONICA Project

CIGARETTE SMOKING AND MORTALITY FROM CORONARY HEART DISEASE AND ALL-CAUSES: A CROSS-CULTURAL PERSPECTIVE

During the baseline surveys of the Seven Countries Study carried out between 1958 and 1964 the prevalence rates of cigarette smokers were high, between 44% in Belgrade professors and 78% in fishermen from Ushibuka. Smoking rates declined substantially during 35 years of follow-up. For cross-cultural comparisons on the relationships between cigarette smoking and mortality, it is necessary to know whether the different cohorts kept to their relative ranks in smokers prevalence. The correlation coefficient describes how strong the prevalence rates of smokers among different cohorts are correlated at different points in time. Around 1970, 10-year follow-up surveys were carried out in 15 of the 16 cohorts. The correlation coefficient for prevalence rates of smokers at baseline versus 10-year follow-up was (r = 0.83, p< 0.001). These results suggest that the cohorts kept their relative ranks in the distribution of the proportion of cigarette smokers.

Keys analyzed the relationships between population rates of smokers, and mortality from CHD and all-causes using 10-year follow-up data (11). He found no relation between the percentage of non-smokers at baseline, and 10-year mortality rates from CHD or all-causes. These analyses were hampered by the very low mortality rates in several southern European and Japanese cohorts. Therefore a longer follow-up period was needed to obtain more stable mortality rates.

The 25-year mortality data also showed no significant relationship between the prevalence of smokers at baseline, and 25-year mortality rates from CHD (Fig 2). However, the high prevalence of smokers and low CHD mortality rates of the two Japanese cohorts, Tanushimaru and Ushibuka, distorted this association. If those two cohorts were excluded, the correlation coefficient increased from r = 0.06 to r = 0.45. This suggests that the low mortality rates from CHD in Japan may be due to other lifestyle and dietary factors that exert a protective effect for coronary mortality in Japanese society. It is therefore of interest to carry out multivariate analyses that adjust for these confounding effects.

Figure 2. Prevalence of cigarette smokers in 1960, and 25-year age-adjusted mortality rates from coronary heart disease.

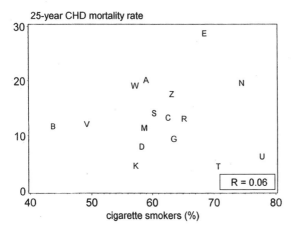

For legend see appendix

Table 3. Regression coefficients (β) for population averages of different exposures, and 25-year age-adjusted coronary heart disease mortality rates (15).

Exposure variable	Univariate	Multivariate[a]		
	β	β	95% CI	P-value
Cigarette smokers (%)	0.045	0.323	0.16, 0.48	0.002
Saturated fat (%E)	0.951	0.905	0.68, 1.13	<0.001
Flavonoids (mg)	-0.161	-0.091	-0.01, -0.17	0.041

a = Multivariate model: Coronary heart disease = smokers + saturated fat + flavonoids

The Seven Countries Study showed by using 5-year mortality follow-up data, that the average population intake of saturated fat was strongly associated with population rates from CHD (14). Later on, using 25-year mortality follow-up data, it was shown that the average population intake of flavonoids was inversely related to 25-year population CHD mortality rates (15). For this reason a multivariate analysis was carried out using 25-year population mortality rates from CHD as the dependent variable, and the prevalence of cigarette smokers and average population intake of saturated fat and flavonoids as independent variables. This analysis showed that the prevalence of cigarette smokers is strongly related to 25-year population mortality rates due to CHD (Table 3). Cigarette smoking in combination with saturated fat, and flavonoid, intake explains 90% of the variance in population mortality rates for CHD.

The Seven Countries Study data suggest that the population prevalence of smokers has a major influence on population CHD mortality rates. The different results obtained in uni- and multivariate analyses were due to the low mortality rates in the two Japanese cohorts. Even though there was a high prevalence of smokers, Japanese were apparently "protected" by their low intake of saturated fat and high intake of flavonoids.

Similar results were obtained for the relationship between cigarette smoking and all-causes mortality. In univariate analyses, the prevalence of cigarette smokers at baseline was not significantly associated with 25-year population all-causes mortality rates (Fig. 3) (16). However, after multivariate analyses, which took the average population intake of saturated fat and vitamin C into account, the prevalence of cigarette smokers also became significantly related to 25-year all-causes mortality rates (Table 4) (16). These variables explain 52% of the variance in population mortality rates from all-causes.

Figure 3. Prevalence of cigarette smokers in 1960, and 25-year age-adjusted mortality rates from all-causes.

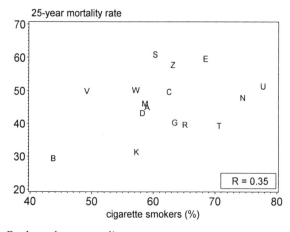

For legend see appendix

Table 4. Regression coefficients (β) for population averages of different exposures, and 25-year age-adjusted all-causes mortality rates (16).

Exposure Variable	Univariate β	Multivariate[a] β	95%CI	P-value
Cigarette smokers (%)	0.37	0.57	0.14, 0.90	0.024
Saturated fat (%E)	0.55	0.94	0.29, 1.59	0.015
Vitamin C (mg)	-0.05	-0.10	-0.20, 0.00	0.062

a = Multivariate model: All-causes mortality = smokers + saturated fat + vitamin C

We conclude from these ecological analyses that the prevalence of cigarette smokers is a major determinant of population mortality rates from both CHD and all-causes. A 10% difference in the prevalence rate of smokers is associated with a 3.2% difference in the 25-year population CHD mortality rate, and a 5.7% difference in 25-year population all-causes mortality rate. The average population prevalence of smokers in the Seven Countries Study at baseline was approximately 60%, and the average population all-causes mortality rate after 25 years of follow-up was about 45%. If the prevalence of smokers is reduced by 50% (from 60 to 30%), a 45 to 28% decrease in 25-year population all-causes mortality rate is predicted; this explains the large public health potential to stop smoking.

CIGARETTE SMOKING AND MORTALITY FROM CORONARY HEART DISEASE AND ALL-CAUSES IN INDIVIDUALS

Individual data of the Seven Countries Study showed that 10-year CHD, and all-causes mortality rates in never-smokers from the U.S., northern and southern Europe were similar (11). Among men who smoked more than 20 cigarettes per day, compared with never-smokers, the 10-year CHD mortality rate was about 4 times higher in northern Europe, about 3 times higher in the U.S., and about 2 times higher in southern Europe. Similar results were obtained for all-causes mortality. This raises the question on whether the health risk of heavy smoking is different among middle-aged men from the U.S. and northern and southern Europe, or whether these results are due to chance. This latter possibility may be the case in relation to CHD mortality rates, because of the low rates observed in the different cohorts.

The question whether differences in harmful effects of cigarette smoking among cohorts are due to chance, was addressed in a paper using the 25-year Seven Countries mortality data (17). The analyses showed on average a 5% difference in 25-year CHD mortality, and a 17% difference in all-causes mortality, comparing men who smoked at least 10 cigarettes per day with never-smokers (Figs. 4 and 5). CHD mortality rates were higher in cigarette smokers in 12 of the 16 cohorts. The negative findings in the other 4 cohorts are probably due to chance, and to the small number of never smokers in some of these cohorts. All-causes mortality was higher among smokers in all 16 cohorts.

An analysis using 15-year mortality data of the two Finnish cohorts showed similar results (9). Relative risk for CHD mortality in current smokers compared to non-smokers was 1.5 in East Finland and 4.1 in West Finland. Using serum thiocyanate levels, we found a relative risk of 2.5 in a multivariate model, in which

Figure 4. Age-adjusted coronary heart disease 25-year difference of smokers of 10 cigarettes per day or more versus never smokers. Error bars represent 95% confidence interval for the death rate difference (17).

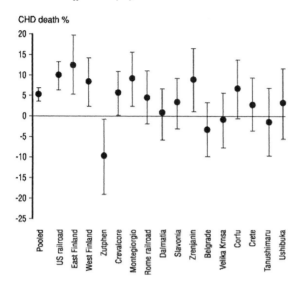

Figure 5. Age- adjusted all-causes 25-year difference of smokers of 10 cigarettes per day or more versus never smokers. Error bars represent 95% confidence interval for the death rate difference (17).

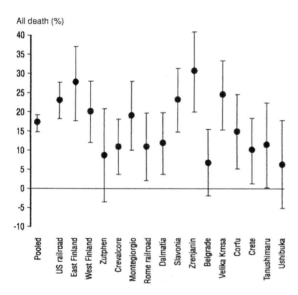

major risk factors including smoking were taken into account, among men with levels above 90 µmol/l compared to men with 50 or less µmol/l. This means that serum thiocyanate level had an "effect" on CHD mortality independent of smoking class. In West Finland, characterized by a relatively low rate of CHD mortality, no relationship was found between serum thiocyanate and coronary deaths. Similar results were found for all-causes mortality. Information on smoking obtained through a questionnaire can be concluded to be an important predictor of CHD and all-causes mortality. Measurement of serum thiocyanate may be of additional value, separate from information collected on smoking history.

In the Finnish cohorts we also studied the effect of the follow-up period on the associations between cigarette smoking, and CHD and all-causes mortality (18). The hazard ratio for CHD mortality in current smokers compared to non-smokers decreased from 6.80 (95%CI 1.64-28.22) after 10 years of follow-up to 1.63 (95%CI 1.24-2.13) after 35 years of follow-up. The 25-year mortality rate for persistent smokers during the first 10 years of follow-up was 1.94 (95%CI 1.36-2.48). For all-causes mortality in relation to 10-, 25- and 35-year risk, these respective risk ratios were 2.16, 1.84 and 1.62. The decreasing strength of the associations with the increasing length of the follow-up period is largely due to the fact that the participants in the study changed their smoking status during the follow-up period. At the end of the 30 years' follow-up, only 15% of the elderly survivors were current smokers, whereas 66% of the baseline population smoked cigarettes.

The predictive power of smoking in old age was studied in Finnish, Dutch, and Italian cohorts of the Seven Countries Study (19,20). Around 1985, 2,170 men aged 65-84 were examined in the 25-year follow-up survey of the Seven Countries Study and followed for 10 years. During that period, 289 men died from coronary heart disease, 545 from cardiovascular diseases and 1033 from all-causes. The odds ratio of current smokers was 1.24 (95%CI 0.91-1.69) for 10-year CHD mortality, and 1.28 (95%CI 1.01-1.63) for cardiovascular diseases mortality (19). For all-causes mortality, the hazard ratio for smokers compared with non-smokers was 1.45 (95%CI 1.22-1.73) (20). After excluding mortality during the first five years of follow-up, the hazard ratio increased to 1.67 (95%CI 1.31-2.14). These results show clearly that if the influence of early mortality, an indicator of pre-morbid conditions, on the association between smoking and mortality is eliminated, a strong association persists between cigarette smoking, and all-causes mortality in old age.

SUMMARY AND CONCLUSIONS

The prevalence of cigarette smokers in middle-aged men at the baseline survey of the Seven Countries Study varied between 44 and 78%. In Europe and elderly men 35 years later, the prevalence varied between 5% and 27%. Cigarette smoking is a strong determinant of CHD, and all-causes mortality rates among populations and risk among individuals. In middle-aged men the risk ratio for long-term all-causes mortality when comparing smokers with non-smokers is about 2. The risk ratio decreases with age, but is still 1.5 in men aged 65-84, followed for 10 years, this increases to 1.7 when early mortality, an indicator of pre-morbid conditions, is eliminated. These results show that smoking is a major health threat into old age. About half of the persistent smokers will eventually be killed by their habit (6).

However, if smokers decide to stop smoking before age 50, as much as 90% of the risk attributable to tobacco can be avoided (4).

REFERENCES

1. Doll R, Hill AB. Smoking and carcinoma of the lung. A preliminary report. BMJ 1950;ii:739-748.
2. Wynder EL, Graham EA. Tobacco smoking as a possible etiologic factor in bronchogenic carcinoma. JAMA 1950;143:329-336.
3. Doyle JT, Dawber TR, Kannel WB, Heslin AS, Kahn HA. Cigarette smoking and coronary heart disease. Combined experience of the Albany and Framingham studies. N Engl J Med 1962;266:796-801.
4. Peto R, Darby S, Deo H, Silcocks P, Whitley E, Doll R. Smoking, smoking cessation and lung cancer in the UK since 1950: Combination of national statistics with two case-control studies. BMJ 2000;321:323-329.
5. Smit HA, Hoeymans N, Bueno de Mesquita HB, Kromhout D. Roken. In: Volksgezondheid Toekomst Verkenning. De gezondheidstoestand van de Nederlandse bevolking in de periode 1950-2010. Ruwaard D, Kramers PGN (Eds). Rijksinstituut voor Volksgezondheid en Milieuhygiëne. Sdu Uitgeverij, Den Haag, 1993:567-572.
6. Doll R, Peto R, Wheatley K, Gray R, Sutherland I. Mortality in relation to smoking: 40 years observations on male British doctors. BMJ 1994;309:901-911.
7. Peto R, Lopez AD, Boreham J, Thun M, Heath C Jr. Mortality from tobacco in developed countries: indirect estimation from national vital statistics. Lancet 1992;339:1268-1278.
8. Keys A, Aravanis C, Blackburn HW, Van Buchem FSP, Buzina R, Djordjevic BS, Dontas AS, Fidanza F, Karvonen MJ, Kimura N, Lekos D, Monti M, Puddu V, Taylor HL. Epidemiological studies related to coronary heart disease: characteristics of men aged 40-59 in seven countries. Acta Med Scand 1967;460 Suppl:1-392.
9. Heliövaara M, Karvonen MJ, Punsar S, Rautanen Y, Haapakoski J. Serum thiocyanate concentration and cigarette smoking in relation to overall mortality and to deaths from coronary heart disease and lung cancer. J Chron Dis 1981;34:305-311.
10. Heliövaara M, Karvonen MJ, Vilhunen R, Punsar S. Smoking, carbon monoxide, and atherosclerotic diseases. BMJ 1978;1:268-270.
11. Keys A, Aravanis C, Blackburn H, Buzina R, Djordjevic BS, Dontas AS, Fidanza F, Karvonen MJ, Kimura N, Menotti A, Mohacek I, Nedeljkovic S, Puddu V, Punsar S, Taylor HL, Van Buchem FSP. Seven countries. A multivariate analysis of death and coronary heart disease. Cambridge, MA; Harvard University Press, ISBN: 0-674-80237-3, 1980:1- 381.
12. Rayner M, Petersen S. Compilers European cardiovascular disease statistics.London: British Heart Foundation, 2000:1-132.
13. Kuulasmaa K, Tunstall-Pedoe H, Dobson A, Fortmann S, Sans S, Tolonen H, Evans A, Ferrario M, Tuomilehto J. Estimation of contribution of changes in classical risk factors to trends in coronary-event rates across the WHO MONICA Project populations. Lancet 2000;355:675-687.
14. Keys A (Ed). Coronary heart disease in seven countries. Circulation 1970;41 Suppl 1:1-211.
15. Hertog MGL, Kromhout D, Aravanis C, Blackburn H, Buzina R, Fidanza F, Giampaoli S, Jansen A, Menotti A, Nedeljkovic S, Pekkarinen M, Simic BS, Toshima H, Feskens EJM, Hollman PCH, Katan MB. Flavonoid intake and long-term risk of coronary heart disease and cancer in the Seven Countries Study. Arch Intern Med 1995;155:381-386.
16. Kromhout D, Bloemberg B, Feskens E, Menotti A, Nissinen A for the Seven Countries Study Group. Saturated fat, vitamin C and smoking predict long-term all-cause mortality rates in the Seven Countries Study. Int J Epidemiol 2000;29:260-265.

17. Jacobs DR, Adachi H, Mulder I, Kromhout D, Menotti A, Nissinen A, Blackburn H for the Seven Countries Study. Cigarette smoking and mortality risk. Twenty-five-year follow-up of the Seven Countries Study. Arch Intern Med 1999;159:733-740.
18. Qiao Q, Tervahauta M, Nissinen A, Tuomilehto J. Mortality from all-causes and from coronary heart disease related to smoking and changes in smoking during a 35-year follow-up of middle-aged Finnish men. Eur Heart J 2000;21:1621-1626.
19. Houterman S, Boshuizen HC, Verschuren WMM, Giampaoli S, Nissinen A, Menotti A, Kromhout D. Predicting cardiovascular risk in the elderly in different European countries. Eur Heart J 2002;23:294-300.
20. Menotti A, Mulder I, Nissinen A, Feskens E, Giampaoli S, Tervahauta M, Kromhout D. Cardiovascular risk factors and 10-year all-cause mortality in elderly European populations. The FINE Study. Eur Heart J 2001;22:573-579.

CHAPTER 2.4

ALCOHOL AND CORONARY HEART DISEASE
IN THE SEVEN COUNTRIES STUDY

Daan Kromhout

Epidemiology has found relationships between alcohol consumption and CHD risk. Many articles have been published on this complex relationship. In a recently published meta analysis, 196 articles on the topic were reviewed, showing that the relationship would depend on the amount of alcohol consumed, on gender and on geographical area (1). Despite the wealth of available data, important questions remain about the health effects of the patterns of drinking and about a possible protective effect of substances, other than alcohol, in red wine (2).

Compared with no alcohol consumption, low to moderate consumption is associated with a lower risk, and may offer protection against CHD. Abstainers and persons with a high alcohol intake run an increased risk of CHD and other vascular diseases (1). This is why a J- or U-shaped relationship is found between alcohol intake and coronary risk. To make the situation more complex, the health effects from a certain amount of alcohol depend on whether it is consumed on one occasion or as moderate daily intake during the week (3). This suggests that not only the amount of alcohol, but also the drinking pattern, is of importance in relation to health. The Seven Countries Study managed to collect information through dietary surveys on the large differences in the drinking pattern between northern and southern Europe.

Baseline dietary information including alcohol intake was collected in detail in small samples of the 16 cohorts. These data provided the possibility to study the ecological association between average alcohol consumption and CHD mortality rates. In the Finnish, Dutch, and Italian cohorts, information on diet and alcohol was collected on all individuals during the course of the follow-up, making it possible to study trends in alcohol consumption and the relationship between alcohol consumption and CHD mortality in individuals.

This chapter summarizes the trends in alcohol consumption during a 35-year period in several European cohorts. The relationship between alcohol consumption and CHD mortality will be described, both at the population and individual levels.

TRENDS IN ALCOHOL CONSUMPTION DURING THE 35-YEAR PERIOD

In the Seven Countries Study, different dietary survey methods were used to quantify alcohol consumption. For the baseline surveys, information on diet and alcohol consumption was collected in small samples of the 16 cohorts using the record method (4). In 14 of the 16 cohorts, food and alcohol consumption was recorded for seven days; in the remaining cohorts this was done for 1 or 4 days. In the Finnish, Dutch, and Italian cohorts, information on food and alcohol was collected at intervals in all individuals using the dietary history method (5). Since 1985, a frequency method has been used to quantify the alcohol consumption of elderly men in Finland and Italy (6). The record method provides information on current alcohol consumption, while the dietary history and food frequency methods provide information on habitual alcohol consumption in the months preceding the interview. The different survey methods provide different answers to the question of how much alcohol is used.

The types of alcoholic beverages used in the different countries varied. In Finland, the commonly used alcoholic beverage is spirits (e.g. vodka). In the Netherlands it is beer and in Italy, wine. An extensive literature review on the effects of specific types of alcoholic beverages on coronary risk concluded that all alcoholic beverages are linked with lower risk, and that a substantial portion of the benefit is from the alcohol, rather than from the other components found in each type of drink (7). To get an estimate of the total amount of alcohol consumed, the alcohol content of the different alcoholic beverages was summed. For 1960, average alcohol intake was, according to reports, based on chemical analysis (8). For the other years, information on the consumption of different alcoholic beverages was converted into absolute alcohol intake by using locally collected data on the alcohol content of different beverages.

Figure 1. Average population absolute alcohol intake in the 16 cohorts in 1960.

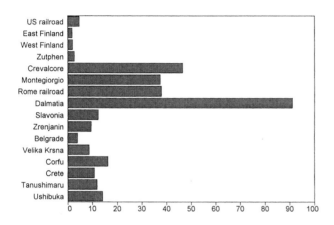

average absolute alcohol intake (g/day)

In the baseline survey around 1960 large differences in the consumption of alcoholic beverages were observed among the different countries (Fig.1). In the U.S., northern Europe and Serbia, beer and spirits were the most commonly consumed beverages. In the southern European cohorts predominantly wine and in Japan sake (rice wine) were consumed. The average absolute alcohol intake in 1960 was very low (2-5 g per day) in the U.S. and northern Europe, moderate (9-16 g per day) in rural Greece, Serbia and Japan, and high (40-90 g per day) in Italy, and Dalmatia (Croatia) (8).

Table 1 provides information on the trend in alcohol intake in the Finnish, Dutch, and rural Italian cohorts during the period, 1970-1995. These data were collected using either the dietary history or food frequency questionnaire. The results show that the average alcohol intake was low and remained stable between 1970 and 1985 in the Finnish cohorts. In Zutphen, The Netherlands, the average alcohol intake doubled between 1970 and 1985 from 9 to 18g per day. The next 10 years the alcohol intake of the Zutphen men decreased and was in 1995 comparable with that of 1970. By far the highest average alcohol intake was observed in 1965 in the rural Italian cohorts of Crevalcore and Montegiorgio, averaging about 85g per day, which corresponds to about seven glasses of wine per day. This high level of intake decreased by about 50% between 1970 and 1985, and by about 40% again between 1985 and 1995, taking 1985 as a reference. In 1995, the average intake was about 25g per day, still about 2.5 times higher than in Zutphen.

Table 1. Trends in average absolute alcohol intake (g per day) for 25 years in five aging European cohorts of the Seven Countries Study from Finland, The Netherlands and Italy.

| Year | 1970 | | 1985 | | 1995 | |
| Age (y) | 50-69 | | 65-84 | | 75-94 | |
Cohort	N	Mean	N	Mean	N	Mean
East Finland	608	5	314	4		
West Finland	683	7	387	6		
Zutphen	615	9	350	18	146	10
Crevalcore	877	88[a]	372	39	144	23
Montegiorgio	662	83[a]	306	47	121	28

a = alcohol intake in 1965

Table 2. Trends in average absolute alcohol intake (g per day) collected in middle-aged men from Finland, The Netherlands, and Italy from 1959 to 1991.

Population	Year	Method	Age (y)	N	Mean
Finland (SCS)	1959	Record	40-59	60	2
FIN MONICA	1982	Record	40-59	441	10
Zutphen (SCS)	1960	Record	40-59	45	3
The Netherlands	1987/88	Record	40-59	661	22
Italy (SCS)	1965	Diet hist	45-64	1541	82
Italy (SCS)	1991	Diet hist	28-53	41	59

SCS = Seven Countries Study

Since the trend in average alcohol intake based on dietary history and food frequency data is confounded by age, we describe the trend in average alcohol intake in independent samples of middle-aged men from Finland, The Netherlands, and Italy who were surveyed about 25 years apart in the period 1959-1991. The data are derived from the dietary surveys described in Chapter 2.1. In Finland and The Netherlands the record method was used and in Italy the dietary history method. These data show an increase in the average absolute alcohol intake in middle-aged men in Finland, a greater increase in the Netherlands and a substantial decrease in Italy. These trends were similar to those observed in aging men between 1970 and 1985.

We conclude that between 1960 and 1985 the average alcohol intake increased in Finland and the Netherlands, and that the increase was largest in the Netherlands. In Italy a continuous decrease in alcohol intake was observed since 1960. Despite these trends, the average alcohol intake in middle-aged men around 1985 was still highest in Italian men.

ALCOHOL INTAKE AND MORTALITY FROM CORONARY HEART DISEASE: A CROSS-CULTURAL PERSPECTIVE

The average intake of alcohol across the population was significantly and inversely associated with 25-year CHD mortality ($r = -0.61$, $p<0.05$) (Fig. 1) (8). Average population intake of alcohol was also inversely associated with average population saturated fat intake ($r = -0.58$, $p<0.05$) and directly with average population flavonoid intake ($r = 0.39$, $p>0.05$). After multivariate analyses, which took into account the confounding effects of average population saturated fat and flavonoid intake, the average population intake of alcohol was found not related to 25-year CHD mortality rates (8).

Figure 2. Logarithm of average population absolute alcohol intake (g/day) at baseline and 25-year age-adjusted coronary heart disease mortality rates (8).

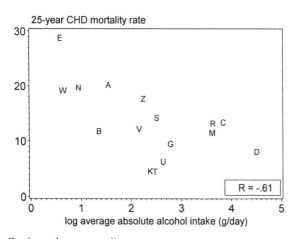

For legend see appendix

Ecological analyses using food disappearance data and CHD mortality from about 20 developed countries found similar results (9-12). The correlation coefficient for per capita wine consumption or alcohol intake, and CHD mortality rates varied between -0.61 and -0.70 for wine, and between -0.39 and -0.70 for alcohol. The relationships remained statistically significant after multivariate analyses.

In univariate analysis, similar relationships between average population intake of alcohol or wine and population CHD mortality rates were found in the Seven Countries Study and in the other ecological studies reviewed. However, after multivariate analyses this association was no longer found present in the Seven Countries Study, but remained in the other ecological studies. This may be due to several factors. The Seven Countries Study is the only truly prospective ecological study. Dietary data were collected in random samples of the middle-aged men who were followed for 25 years. In the other studies, national food disappearance data were correlated with national CHD mortality data.

In the Seven Countries Study the average population intake of alcohol and different nutrients was chemically analyzed in one laboratory. In the other studies food balance sheet data were used. These data represent the availability of foods per country and not foods actually consumed; they can not be broken down by age and gender. Fatty acid intake was calculated from food tables (9,11), or dairy or animal fat was taken as a proxy for saturated fat (10,12). Probably for these reasons, a stronger association was found between saturated fat intake and CHD mortality in the Seven Countries Study. Finally, besides alcohol intake, the full multivariate model included the intake of saturated fat, flavonoids and the prevalence of cigarette smokers. Control for confounding was therefore more rigid in the Seven Countries Study than in the other ecological studies.

"THE FRENCH PARADOX"

Based on the low reported mortality rate for CHD in France and its relatively high intake of saturated fat, Renaud proposed the French paradox (10). He suggested that the high alcohol intake, especially from wine, in France might explain this paradox. His ecological study showed that the combination of a high animal fat intake and high wine intake was associated with a low mortality rate due to CHD (10).

There are other such paradoxes, if only one correlate of CHD is taken into account. Finland, for example, has a higher than expected mortality from CHD based on its dietary cholesterol and saturated fat index (11). In the Seven Countries Study, Japan shows lower mortality from CHD than expected according to its high prevalence rate of smokers. Taking other risk factors (saturated fat and flavonoid intake) into account, however, we find that Japan follows the line for predicted CHD mortality (13).

Much evidence indicates that CHD mortality rates are determined by several risk factors. Taking only one factor into account, and proposing a paradox in this context, is a questionable strategy. The multifactorial nature of the disease must be considered. For example, the relatively low CHD mortality rate of France is, despite a relatively high intake of saturated fat, not only associated with a high level of wine consumption but also with a high intake of fresh vegetables and fruits (10,14). Ducimetiére and coworkers showed that the coronary event rates in men aged 35-64 in the French, Italian, and Catalonian regions of the WHO-MONICA Project were similar (15). They concluded that "the time has come to relieve epidemiology of the French paradox. Much more attention should be paid to collecting reliable data to produce more satisfactory explanations for the complex causes of heart disease."

INDIVIDUAL ALCOHOL CONSUMPTION AND MORTALITY FROM CORONARY HEART DISEASE

A detailed meta analysis, based on 28 cohort studies, concluded that a low alcohol intake (20g per day) compared with non-drinking was associated with a 20% lower CHD risk (1). Significant excess risk began from higher intakes ($\geq$ 89 g per day or seven drinks per day). The results differed according to gender. A major protective effect occurred in men at 25 g (=two drinks) per day and in women at 10 g (less than one drink per day). Significant excess risk was observed beyond 114 g per day in men and 52 g per day in women. These results suggest a small protective effect of alcohol at a low level of intake and a higher susceptibility of women to negative alcohol effects.

In the Seven Countries Study also the association between individual alcohol intake and coronary risk in the Finnish and Italian cohorts have been studied. In Finland, mostly beer and spirits are consumed and binge-drinking is common. In Italy, most wine is consumed daily with the meal. The cohort studies from Finland and Italy provide evidence on the relationship between drinking pattern and CHD mortality.

Finnish data on alcohol consumption were collected in 1178 men aged 55-74 in 1974 and in 716 men aged 65-84 in 1984 (16). Alcohol consumption was quantified by frequency of consumption (bottles of beer) during the week prior to collecting the data and bottles of spirits and wine during the prior 30 days. The amount of absolute alcohol consumed during the 30 days previous was calculated. In 1974, 30% of the men in east Finland and 40% of the men in west Finland were abstainers (17); the average absolute alcohol intake was very low (5g per day in east Finland and 6 g per day in west Finland). Only 16% of men consumed more that 9g absolute alcohol per day. Men who drank more than the mean were called "heavy drinkers." This is not more than half a "drink" per day. However, with the Finnish drinking pattern, it is possible that on one occasion, more than 3 drinks, or during the course of a month, more than 15 drinks were consumed. This type of binge drinking was predicted to go with heavy smoking (16).

Men examined in 1974 in Finland were followed for mortality for 10 years (17). At the low levels of alcohol intake of these elderly men, CHD mortality was unrelated to "heavy" alcohol consumption (RR= 1.2, 95%CI 0.7-2.2) (16). In spite of a small number of violent deaths (n= 15), heavy alcohol intake was strongly associated with violent death (RR= 16.0, 95%CI 1.6-156.2). This may be viewed as an indicator for binge-drinking.

The disease associations of alcohol consumption in a Mediterranean food pattern was studied in two rural cohorts of the Seven Countries Study (19). In 1965, 1,536 men aged 45-64 from Crevalcore and Montegiorgio, participated in a dietary survey. Data on food and alcohol consumption were collected using the dietary history method and the men were followed for mortality for 15 years.

The men in rural Italy had a high daily alcohol consumption in 1965 and consumed mostly wine and some spirits. The average alcohol consumption was 88 g per day in Crevalcore and 84 g per day in Montegiorgio. About 15% of the men did not drink alcohol. The average alcohol intake of men in the highest quintile was 165 g per day, equivalent to about 1.5 liter of wine per day.

In men free from cardiovascular diseases at the entry examination, a J-shaped relationship was observed between alcohol intake and 15-year CHD mortality (Fig.3). The lowest quintile of alcohol intake was the reference category (with RR= 1.00). The third quintile had an adjusted relative risk of 0.67 (95%CI 0.29-1.58) and the fifth quintile an adjusted relative risk of 1.61 (95%CI 0.79-3.31). Similar but lower relative risks were observed for the relationship between alcohol intake and 15-year all-causes mortality.

These results, occurring among rural Italian cohorts, provide evidence that the association between alcohol intake and CHD mortality differs per region. Studies performed in Mediterranean countries tended to report a higher "protective effect"

Figure 3. Relationship between alcohol intake in 1965 and 15-year age-adjusted mortality rates due to coronary heart disease (18).

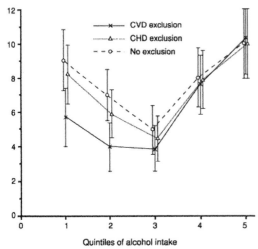

CHD mortality rate (%)

Quintiles of alcohol intake

CVD = cardiovascular diseases
CHD= coronary heart disease

Figure 4. Relationship between alcohol consumption and relative risk for coronary heart disease in men by region (1).

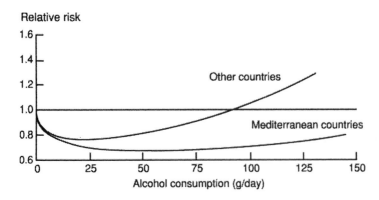

Relative risk

Alcohol consumption (g/day)

of alcohol than in countries outside the Mediterranean (Fig. 4). This may be due in part to a difference in pattern of consumption. In the Mediterranean areas, for example, drinking habits are characterized by constant daily amounts of alcohol in the form of wine consumed with meals. In northern Europe and the U.S. alcohol was commonly consumed during the weekend in the form of beer and spirits, and outside meals. It is only a more recent habit in these countries to consume wine with meals.

COMMENTS

The accuracy of the quantification of alcohol intake through self-reports can be questioned. The actual alcohol intake may be under- or overreported depending on the culture studied. However, generally the reproducibility of questions on alcohol consumption is high (19). This means that questionnaire data can be used to rank individuals in the distribution of alcohol consumption. This makes a reliable estimation of the association between alcohol consumption and the occurrence of CHD possible. Information on the validity of the alcohol consumption estimate is more difficult to obtain. In the cohorts from Finland, The Netherlands and Italy we found strong correlations between alcohol consumption and HDL cholesterol levels (6), suggesting that the differences in alcohol consumption level between different countries are probably real.

The studies carried out in Finland suggested that even at a low average alcohol intake binge-drinking is detrimental to health (16, 17). The relationship between beer binging and mortality at higher levels of alcohol intake than that in elderly men, was studied outside the Seven Countries Study in 1641 beer drinkers of 42-60 years from Kuopio, Finland (20). The mean follow-up time was 5.6 years for acute myocardial infarction and 7.7 years for all-causes mortality. The risk of fatal acute myocardial infarction was substantially greater (RR= 6.50, 95%CI 2.05-20.61) in men whose usual "dose" of beer was 6 or more bottles per occasion, compared with men who usually consumed less than 3 bottles. Similar results were found for all-causes mortality (RR=7.10, 95%CI 2.01-25.12). Such an association was not observed for fatal and non-fatal myocardial infarction taken together. These associations changed only slightly when potential confounders were taken into account. Beer binging was associated with an increased risk of fatal myocardial infarction, and all-causes mortality, independent of the average consumption of alcohol.

Studies performed in Mediterranean countries reported a stronger "protective effect" of alcohol than those from other countries. In the Mediterranean countries wine is taken with meals. It is known that alcohol taken with a meal is absorbed at a slower rate, and blood alcohol tends to peak at a lower level (21). This is probably of benefit since alcohol spikes promote intoxication. There is some suggestion that the consumption of wine with meals might have a favorable effect on post-prandial hyperlipidemia (22). These suggestions need further exploration before definite statements can be made about a larger protective effect of alcohol or wine on CHD in the context of a Mediterranean dietary pattern.

An important issue to be addressed here is whether the lower risk for CHD of consuming a small amount of alcohol is causal. In men, the consumption of 25 g of alcohol per day was associated with a 23% lower relative risk compared with non-drinkers (1). If the association is causal, the most likely candidates for this protective effect are blood lipid levels, especially HDL cholesterol, and hemostatic factors such as fibrinogen and platelet aggregation (23).

We examined in the Finnish, Dutch, and Italian cohorts of the Seven Countries Study the association between alcohol intake and HDL cholesterol level (6). This study was carried out in 2,255 men aged 65-84. A strong dose–response association was observed between habitual alcohol intake and HDL cholesterol level (Table 3). The difference between men who consumed an average of 25 g of alcohol per day compared with non-drinkers was 0.12 mmol/l. This is in the same order of magnitude as the 0.10 mmol/l difference in HDL cholesterol level for a 30-g per day difference in alcohol observed in short-term experimental studies (23). Rimm and co-workers calculated that this difference might reduce CHD risk by 16.8% (21). Because of the similarity of results of our observational study and the meta analysis of the experimental studies by Rimm and co-workers , it is concluded that a large part (at least 75%) of the observed lower CHD risk among alcohol consumers is due to an increase in HDL cholesterol level.

Table 3. Relationship between alcohol intake and average HDL cholesterol level (mmol/l) in 2,173 elderly men from Finland, The Netherlands and Italy (6).

Alcohol (g per day)	N	HDL cholesterol (mmol/l)	
		Crude Mean	Adjusted[a] Mean
0	560	1.13	1.12
1-9	573	1.15	1.14
10-19	197	1.19	1.21
20-29	422	1.24	1.24
≥ 30	421	1.38	1.39
		F = 43.4	F = 35.9
		P < 0.001	P < 0.001

a = Adjusted for age and cohort

Besides an apparently favorable effect of a moderate amount of alcohol intake, there are also favorable effects on fibrinogen (23), platelet aggregation (24), and insulin resistance (21). There are, however, detrimental effects of moderate amounts of alcohol on triglycerides and blood pressure (21, 23). It is hard to predict the net effect of alcohol on all these biological risk factors. However, because of the strong effect of alcohol on HDL cholesterol level, it is likely that the apparent protective effect of a moderate amount of alcohol on coronary risk is causal.

SUMMARY AND CONCLUSIONS

The Seven Countries Study showed large differences in alcohol intake among the cohorts. Intakes in 1960 tended to be low in the U.S. and in northern Europe, moderate in Greece, Serbia and Japan, and high in Italy and Dalmatia. During 35 years of follow-up, alcohol intake increased in Finland and the Netherlands but did not reach the high Italian level of intake. Average population alcohol intake was inversely related to 25-year CHD mortality rates. This association was no longer present after multivariate analysis with dietary variables. Individual data from the Finnish and the Italian cohorts suggest that not only the amount, but the pattern, of drinking is important in CHD risk. Binge drinking increases the risk of fatal CHD, and all-causes mortality. Alcohol consumed with meals as in the Mediterranean countries, provided a stronger "protective effect" than alcohol consumed in other countries. The strong relationship between alcohol intake and HDL cholesterol level (seen in many observational studies including the Seven Countries Study, as well as in experimental studies) is in accordance with a causal relationship between

106

moderate alcohol intake and protection from coronary risk. Currently we are unable to contribute information on any specific effect of red wine.

REFERENCES

1. Corrao G, Rubbiati L, Bagnardi V, Zambon A, Poikolainen K. Alcohol and coronary heart disease: a meta-analysis. Addiction 2000;95:1505-1523.
2. Grobbee DE, Rimm EB, Keil U, Renaud S. Alcohol and the cardiovascular system. In: Health issues related to alcohol consumption. Second edition, MacDonald I (Ed). ILSI Europe, Blackwell Science Ltd 1999:125-179.
3. Poikolainen K. It can be bad for the heart too: drinking patterns and coronary heart disease. Addiction 1998;93:1757-1759.
4. Kromhout D, Keys A, Aravanis C, Buzina R, Fidanza F, Giampaoli S, Jansen A, Menotti A, Nedeljkovic S, Pekkarinen M, Simic BS, Toshima H. Food consumption patterns in the nineteen sixties in Seven Countries. Am J Clin Nutr 1989;49:889-894.
5. Huijbregts PPCW, Feskens EJM, Räsänen L, Alberti-Fidanza A, Mutanen M, Fidanza F, Kromhout D. Dietary intake in five aging cohorts of men in Finland, Italy and the Netherlands. Eur J Clin Nutr 1995;49: 852-860.
6. Kromhout D, Nissinen A, Menotti A, Bloemberg B, Pekkanen J, Giampaoli S. Total and HDL cholesterol and their correlates in elderly men in Finland, Italy and the Netherlands. Am J Epidemiol 1990;131:855-863.
7. Rimm EB, Klatsky A, Grobbee D, Stampfer MJ. Review of moderate alcohol consumption and reduced risk of coronary heart disease: Is the effect due to beer, wine or spirits? BMJ 1996;312:731-736.
8. Kromhout D, Bloemberg BPM, Feskens EJM, Hertog MGL, Menotti A, Blackburn H, for the Seven Countries Study Group. Alcohol, fish, fiber and antioxidant vitamins do not explain population differences in CHD mortality. Int J Epidemiol 1996;25(4):753-759
9. St Leger AS, Cochrane AL, Moore F. Factors associated with cardiac mortality in developed countries with particular reference to the consumption of wine. Lancet 1979;i:1017-1020
10. Renaud S, De Lorgeril M. Wine, alcohol, platelets and the French paradox for coronary heart disease. Lancet 1992;339:1523-1526.
11. Artaud-Wild SM, Connor SL, Sexton G, Connor WE. Differences in coronary mortality can be explained by differences in cholesterol and saturated fat intakes in 40 countries but not in France and Finland. A paradox. Circulation 1993;88:2771-2779.
12. Criqui MH, Ringel L. Does diet or alcohol explain the French paradox? Lancet 1994;344:1719-1723.
13. Kromhout D. Diet-heart issues in a pharmacological era. Lancet 1996;348 Suppl 1:S20-S22.
14. Drewnowski A, Ahlstrom-Henderson S, Shore AM, Fischler C, Preziosi P, Hercberg S. Diet quality and diet diversity in France: Implications for the French paradox. J Am Diet Assoc 1996;96:663-669.
15. Ducimetière P, Lang T, Amoyel P, Arveiler D, Ferrières J. Rates of coronary events are similar in France and Southern Europe. BMJ 2000;320:249.
16. Kivelä SL, Nissinen A, Punsar S, Puska P, Karvonen M. Determinants and predictors of heavy alcohol consumption among aging Finnish men. Compr Gerontol B 1988;2:103-109.
17. Kivelä SL, Nissinen A, Ketola A, Punsar S, Puska P, Karvonen M. Alcohol consumption and mortality in aging or aged Finnish men. J Clin Epidemiol 1989;42:61-68.
18. Farchi G, Fidanza F, Mariotti S, Menotti A. Alcohol and mortality in the Italian cohorts of the Seven Countries Study. Int J Epidemiol 1992;21:74-82.

19. De Vries JHM, Lemmens PHHM, Pietinen P, Kok FJ. Assessment of alcohol consumption. In: Health issues related to alcohol consumption. Second edition, MacDonald I (Ed). ILSI Europe, Blackwell Science Ltd. 1999:27-62.
20. Kauhanen J, Kaplan GA, Goldberg DE, Salonen JT. Beer binging and mortality: results from the Kuopio Ischaemic Heart Disease Risk Factor Study, a prospective population based study. BMJ 1997;315:846-851.
21. Criqui MH. Do known cardiovascular risk factors mediate the effect of alcohol on cardiovascular disease? In: Alcohol and cardiovascular diseases. Willey, Chichester 1998:159-172.
22. Veenstra J. Ockhuizen T, Pol M van de, Wedel M, Schaafsma G. Effects of a moderate dose of alcohol on blood lipids and lipoproteins postprandially and in fasting state. Alcohol & Alcoholism 1990;25:371-377.
23. Rimm EB, Williams P, Fosher K, Criqui M, Stampfer MJ. Moderate alcohol intake and lower risk of coronary heart disease: meta-analysis of effects of lipids and haemostatic factors. BMJ 1999;319:1523-1528.
24. Renaud SC, Beswick AD, Fehily AM, Sharp DS, Elwood PC. Alcohol and platelet aggregation: the Caerphilly Prospective Heart Disease Study. Am J Clin Nutr 1992;55:1012-1017.

CHAPTER 2.5

PHYSICAL ACTIVITY, PHYSICAL FITNESS AND CORONARY HEART DISEASE IN THE SEVEN COUNTRIES STUDY

Alessandro Menotti

An adequate level of physical activity is considered by scientists and lay-people alike to be important to preserve health and prevent disease, along with other lifestyle patterns such as eating, drinking, and smoking habits, and psycho-social adjustment. However, the measurement of habitual physical activity is complex and uncertain. Measuring physical activity is needed to characterize both populations and individuals.

Misunderstandings persist in this field among terms and concepts, which appear similar, such as physical activity, exercise, and fitness. Physical activity is defined as "any bodily movement produced by skeletal muscles that results in energy expenditure" (1). Physical exercise has been defined as " a peculiar type of physical activity that is planned, structured, repetitive and purposive, in the sense that improvement and maintenance of one or more components of physical activity is an objective" (1). Physical fitness, on the other hand, related to the ability to perform work, represents the result of genetically determined characteristics, the structure and function of muscular masses and the nervous, and circulatory and respiratory systems, along with the influence on these of physical activity and exercise. Thus fitness is the consequence of genetic characteristics modified by type and amount of physical activity or exercise.

A hypothesis under investigation for many decades was that high levels of all types of physical activity and of physical fitness were associated with lower risk of CHD and other cardiovascular diseases. Difficulties in properly measuring physical activity and energy expenditure were, and are, still notable, particularly when large numbers of individuals are required. Measurement of physical fitness, as derived from exercise testing, has rarely been made in large population studies.

In the Seven Countries Study, job-related physical activity was ascertained by questionnaire during the first 10 years of follow-up. Because of continuous automatization and mechanisation the importance of job-related physical activity decreased and leisure time physical activity increased. In the elderly men examined since 1985 both job and leisure time related physical activity were measured by a questionnaire. Resting heart rate was used as a simple indicator of physical fitness. This chapter reports trends in physical activity and the relationships among physical activity and physical fitness, and CHD.

MEASURING PHYSICAL ACTIVITY AND PHYSICAL FITNESS

Manuals dealing with the measurement of habitual physical activity have suggested a number of procedures: food consumption representing energy expenditure, measured maximal oxygen uptake or work capacity, recording of heart rate at work, time-task determinations, and retrospective physical activity questionnaires. Most of these are complex, time-consuming, expensive, and often result in uncertain interpretation.

At the beginning of the Seven Countries Study neither the tools, time, nor financial support were available for any sophisticated method of physical activity measurement. Moreover, the majority of men enrolled in the study lived in rural areas where heavy physical activity related to work was usual. Physical activity among men in the heaviest activity classes was rarely of the aerobic type of recreational physical exercise to increase fitness. The influence of the sociocultural environment, and fashion, meant that almost none of Seven Countries Study participants took leisure time exercise in any substantial amount, as now common

110

in many cultures where the majority of jobs are sedentary. Therefore a rough classification of habitual physical activity could be made based entirely on occupation.

Physical activity classification in the Seven Countries Study was based on responses to questions about occupation and usual activities, including part-time jobs and non-occupational exercise. In addition, the U.S. railroad men answered a detailed questionnaire about leisure time and recreational activity (but only their occupational activity is considered here). A list of almost 100 occupations was used for final classification (2). Classification of railroad employees in the U.S. and Rome was facilitated by the availability of working profiles for different occupations. In most analyses, three categories were considered: class 1, corresponding to sedentary people or those taking very little physical activity; class 2, corresponding to moderately active people (during a substantial part of the day); and class 3, corresponding to active or very active people, classified as heavy workers, who performed hard physical work much of the time.

A rough estimate of energy expenditure corresponding to these three physical activity classes was made on the basis of ergonometric procedures carried out in another study of Italian railroad employees. Here, the same three levels were adopted to classify the men. For sedentary men, the energy expenditure was less than 2,400 kcal ($<$ 10.0 MJ) per day; for the moderately active it was between 2,400 and 3,000 kcal (10.0 – 12.6 MJ) per day. The heavy workers, however, showed an estimate of more than 3,000 kcal ($>$12.6 MJ) per day. (3,4)

More detailed measurements were occasionally obtained. In the U.S. railroad cohort a precursor of the Minnesota Leisure Time Physical Activity Questionnaire (LTPA) was administered (5). In the cohort of West Finland a detailed questionnaire on physical activity, for both working and leisure time, was used at the time of the 5-year re-examination in 1964 (6). In the Zutphen Elderly Study among men aged 65 to 84 years, a detailed questionnaire on habitual physical activity (including leisure time) was administered at the entry examination and a careful classification of time spent in heavy activity was obtained (7-11). Most items in the questionnaire included the description of leisure time activity (among retired men). This was extended five years later to the cohorts of elderly men in Finland and Italy.

Simple measurements related to physical fitness such as resting heart rate derived from the ECG were taken in all cohorts. In some cohorts information on indicators of physical fitness was collected through a spirometric test and mid-arm circumference. An objective procedure (a sub-maximal) treadmill test to measure physical fitness was applied only in the U.S. railroad cohort at entry examination (12).

DISTRIBUTION OF PHYSICAL ACTIVITY AT ENTRY EXAMINATION AND DURING 10-YEARS OF FOLLOW-UP

A complex picture is shown for the proportion of men placed in one of the three physical activity classes at entry examination (Fig. 1). There were no men doing heavy physical work in the U.S. railroad and the Belgrade professors cohorts, while they made up a large majority in all the rural areas of Finland, Italy, Croatia, Velika Krsna, Crete and Japan, except for Corfu. Men with moderate activity represented the majority in Zutphen, whereas a balanced distribution among the three activity

Figure 1. Proportion of men in three physical activity levels at work in the 16 cohorts as measured at entry examination.

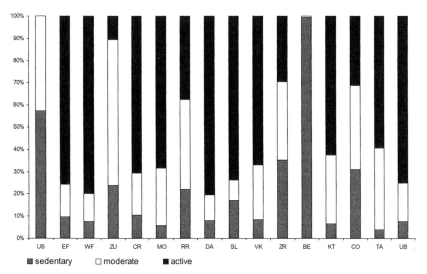

For legend see appendix.

Table 1. Changes in the proportion of sedentary men based on job-related physical activity between baseline and 10 years of follow-up in 16 cohorts.

Cohort	Sedentary men Year 0 (%)	Sedentary men Year 10 (%)	Changes %
U.S. railroad	57	n.a.	n.a.
East Finland	10	49	+410
West Finland	8	30	+300
Zutphen	24	13	-45
Crevalcore	11	35	+233
Montegiorgio	6	21	+262
Rome railroad	22	77	+250
Dalmatia	8	17	+115
Slavonia	17	19	+11
Velika Krsna	9	20	+135
Zrenjanin	35	59	+68
Belgrade	99	96	-3
Crete	7	17	+158
Corfu	31	25	-19
Tanushimaru	4	19	+387
Ushibuka	8	n.a.	n.a.

n.a. = not available

classes was found in the Rome railroad cohort, Zrenjanin and Corfu. It is probable, however, that heavy physical activity is not interpreted the same across the different

112

cultures, in Finland, for example, where workers doing heavy work alternated work as lumberjacks and farmers.

During the 10 years of follow-up, the proportion of men doing heavy work declined everywhere with a corresponding increase in the proportion of sedentary men (13). In Table 1, changes in the proportion of sedentary men are given for most cohorts, which shows an almost universal increase in sedentary life. This is due to aging of the populations but also to the increasing proportion of people who have retired from active jobs.

PHYSICAL ACTIVITY AND CORONARY HEART DISEASE RISK FACTORS

It is a popular belief that levels of habitual physical activity influence the levels of other risk factors. An analysis using the baseline data gave some indication of how high levels of some risk factors (identified by age and cohort-specific values in deciles 8 to 10 of the distribution) were distributed, and how they corresponded, or not, to expectations based on the null hypothesis of no relationship to activity (2). The risk factors considered were relative body weight (against an arbitrarily selected standard), the sum of triceps and subscapular skinfold thickness, systolic and diastolic blood pressure, and serum cholesterol, measured at entry examination in selected northern and southern European areas. The ratio (observed / expected = O/E x 100) was generally highest in sedentary men, intermediate among moderately active men, and lowest among heavy workers. This was true in both northern and southern Europe, with small irregularities only for systolic blood pressure and serum cholesterol in northern Europe. These results suggest that high levels of physical activity are associated with favorable levels of CHD risk factors.

PHYSICAL ACTIVITY AND CORONARY HEART DISEASE IN CROSS-CULTURAL COMPARISONS

Figure 2. The association of the average Physical Activity Index at baseline with 25-year coronary heart disease death rates.

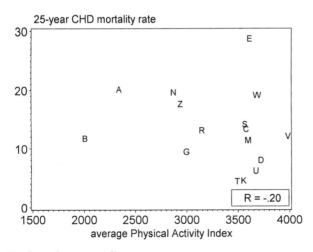

For legend see appendix

The 10-year CHD incidence rates for each cohort were plotted against indicators of physical activity (13). In not one instance did the ecological correlation coefficient reach statistical significance. The correlation coefficient was 0.16 for CHD incidence versus the proportion of sedentary men, and -0.18 for the proportion of active men. The correlation between baseline average population physical activity index (see chapter 3.3) and 25-year CHD death rates was –0.20 (Fig. 2).

PHYSICAL ACTIVITY AND CORONARY HEART DISEASE INCIDENCE IN INDIVIDUALS

Data on the 5-year follow-up could be analyzed only in some cohorts and in univariate fashion only. When numbers of events were large enough, the hard diagnosis of CHD was the endpoint considered, otherwise any CHD events was used (14). An analysis of the first 5-year follow-up reported the observed/expected ratio (O/E) of events in three physical activity categories after adjustment for age distribution. This approach was needed since lower physical activity levels are typical of relatively older people who produce the most disease events. The picture was not uniform; the highest ratios were not always seen in the sedentary group. On the other hand, all the O/E ratios for the heavy physical activity group were smaller than 1, suggesting some "protection" for the more active men. No statistical tests were made due to the small number of cases in all classes. The regularly decreasing trend in CHD incidence from sedentary to moderate to heavy work was pronounced in Montegiorgio and Croatia, and, also in the U.S. railroad for its two available activity classes.

After 10 years of follow-up an analysis was done in cohorts pooled by country (13). A decreasing regular trend in CHD incidence was very clear from sedentary to moderate to heavy workers in rural Italy, Greece and Japan (where the sedentary class was pooled with the moderate one). In general, the heavy activity class carried the lowest rate for hard CHD, but this was not true in the Netherlands. A few differences between pairs of rates were statistically significant.

Table 2. Physical activity at entry examination and 10-year CHD deaths or incidence in groupings of the cohorts. Reconstructed and modified from reference (13).

Areas	Endpoint	β	SE	RR	95 %CI
U.S. railroad	CHD deaths	+0.0248	0.2266	1.02	0.66 – 1.60
Northern Europe	CHD deaths	-0.2433	0.1502	0.78	0.58 – 1.05
Northern Europe	Any CHD	-0.0759	0.1126	0.93	0.74 – 1.16
Southern Europe	CHD deaths	-0.4021	0.1596	0.67	0.49 – 0.91
Southern Europe	Any CHD	-0.0683	0.1108	0.94	0.75 – 1.16

β = Coefficient for physical activity derived from the multiple logistic function.
SE = Standard Error. Relative Risk (RR) for the difference of one class of physical activity (1 = sedentary; 2 = moderate; 3 = active), CI = Confidence interval. The model included age, systolic blood pressure, serum cholesterol, smoking habits, and resting heart rate as possible confounders.

Again using the 10-year data (CHD death or any CHD), multivariate coefficients derived from the multiple logistic function were calculated, and

114

adjusted for five possible confounding factors (13) (Table 2). For the U.S. railroad workers, the pool of northern, and separately taken, southern European areas, all coefficients were negative (except the one for the U.S. cohort). However, only the coefficient for southern Europe predicting CHD deaths was statistically significant. The relative risk for a difference of one class of physical activity varied between 0.67 and 1.02.

PHYSICAL ACTIVITY AND LONG-TERM MORTALITY FROM CORONARY HEART DISEASE IN INDIVIDUALS

Multivariate coefficients for physical activity in the prediction of CHD deaths during 20 years of follow-up are summarized in Table 3 (15). All data are derived using Cox proportional hazards models. In general, the picture does not differ from that seen with the 10-year univariate analyses. Generally a protective effect of high levels of physical activity was observed. On the other hand, this association was statistically significant in only a few cases. The relative risk ranged between 0.54 and 1.04.

Table 3. Physical activity at entry examination and 20-year CHD deaths in groupings of the cohorts. Reconstructed and modified from reference (15).

Areas	β	SE	RR	95 % CI
East and West Finland	-0.2654	0.0834	0.77	0.65 – 0.90
Zutphen	+0.0422	0.1623	1.04	0.76 – 1.43
Crevalcore, Montegiorgio and Rome railroad	-0.2982	0.0947	0.74	0.62 – 0.89
Velika Krsna, Zrenjanin	-0.0202	0.1554	0.98	0.72 – 1.33
Crete and Corfu	-0.4529	0.2461	0.64	0.39 – 1.03
Tanushimaru and Ushibuka	-0.6245	0.2826	0.54	0.31 – 0.93
Pool of all groups	-0.2360	0.0520	0.79	0.71 – 0.88

β = coefficients for physical activity derived from the Cox proportional hazards model, with age, average blood pressure, serum cholesterol, cigarette consumption, and Body Mass Index as covariates. SE = Standard Error, RR = Relative Risk, for the difference of one class of physical activity (1 = sedentary; 2 = moderate; 3 = active). CI = Confidence interval

Findings reported in table 3 were compiled from a systematic analysis dealing with the 20-year follow-up (15), although in that preliminary analysis some cohorts could not be considered (e.g. U.S. railroad, and two cohorts from Croatia and Belgrade). This set of data was used to produce a meta-analytical estimate for physical activity, following a technique developed by Dyer (16). The pooled estimate provided a relative risk (for 1 class difference in physical activity) of 0.79 (95% CI 0.71-0.88). Taking a 2 class difference, i.e. comparing the men with sedentary jobs to those with the heavy jobs, the relative risk was 0.62 (95% CI 0.51-0.77). Following the suggested procedure that must precede the pooled estimate of coefficients, the test for heterogeneity was computed and was not statistically significant (p> 0.10 and < 0.20). Similar analysis using the 25-year mortality data was not systematically produced (17-19) but in some instances, such as in the case of the pool of the Finnish, Dutch and Italian data, the relative risks were similar to those shown for the 20-year follow-up analysis.

DETAILED STUDIES ON PHYSICAL ACTIVITY AND CORONARY HEART DISEASE IN SPECIFIC COHORTS

Special analyses based on more accurate measurement of habitual physical activity were carried out for some cohorts. In the U.S. railroad cohort a precursor of the Minnesota Leisure Time Physical Activity Questionnaire (LTPA) was administered (5). A high level of caloric expenditure by the LTPA was "protective" for CHD death. For example, the relative risk for CHD death in a follow-up of about 20 years for sedentary men who expended < 250 kcal/wk in leisure time physical activity versus those who expended > 2000 kcal / wk was 1.39. This relationship was attenuated after adjusting for other risk factors but remained independent and statistically significant.

In the cohort of West Finland a detailed questionnaire on physical activity, including working and leisure time, was administered at the time of the 5-year re-examination in 1964 (6). After exclusion of prevalent CHD cases or severe ECG findings, or the inability to complete the single step test for the post-exercise ECG, a total of 636 healthy men were considered in follow-up during the next 20 years. Two major classes of physical activity (high and low) were used in most analyses. During the first two-thirds of the follow-up period, men with a high level of physical activity had a lower death rate than those with a low level; however, during the last third of the follow-up period the two curves gradually converge. Overall, among those who died, the ones with a high level of physical activity lived 2.1 years longer (p = 0.002, after adjustment for age, systolic blood pressure, serum cholesterol, and Body Mass Index) than those with a low level of physical activity. The difference was mainly due to a higher death rate from CHD among the men with a low level of physical activity, with a relative risk of 1.4 (unadjusted) and 1.3 (after adjustment for major risk factors).

In the elderly men from Zutphen aged 65 to 84 years, a detailed questionnaire on habitual physical activity (including leisure) was administered at entry examination and a careful classification of time spent in heavy activities was obtained (7-11). The relative risk for CHD and cardiovascular deaths was then computed for each tertile, taking the lowest as reference and producing adjustments in three steps. In general, all relative risks in tertile 2 and 3 of the distribution (the two highest) were smaller than 1.0 but only for tertile 3 (the highest) and for the cardiovascular endpoint, did the 95% confidence intervals not include 1.0 (after multiple adjustments) for age, for age and baseline presence of the considered disease, and for age, disease and lifestyle factors, e.g. cigarette smoking and alcohol consumption).

A similar classification of elderly men in the cohorts from Finland, The Netherlands, and Italy was possible only at the 5-year follow-up examination of the FINE Study. Levels of physical activity were cross-sectionally related, with more favorable levels of some risk factors and especially with lower average levels of resting heart rate (9). In the Zutphen Elderly Study it was also shown that change in physical activity levels was associated with lower all-causes mortality if the change, represented an increase of the habitual level during the past few years (11).

At baseline examination there were differences in average population levels of resting heart rate, but some were judged to be non-comparable due to different environmental situations at the time of the measurement (13). The inverse relationship of average population resting heart rate to the proportion of very active men was not statistically significant (r = –0.28). Average population resting heart rate was also not related to 10-year CHD incidence (r = 0.10) (13).

A similar analysis relating baseline average resting heart rate with 25-year CHD deaths gave a non-significant correlation coefficient of 0.26 (Fig. 3). When the Finnish cohorts were excluded, the correlation coefficient became larger (r = 0.58), suggesting that the Finns were outliers.

Figure 3. Relationship of population average resting heart rate (beats/min) with age-adjusted 25-year coronary heart disease death rates per 1,000.

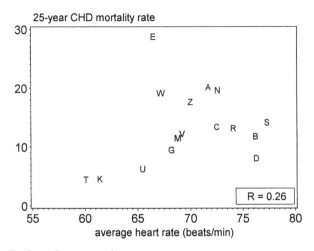

For legend see appendix.

Analyses at the individual level showed that within each cohort average resting heart rate was always higher among sedentary men compared to heavy workers (Table 4). In 13 cohorts the difference was statistically significant. Average resting heart rates among moderately active men were in between sedentary and heavy workers.

In the rural Italian areas standard physical activity class was explored in relation to possible indicators of physical fitness, i.e. resting heart rate, vital capacity, forced respiratory volume in ¾ second, and mid-arm circumference (an indicator of muscular mass) (20). At entry examination average resting heart rate was higher in sedentary subjects, whereas all other risk factors were greater among heavy workers, with intermediate levels among moderately active men (Table 5). Differences in the levels of these factors between sedentary and heavy workers were all statistically significant.

Table 4. Average levels of resting heart rate (beats/min) in cardiovascular disease free men with sedentary and heavy jobs at entry examination in 16 cohorts. Reconstructed and modified from reference 13.

Cohort	Sedentary activity Mean	SD	Heavy activity Mean	SD	P for difference
U.S. railroad	71.8	12.2	70.4[a]	12.0	0.009
East Finland	74.4	14.2	65.2	12.4	< 0.001
West Finland	74.8	16.0	66.5	11.5	< 0.001
Zutphen	72.8	12.5	68.9	11.4	0.016
Crevalcore	77.9	14.5	70.8	12.3	< 0.001
Montegiorgio	75.8	18.2	67.0	10.6	< 0.001
Rome railroad	75.8	13.6	73.9	13.1	0.155
Dalmatia	80.6	16.7	75.8	16.9	0.058
Slavonia	79.8	13.7	76.1	13.2	0.008
Velika Krsna	70.4	10.9	68.5	10.9	0.351
Zrenjanin	70.3	10.4	69.9	12.3	0.768
Belgrade	76.3	11.4	63.3[a]	10.1	0.049
Crete	64.9	10.8	60.2	11.2	0.012
Corfu	70.6	14.1	66.2	11.9	0.003
Tanushimaru	66.9	10.5	59.3	10.5	0.009
Ushibuka	70.0	11.3	64.4	10.8	0.006

a = Moderate instead of heavy activity.

Table 5. Average levels of some indicators of physical fitness at baseline to physical activity classes in the rural Italian areas. Reconstructed and modified from reference 20.

Indicator of physical fitness	Physical activity Sedentary Mean	SD	Moderate Mean	SD	Heavy Mean	SD
Resting heart rate (b/min)	77.2	14.6	74.0	13.2	69.6	11.8*
Vital capacity/height (dl/m)	22.3	4.0	22.6	3.4	23.3	3.3*
FEV/height (dl/ m)	13.4	3.2	13.8	3.1	14.1	3.0**
Mid-arm circumference (cm)	26.0	2.6	26.8	2.5	36.9	2.1*

FEV = Forced Expiratory Volume
* p < 0.05; ** p <0.01 for differences between sedentary and heavy physically active men.

In univariate analyses dealing with selected cohorts, a positive and significant association between resting heart rate and 10-year CHD death was observed in the U.S.A.(13). Resting heart rate was related to both CHD death and incidence in the pool of the Greek and rural Italian areas (13). A difference of 10 beats per minute was associated with a 25% difference in 10-year risk for CHD death. This association persisted after multivariate analysis. In the other cohorts resting heart rate was not related to either CHD death or incidence (13). In a multivariate model predicting 25-year CHD death, including the Finnish areas, the two rural Italian areas and the Dutch cohort, resting heart rate was positively associated with CHD death although not significantly (t-value = 1.42) (21).

Another analysis on resting heart rate and 10-year CHD and cardiovascular mortality was recently carried out in the five European cohorts of the FINE Study (22). The subjects were aged 65-84 years at entry examination and were living in two rural Finnish areas, two rural Italian areas and the town of Zutphen. Prevalent cases with cardiovascular diseases and subjects with ECG abnormalities were excluded from the analysis. The Cox proportional hazards model was used and adjustments were made for several risk factors and for cohort. Relative risks for CHD and cardiovascular diseases were greater for the highest resting heart rate class compared to the lowest. The analysis was replicated excluding the first 2 years of follow-up showing similar results (Table 6).

Table 6. 10-year coronary and cardiovascular disease mortality in elderly men as a function of baseline resting heart rate in the pool of all FINE cohorts. Estimates adjusted for major risk factors and cohort. Derived from reference 22.

Mortality	Resting heart rate (b/min)				
	< 60	60 – 70	70 – 80	> 80	P for trend
Coronary heart disease					
Death rate per 1,000	105	122	121	129	
RR	1.0	0.9	1.2	1.4	0.025
95 % CI		0.6 – 1.4	0.8 – 1.9	0.9 – 2.2	
RR[a]	1.0	0.9	1.2	1.4	0.044
95 % CI		0.7 – 1.5	0.8 – 2.0	0.8-2.3	
Cardiovascular diseases					
Death rate per 1,000	225	230	227	262	
RR	1.0	1.1	1.2	1.5	0.003
95 % CI		0.8 – 1.4	0.9 – 1.6	1.1 – 2.1	
RR[a]	1.0	1.1	1.2	1.4	0.048
95 % CI		0.8 – 1.5	0.8-1.7	1.0 – 2.0	

RR = Relative Risk   CI = Confidence interval
a = after excluding mortality during first 2 years of follow-up.

In the U.S. railroad cohort a sub-maximal treadmill test was administered (12). The exercise heart rate of individuals was directly and significantly related to 20-year CHD, cardiovascular and all-causes mortality risk, when adjusted for age, but largely attenuated when adjusting also for blood pressure, serum cholesterol and smoking habits. For example, an exercise test ending with a heart rate of 135 beats per minute had a relative risk of 1.20 for CHD death compared to one with a heart rate of 105.

COMMENTS

The evidence about beneficial effects of physical activity on CHD suffers the usual problems of most population studies - the weakness of methodology in ascertaining

Table 7. Summary of findings on the relation between physical activity, physical fitness and cardiovascular diseases in three reviews (1, 23, 26).

Source	Number and type of studies	Investigated variable	Endpoint	Number with inverse relationship	Dose-Response relationship
Lange Andersen et al (23)	20 Epidemiologic studies	Physical activity	CHD	16 / 20	n.a.
Powell et al (1)	20 Occupational cohorts	Physical activity at work	CHD incidence	21 / 35	n.a.
	16 Population cohorts	Physical activity	CHD Incidence	25 / 49	n.a.
	3 Occupational groups	Job-related physical activity	CHD mortality	3 / 3	n.a.
	4 Case-control studies	Job and leisure time related physical activity	CHD Incidence	6 / 9	n.a.
U.S. DHHS Report (26)	6 Population or occupational groups	Physical activity	CVD	4 / 6	3 / 6
	5 Population or occupational groups	Physical fitness	CVD	5 / 5	4 / 5
	36 Population or occupational groups	Physical activity	CHD	32 / 36	15 / 36
	7 Population or occupational groups	Physical fitness	CHD	7 / 7	6 / 7

n.a. = not available
Note: In the analysis of Powell et al (1) more than one outcome or comparison may be presented in each study.

physical activity. Moreover, these levels may be affected by socioeconomic status, that could play an important confounding role. Despite these limitations in the majority of analyses, the relative risk for CHD events in the active men was less than 1.0 although not always statistically significant. Similar findings were obtained in the Dutch section of the FINE Study, where the baseline dealt with men aged 65 to 84 years, instead of 40 to 59 years.

The association between high levels of job-related physical activity and more favorable levels of other risk factors was found in the baseline data of the Seven Countries Study. It was also observed for a more detailed classification of physical activity estimated in the FINE Study among elderly men. The limited analyses of different indicators of physical fitness such as resting heart rate and sub-maximal treadmill test, suggested a protective role of higher degrees of physical fitness in univariate analyses. These associations were however not independent of physical activity and not statistically significant in multivariate analyses.

Cross-cultural analyses, correlating population average job-related physical activity with CHD incidence or mortality did not show significant relationships. Similar results were found for the cross-cultural association between average resting heart rate and CHD death. These results suggest that physical activity and resting heart rate do not play an important role in explaining cross-cultural differences in CHD mortality rates. We conclude that at the population level physical activity does not in contrast to the situation in individuals, independently contribute to CHD mortality rates in populations.

A number of careful reviews on the relationship between habitual physical activity and disease, in particular CHD, in individuals appeared during the past 25 years (1, 23-26). In those reviews a large number of studies were analyzed and compared for the possible beneficial effects of physical activity in preventing or delaying CHD events. In each of the reviews, mention was made of contributions to the problem of data from the Seven Countries Study.

A summary of analytical findings from three reviews depicts the general situation derived from population studies conducted the last few decades (Table 7). A majority of studies showed an inverse association of physical activity levels with CHD occurrence, and in roughly two-thirds of them a significant association was shown. The relative risk for sedentary versus active subjects was variable but found frequently in the range of 1.5 to 2.4, depending on the type of disease manifestation, adjustment for other variables, and type of measurements. The reviewers noted that the relative risks are similar in magnitude to those obtained for differences in the levels of risk factors measured with greater precision, such as blood pressure, serum cholesterol, and smoking habits. Again it is impressive that agreement is substantial in these conclusions derived from studies in many different groups in terms of gender, age range, methodology in measuring habitual physical activity, different range in caloric expenditure between the extreme groups, different endpoints, duration of follow-up, and type of analysis. In the review of Powell and coworkers (1), where the contributions in the literature were graded for quality, the best studies were more likely to provide an inverse association between physical activity and CHD, that is, a favorable "effect."

All the reviews recognize the observational nature of the association between physical activity and CHD risk, but intervention studies are practically impossible to conduct. Moreover, it is proposed that the apparent protective effects of physical activity with respect to CHD are due to

- reduced severity or progression of coronary lesions;
- a reduced risk of coronary thrombosis;

- an increased myocardial vascularization and coronary blood flow;
- an improved metabolic capacity, mechanical performance, and cardiovascular efficiency;
- a reduced risk of ventricular fibrillation.

All these effects go beyond the impact that regular physical activity may have in beneficially influencing the levels of coronary risk factors. In most population studies there is no way to study quantitatively the factors associated with those mechanisms but studies measuring plasma fibrinogen and other coagulation factors have produced evidence in relation to a reduced risk of coronary thrombosis (27-30). An increased myocardial vascularization and coronary blood flow was partly considered in studies measuring physical fitness, but in the majority of studies only resting heart rate is the available measurement. Population studies using exercise testing are rare; however, they are suggestive for a protective role of physical fitness for CHD (31-34).

SUMMARY AND CONCLUSIONS

The measurement of physical activity in the Seven Countries Study was based on simple criteria that allowed participants to be classified into three broad classes based on occupation. Baseline analyses showed an association between high levels of physical activity, and lower levels of other CHD risk factors. Analyses made on short- and long-term follow-up showed inverse associations of physical activity level with incidence and mortality from CHD. The advantage of being physically active corresponded to a relative risk of about 0.80 for a difference of one class in physical activity and of about 0.60 when comparing very active with sedentary men. Even the measurement of physical activity in elderly men allowed identification, in limited analyses, of an inverse association of activity class with the risk of CHD death.

Cross-cultural analyses showed that at the population level physical activity and resting heart rate were not related to CHD incidence and mortality.

In individuals physical activity was directly related to resting heart rate, an indicator of physical fitness. In univariate analyses resting heart rate was positively associated with CHD mortality especially in elderly men. In multivariate analyses taking physical activity and other risk factors into account resting heart rate was generally not significantly associated with CHD mortality.

These conclusions do not answer the question whether the current fashion of engaging in strenuous leisure time physical exercise is beneficial to reducing CHD risk. In fact, in the Seven Countries Study, populations were classified on physical activity in relation to manual labor, which was typical of agricultural environments in many parts of the world in the 1950s and the 1960s. Substantial changes in working habits have occurred in subsequent decades, with more people becoming sedentary. This represents a new situation that could not be explored using this material. Valuable indications emanated however, from data on elderly men showing that moderate leisure activities also seem beneficial.

We conclude that physical activity is an independent predictor of CHD risk in individuals but not of population differences in CHD mortality rates.

REFERENCES

1. Powell KE, Thompson PD, Caspersen CJ, Kendrick JS. Physical activity and the incidence of coronary heart disease. Ann Rev Publ Hlth 1987; 8: 253-287.
2. Keys A, Aravanis C, Blackburn HW, Van Buchem FSP, Buzina R, Djordjevic BS, Dontas AS, Fidanza F, Karvonen MJ, Kimura N, Lekos D, Monti M, Puddu V, Taylor HL. Epidemiological studies related to coronary heart disease: characteristics of men aged 40-59 in seven countries. Acta Med Scand 1967;460:Suppl 180:1-392.
3. Menotti A, Puddu V. Ten-year mortality from coronary heart disease among 172,000 men classified by occupational physical activity. Scand J Work Environ Hlth 1979; 5: 100-108.
4. Menotti A, Seccareccia F. Physical activity at work and job responsibility as risk factors for fatal coronary heart disease and other causes of death. J Epidemiol Comm Hlth 1985; 39 : 325-329.
5. Slattery ML, Jacobs DR jr, Nichaman NZ. Leisure time physical activity and coronary heart disease death. The US Railroad Study. Circulation 1989; 79: 304-311.
6. Pekkanen J, Marti B, Nissinen A, Tuomilehto J, Punsar S, Karvonen MJ. Reduction of premature mortality by high physical activity in 20 year follow-up of middle-aged Finnish men. Lancet 1987; 1: 1473-1477.
7. Caspersen CJ, Bloemberg BPM, Saris WHM, Merrit RK, Kromhout D. The prevalence of selected physical activities and their relation with coronary heart disease risk factors in elderly men: the Zutphen Study, 1985. Am J Epidemiol 1991; 133: 1078-1092.
8. Westerterp KR, Saris WHM, Bloemberg BPM, Kempen K, Caspersen CJ, Kromhout D. Validation of the Zutphen Physical Activity Questionnaire for the Elderly with doubly labeled water [abstract]. Med Sci Sports Exerc 1992; 24: S68.
9. Bijnen FC, Feskens EJ, Caspersen CJ, Giampaoli S, Nissinen AM, Menotti A, Mosterd WL, Kromhout D. Physical activity and cardiovascular risk factors among elderly men in Finland, Italy, and the Netherlands. Am J Epidemiol 1996;143:553-561.
10. Bijnen FCH, Caspersen CJ, Feskens EJM, Saris WHM, Mosterd WL, Kromhout D. Physical activity and 10-year mortality from cardiovascular diseases and all causes: the Zutphen Elderly Study. Arch Intern Med 1998; 158: 1499-1505.
11. Bijnen FC, Feskens EJ, Caspersen CJ, Nagelkerke N, Mosterd WL, Kromhout D. Baseline and previous physical activity in relation to mortality in elderly men: the Zutphen Elderly Study. Am J Epidemiol 1999; 150: 1289-1296.
12. Slattery K, Jacobs DR. Physical fitness and cardiovascular disease mortality. The US Railroad study. Am J Epidemiol 1988; 127: 571-580.
13. Keys A, Aravanis C, Blackburn H, Buzina R, Djordjevic BS, Dontas AS, Fidanza F, Karvonen MJ, Kimura N, Menotti A, Mohacek I, Nedeljkovic S, Puddu V, Punsar S, Taylor HL, Van Buchem FSP. Seven countries. A multivariate analysis of death and coronary heart disease. Cambridge MA: Harvard University Press; 1980:1-381.
14. Keys A (Ed). Coronary heart disease in seven countries. Circulation 1970; 41 Suppl 1: 1-211.
15. Menotti A, Keys A, Aravanis C, Blackburn H, Dontas A, Fidanza F, Karvonen MJ, Kromhout D, Nedeljkovic S, Nissinen A, Pekkanen J, Punsar S, Seccareccia F, Toshima H. Seven Countries Study. First 20 year mortality data in 12 cohorts of the Seven Countries. Ann Med 1989; 21: 175-179.
16. Dyer AR. A method for combining results from several prospective epidemiologic studies. Stat Med 1986; 5: 303-317.
17. Menotti A, Seccareccia F, Blackburn H, Keys A. Coronary mortality and its prediction in samples of US and Italian railroad employees in 25 years within the Seven Countries Study of Cardiovascular Diseases. Int J Epidemiol 1995;24: 515-512.
18. Menotti A, Keys A, Kromhout D, Nissinen A, Blackburn H, Fidanza F, Giampaoli S, Karvonen M, Pekkanen J, Punsar S, Seccareccia F. Twenty-five year mortality from

coronary heart disease and its prediction in five cohorts of middle aged men in Finland, the Netherlands and Italy. Prev Med 1990; 19: 270-278.

19. Buzina R, Mohacek I, Menotti A, Seccareccia F, Lanti M, Kromhout D, Keys A. Twenty-five year mortality from coronary heart disease and its prediction in two Croatian cohorts of middle-aged men. Eur J Epidemiol 1995; 11: 259-267.

20. Seccareccia F, Menotti A. Physical activity, physical fitness and mortality in a sample of middle aged men followed-up for 25 years. J Sports Med Phys Fit 1992; 28 : 335-341.

21. Menotti A, Keys A, Kromhout D, Nissinen A, Blackburn H, Fidanza F, Giampaoli S, Karvonen M, Pekkanen J, Punsar S, Seccareccia F. Twenty-five year mortality from coronary heart disease and its prediction in five cohorts of middle-aged men in Finland, the Netherlands and Italy. Prev Med 1990; 19: 270-278.

22. Schuit AJ, Menotti A, Feskens EJM, Nissinen A, Tervahauta M, Giampaoli S, Kromhout D. Resting heart rate is a predictor of 10-year mortality in elderly men: findings from the FINE Study. Submitted.

23. Lange Andersen K, Masironi R, Rutenfranz J, Seliger V, Degré S, Trygg K, Orgim M. Habitual physical activity and health. WHO Regional Publications, European Series No. 6. Copenhagen, World Health Organization, Regional Office for Europe, ISBN 92 9020 106 1. 1978:1-188.

24. Special Section: Public health aspects of physical activity and exercise. Public Health Reports (11 articles). J US Publ Hlth Serv 1985; 100: 118-124.

25. Leon AS. Physical activity and risk of ischemic heart disease- an update 1990. In: Sport for All. Oja P, Telama R (Eds). Elsevier Science Publishers BV, 1991: 251-264.

26. US Department of Health and Human Services. Physical Activity and Health. A Report of the Surgeon General. Atlanta GA, US Department of Health and Human Services, Centers for Disease Control and Prevention. National Center for Chronic Disease Prevention and Health Promotion 1996:1-278

27. Connelly JB, Cooper JA, Meade TW. Strenous exercise, plasma fibrinogen, and factor VII activity. Br Heart J 1992; 67: 351-354.

28. Rankinen T, Rauramaa R, Vaisanen S, Penttila IM, Uusutupa M. Relation of habitual diet and cardiorespiratory fitness to blood coagulation and fibrinolitic factors. Thromb Haemost 1994; 71: 180-183.

29. Lakka TA, Salonen JT. Moderate to high intensity conditioning leisure time physical activity and high cardiorespiratory fitness are associated with reduced plasma fibrinogen in eastern Finnish men. J Clin Epidemiol 1993; 46: 1119-1127.

30. Elwood PC, Yarnell JWG, Pickering J, Fehily AM, O'Brien JR. Exercise, fibrinogen, and other risk factors for ischemic heart disease. Caerphilly Prospective Heart Disease Study. Br Heart J 1993; 69: 183-187.

31. Ekelund IG, Haskell WL, Johnson JL, Whaley FS, Criqui MH, Sheps DS. Physical fitness as a predictor of cardiovascular mortality in asymptomatic North American men: the Lipid Research Clinics Mortality Follow-up Study. N Engl J Med 1988; 319: 1379-1384.

32. Hein HO, Suadicani P, Gyntelberg F. Physical fitness or physical activity as predictor of ischaemic heart disease: a 17-year follow-up in the Copenhagen Male Study. J Intern Med 1992; 232: 471-479.

33. Sobolski J, Kornitzer M, DeBacker G, Dramaix M, Abramowicz M, Degre S , Denolin H. Protection against ischemic heart disease in the Belgian Physical Fitness Study: physical fitness rather than physical activity ? Am J Epidemiol 1987; 125: 601-610.

34. Blair SN, Kohl HW, Paffenbarger RS jr, Clark DG, Cooper KH, Gibbons LW. Physical fitness and all-cause mortality: a prospective study of healthy men and women. JAMA 1989; 262: 2395-2401.

PART III: BIOLOGICAL RISK FACTORS AND CORONARY HEART DISEASE

CHAPTER 3.1

SERUM CHOLESTEROL AND CORONARY HEART DISEASE IN THE SEVEN COUNTRIES STUDY

Daan Kromhout

In the past century cholesterol played a predominant role in research on the etiology of CHD. On the basis of largely experimental work in rabbits and on cross-cultural comparisons of serum cholesterol levels in humans, the hypothesis was formed that arteriosclerosis and its complications were associated with hypercholesterolemia (1). Cholesterol is transported in the blood in lipoprotein fractions. In the 1950s it was shown in clinical studies that the Low Density Lipoprotein (LDL) fraction in cardiac patients was higher, and the High Density Lipoprotein (HDL) fraction lower, when compared with controls (2). Advances in the genetics and cellular biology of cholesterol increased understanding about the role of mechanisms by which genes, hormones, and diet regulate serum cholesterol levels (3). Critical components of this system are lipoprotein receptors in the liver and extra-hepatic tissues that mediate the uptake and degradation of cholesterol-carrying lipoproteins.

By the 1960s, prospective epidemiological studies showed that serum total cholesterol levels were positively associated with CHD risk (4). In the 1970s epidemiological studies showed that HDL cholesterol levels were protective, in contrast to LDL cholesterol (5). This is because HDL is involved in reverse cholesterol transport from the peripheral tissues to the liver, where cholesterol is catabolized to bile acids. In the late 1980s, experimental work suggested that modified LDL, (e.g. oxidized LDL) could play a prominent role in the development of atherosclerosis (6). In summary, half a century of research on cholesterol has made clear that total cholesterol, as an indicator of LDL cholesterol levels, and HDL cholesterol play an important role in causing and predicting risk for CHD.

In this chapter, we will summarize the findings on total and HDL cholesterol from the Seven Countries Study. We also discuss trends in serum total cholesterol levels over a 35-year period, dietary determinants of serum total cholesterol, and serum total cholesterol levels and CHD risk from both cross-cultural and within-population perspectives. Finally, we will discuss the role of HDL cholesterol in CHD risk.

TRENDS IN SERUM CHOLESTEROL LEVELS OVER 35 YEARS

Determination of serum cholesterol level under field conditions was a major problem for the Seven Countries Study, and blood had to be collected in remote areas in northern and southern Europe. Valid cholesterol values were essential to cross-cultural comparisons. The Abell-Kendall method was used as the reference method. It provides similar cholesterol values to the enzymatic methods currently used (7,8). Anderson and Keys developed a simple method based on the Abell-Kendall method (9), and found that small samples (0.1 ml) of serum could be preserved for several months at temperatures of 25-30°C by air drying on filter paper. This allowed transportation to central laboratories in Minneapolis and Naples, where the dried serum samples were extracted from the filter paper by hydrolysis. This method was reproducible and valid compared to results of cholesterol determinations in fresh samples.

Standardization of serum cholesterol determinations was not always easy according to Keys in his memoirs (10). In a 1957 pilot study in Nicotera in southern Italy, the dried serum samples were sent for analysis to the University of Minnesota laboratory, where extremely high values were found in some samples. Keys wrote: "Detective work found the reason. Our Nicotera laboratory was full of flies and some of the filter paper samples showed flyspecks. We found that flyspecks contain cholesterol, or something that acts like it in the analysis! Putting screens on the windows solved the problem" (10).

Later in the 1960s, the Centers for Disease Control (CDC) in Atlanta, Georgia developed a Cooperative Cholesterol Standardization Program headed by Dr. Gerald Cooper, which developed into a worldwide service supported by the World Health Organization (11). It became possible to standardize not only total cholesterol, but also HDL cholesterol determinations for multi-center studies and trials internationally.

When the Seven Countries Study started little was known about population levels of serum cholesterol in different parts of the world. Pilot studies by Keys and co-workers in specific population groups had shown that cholesterol levels were low in Southern Europe and Japan and high in the U.S.A. and Finland (12). However, systematic comparative population data were not available.

Figure 1. Average population serum cholesterol level in 16 cohorts around 1960.

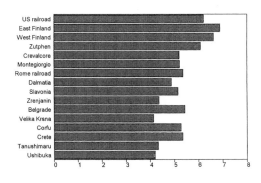

average serum cholesterol (mmol/l)

Figure 2. Serum cholesterol distribution in men aged 40-59 in East Finland and Velika Krsna (Serbia) during the baseline survey of the Seven Countries Study.

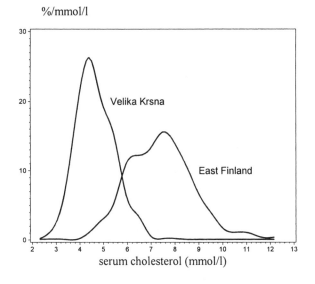

129

The data from the first-round surveys of the Seven Countries Study carried out from 1958-1964, showed that the highest average cholesterol levels in men aged 40-59 were found in Finland (about 7 mmol/l) and the lowest in Velika Krsna (Serbia) and Japan (about 4 mmol/l) (Fig. 1). Figure 2 shows that there is only a small overlap between the serum cholesterol distribution of middle-aged men in East Finland and Velika Krsna. This indicates that around 1960 there were large differences in serum cholesterol distribution within Europe. The implication is that the whole population of East Finland is at high risk regarding CHD, compared with that of Velika Krsna (13).

Table 1. Trends in average serum cholesterol level (mmol/l) in men aged 40-59 at baseline among several European cohorts of the Seven Countries Study in the 1960-1995 period.

| Year | 1960 | | 1970 | | 1985 | | 1995 | |
| Age (y) | 40-59 | | 50-69 | | 64-84 | | 75-94 | |
Cohort	N	Mean	N	Mean	N	Mean	N	Mean
East Finland	803	6.87	655	7.11	312	6.15	117	5.51
West Finland	857	6.61	717	6.78	381	6.06	151	5.42
Zutphen	829	6.09	625	6.18	362	6.13	132	5.46
Crevalcore	962	5.21	735	5.82	373	5.80	143	5.54
Montegiorgio	710	5.22	533	5.61	307	5.94	113	5.40
Zrenjanin	516	4.36	418	5.94	150	6.29	50	5.90
Belgrade	538	5.44	433	6.37	199	6.35	123	5.78
Velika Krsna	510	4.14	410	4.92	168	5.41	67	5.27

Table 2. Trends in average levels of serum cholesterol in men with an average age of 50 years in the 1960-1995 period in several European populations (13,15,16).

| Place | Cholesterol (mmol/l) | | |
	1960	1985	1995
North Karelia (SF)	6.8	6.4	6.0
Turku/Loimaa (SF)	6.5	6.2	5.9
Zutphen (NL)	6.0		
Ghent (B)		6.1	6.0
Crevalcore (I)	5.1		
Friuli (I)		6.3	5.9
Montegiorgio (I)	5.1		
Brianza (I)		5.6	5.9
Zrenjanin (S)	4.3		
Novi Sad (S)		-	6.4

The 1960 data are baseline data from the Seven Countries Study.
The 1985 and 1995 data are from the WHO-MONICA project

Long-term follow-up surveys were carried out in the Finnish, Dutch, Italian, and Serbian cohorts; the results over a 35-year period among these aging cohorts are summarized in Table 1. These show that in 1985 the average population cholesterol levels were about 6 mmol/l in seven of the eight cohorts (11,14). The average values had decreased in Finland, remained stable in the Netherlands, and increased in Italy and especially in Serbia. Later, between 1985 and 1995, average cholesterol levels (varying between 5.3 and 5.9 mmol/l) decreased in elderly men of all cohorts.

These trends in serum cholesterol levels are confounded by aging of the population. We therefore examined the trends in average serum cholesterol level in men with an average age of 50 years for the 1960-1995 period. Insights were obtained by comparing data collected at baseline in the Seven Countries Studies with those from the WHO-MONICA project (13,15,16) (Table 2). These data show the same general trend in average serum cholesterol level in middle-aged men in different European countries as in the aging populations of the Seven Countries Study. We conclude that in the period, 1960-1995, large changes occurred in average population cholesterol levels. Generally, the original high values in northern European countries decreased and the low values in southern and continental European countries increased. Nowadays, population differences in cholesterol level within Europe are small.

These findings indicate the dynamic nature of cholesterol values in populations. The country with the highest value in 1960 (Finland) had one of the lowest values in 1995, and the one with the lowest in 1960 became the highest in 1995 (Zrenjanin, Serbia). We find that mainly lifestyle changes, especially dietary changes, account for these trends in cholesterol levels. For example, national food balance-sheet data and dietary surveys carried out in Finland showed changes in fat consumption, that is, low-fat and polyunsaturated fat-rich margarine, and low-fat milk products, replaced butter and high-fat milk products (17). The change from boiled to filtered coffee may also partly be responsible for these changes. Food balance-sheet data from Yugoslavia suggest that an increased consumption of meat, milk products, edible fats, and eggs attributed to the strong increase in average serum cholesterol level in Serbia (17).

FATTY ACIDS, BODY WEIGHT AND SERUM TOTAL CHOLESTEROL

With the exception of the cohorts in Finland, The Netherlands and Italy, detailed individual dietary data were not collected in the different cohorts of the Seven Countries Study. During the period 1960-1995, however, individual dietary data were collected repeatedly in the Zutphen cohort in the Netherlands. These data were used to study associations between diet and serum total cholesterol level in free-living men. Because of the availability of repeatedly collected information it was possible to study changes in the intake of fatty acids, dietary cholesterol, and body weight in relation to changes in serum total cholesterol level. For a proper perspective on these results of the analyses using observational data we summarize here the results of controlled dietary experiments on the effect of fatty acids and dietary cholesterol on serum total cholesterol levels.

Classic controlled dietary experiments carried out by Keys and co-workers, by Hegsted and co-workers, and by others in the 1960s, showed that, compared with carbohydrates, saturated fatty acids and dietary cholesterol increased serum total cholesterol levels; monounsaturated fatty acids were neutral in effect, and polyunsaturated fatty acids decreased levels (18,19). The cholesterol-increasing effect of saturated fatty acids was twice as strong as the decreasing effect of polyunsaturated fatty acids, and much stronger than the dietary cholesterol effect. The saturated fatty acid effect was due to fatty acids with 12-16 carbon atoms. The saturated fatty acid with 18 carbon atoms, stearic acid, had a neutral cholesterol effect comparable with carbohydrates (18). These results were confirmed by later controlled dietary experiments (20,21), which showed that the cholesterol-lowering effect of polyun-saturated fatty acids was smaller than in the early experiments (18,19).

Monounsaturated *trans* fatty acids are formed when vegetable and fish oils are partially hydrogenated, as in margarine production to give margarine better texture and stability. Studies carried out in the 1970s produced conflicting results for the effect of *trans* fatty acids on serum total cholesterol level. However, in the early 1990s, controlled dietary experiments showed that *trans* fatty acids increased serum total cholesterol level, especially LDL cholesterol (22). We conclude that saturated fatty acids, especially those with 12-16 carbon atoms, and *trans* fatty acids increase total and LDL cholesterol. *Cis* monounsaturated and polyunsaturated fatty acids lower both total and LDL cholesterol levels compared to saturated and *trans* fatty acids.

Controlled dietary experiments are generally done in isocaloric states, with a maximum variation of + or − 2 kg, because weight changes themselves cause changes in serum total cholesterol levels (23). However, in free-living populations body weight increases over time in middle-aged men, with only small changes in fatty acids and dietary cholesterol intake. This hampers the study of the effect of *changes* in fatty acids and dietary cholesterol among free-living populations.

We studied changes in body weight, fatty acids, and dietary cholesterol in relation to serum cholesterol levels in the Zutphen Study (24,25). Data repeatedly collected in 1960, 1965, and 1970, and in 1985, 1990, and 1995, were used for these analyses. The 1960-1970 data showed that changes in body weight were the strongest correlates of changes in serum total cholesterol. In Zutphen men, a change in body weight of 1 kg was associated with a change of 0.05 mmol/l serum total cholesterol (24). This association was independent of initial body weight from the baseline survey. Changes in individual dietary fatty acid intake were not related to changes in serum total cholesterol level. A weak positive association was observed between individual changes in dietary cholesterol intake and serum total cholesterol level.

These associations were also studied in the Zutphen Elderly Study among men aged 65-84 in 1985 (25). For these analyses repeatedly collected data in the 1985-1995 period were used, because much more detailed information on the fatty acid composition was available. A positive association was observed between changes in body weight and changes in serum total cholesterol level. This association was, however, weaker than in middle-aged men.

Changes in individual intakes of saturated and *trans* fatty acids and dietary cholesterol were positively related to individual changes in serum total cholesterol level (25). However, these associations were not statistically significant. The strength of these associations was similar to those found in controlled dietary experiments for change in *trans* fatty acids and dietary cholesterol, but was weaker than those for saturated fatty acids. Changes in individual polyunsaturated fatty acids intake were strongly inversely associated with changes in serum total cholesterol level. This association was comparable to that obtained in controlled dietary experiments.

We conclude that in free-living populations, changes in body weight are an important determinant of changes in serum total cholesterol level, especially in middle-aged men. With the exception of changes in dietary cholesterol, the

132

associations between changes in fatty acids and serum total cholesterol levels were not observed in middle-aged men in the 1960-1970 period. However, in elderly men examined in the 1985-1995 period, several associations were observed. The association between changes in dietary saturated fatty acids and changes in serum total cholesterol level is weaker than in controlled dietary experiments. For changes in *trans* fatty acids, dietary cholesterol, and polyunsaturated fatty acids, similar changes in serum total cholesterol were observed as those in controlled dietary experiments. These results suggest that if detailed information on the fatty acid content of foods is available in free-living populations, similar associations to those in controlled dietary experiments will exist between changes in the intake of fatty acids, and changes in serum total cholesterol level. The only exception is the weaker association between changes in saturated fatty acids, and changes in serum total cholesterol level.

SERUM TOTAL CHOLESTEROL AND CORONARY HEART DISEASE FROM A CROSS-CULTURAL PERSPECTIVE

One of the hypotheses studied in the Seven Countries Study was that differences in population rates of CHD were related to mode of life, including composition of the diet. Within this context a prominent place was given to the role of serum cholesterol in explaining different population rates of CHD. The hypothesis that average population serum cholesterol levels were related to population CHD rates was tested for the first time using baseline average population serum cholesterol levels and 5-year fatal, and non-fatal, CHD rates. The coefficients for these ecological correlations were about 0.8 (26).

Similar associations were observed using 10- and 25-year mortality follow-up data (13,27). Menotti and coworkers showed that the coefficient for ecological correlations between average population serum cholesterol values at baseline, and population CHD mortality rates, decreased with increasing follow-up period from 0.81, using 10-year mortality, to 0.73, using 25-year mortality data. This was explained by the relatively weak contribution of the coefficient for entering average population serum cholesterol levels into late CHD mortality rates. They also showed that not only were baseline average population serum cholesterol levels significantly related to 25-year population CHD mortality rates, but also the *changes* in population average serum cholesterol levels during the first 10 years of follow-up. There was also a negative interaction between average population serum cholesterol levels at baseline and changes during a 10-year period. This means that populations having low average serum cholesterol levels and increased their average level during 10 years of follow-up are at increased risk of CHD mortality. This is shown in the Serbian cohorts, Zrenjanin and Velika Krsna.

The association between baseline average serum cholesterol levels and population CHD mortality rates during different follow-up periods, is non-linear (Fig. 3). For average population serum cholesterol levels below 5.5 mmol/l, the data show no relationship with population CHD mortality rates and above this level a dose-response relationship is noted. This suggests that the public health goal should be to reduce average population serum cholesterol levels below 5.5 mmol/l.

Figure 3. Average population serum cholesterol levels at baseline versus 25-year age-adjusted coronary heart disease mortality rates.

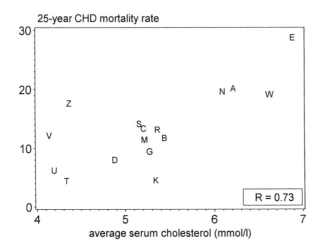

For legend see appendix

SERUM TOTAL CHOLESTEROL AND CORONARY HEART DISEASE WITHIN POPULATIONS

One of the goals of the Seven Countries Study was to investigate the strength of risk factors in different cultures. Differences could have large implications for prevention and treatment of CHD in individuals.

To answer these questions with conviction, a large number of coronary events are needed. The associations between *individual* concentrations of serum cholesterol and CHD mortality in the different cohorts were investigated after 10 and 25 years of follow-up (13,28). After 10 years of follow-up, clear dose-response relationships were observed between serum cholesterol levels at baseline, and 10-year CHD mortality in the U.S.A., Finland and the Netherlands. Numbers of coronary cases were too small to make pronouncements about the form of the relationship between serum cholesterol and CHD in the individual cohorts from southern Europe and Japan. Therefore a much longer follow-up period was needed. After obtaining 25-year mortality data, and repeat measurements of serum cholesterol, it was possible to answer questions about:

- Differences in the strength of the association between serum cholesterol, and CHD mortality, in different cultures.
- The effect of regression dilution bias on the strength of the association between serum cholesterol, and CHD (see definition below).
- Differences in absolute risk for CHD mortality in relation to serum cholesterol in different cultures.

Analyses of the relationship between serum cholesterol at baseline and long-term CHD mortality showed that a difference of 0.50 mmol/l in serum cholesterol is associated with a 12% additional risk for 25-year CHD mortality (RR = 1.12, 95%CI

= 1.09-1.16). These data suggest that the strength of the association between serum cholesterol and CHD is similar in different populations (26).

Biological risk factors are subject to random fluctuations due to measurement error and day-to-day biological fluctuations. When subjects are characterized according to their serum cholesterol level on the basis of a casual cholesterol measurement, the bottom category contains disproportionately many persons whose baseline cholesterol has been underestimated and the top category contains disproportionately many persons whose baseline cholesterol was overestimated. Therefore the observed cholesterol difference between the bottom and the top categories is larger than the "true" difference. This weakens the estimate of the relationship between serum cholesterol and CHD mortality. This phenomenon is often referred to as regression dilution bias.

The magnitude of dilution bias, the so-called dilution factor, can be calculated when more than one measurement of serum cholesterol is available from the same subjects. With the exception of measurements on the Japanese cohorts, cholesterol measurements were repeated five years after the baseline survey. This provided the possibility to calculate dilution factors for the different populations. As a result, the strength of the association between serum cholesterol and 25-year mortality from CHD increased 45%, taking regression dilution into account. After adjustment for regression dilution, the risk ratio amounted to 1.17 per 0.50 mmol/l of serum cholesterol as opposed to the previously mentioned risk ratio of 1.12 before adjustment. The regression dilution factor was similar in the different populations.

These results show that serum cholesterol is a strong predictor of CHD mortality. The longitudinal data of the rural Italian cohorts were used to study the effect of changes in serum cholesterol during the first 10 years of follow-up on CHD incidence during the next 15 years (29). This analysis showed that both baseline serum cholesterol and changes in serum cholesterol during 10 years of follow-up were independent predictors of coronary risk.

Data from the Dutch and Finnish cohorts of the Seven Countries Study were used to study the relationship between baseline serum cholesterol level, and long-term myocardial infarction incidence and coronary mortality (30,31). Both studies showed that baseline serum cholesterol levels predict myocardial infarction incidence (30) and coronary mortality (31) during a follow-up period of 25 years. The Zutphen data showed that this association was due to a strong relationship between baseline serum cholesterol and myocardial infarction incidence during the first 15 years of follow-up (30). Baseline serum total cholesterol was, however, not related to myocardial infarction incidence after 15-25 years of follow-up. The Finnish data, using mortality instead of incidence, showed that the strength of this association was stronger during the first 10 years of follow-up (RR= 1.87) compared with the next 15 years (RR= 1.39) (31). However, this later relationship was still borderline, as far as statistical significance was concerned. On the basis of the results of these two studies, we conclude that a casual baseline serum cholesterol measurement serves as a strong individual predictor of myocardial infarction incidence, and coronary mortality, till about 15 years of follow-up. Thereafter, the strength of the association diminishes, probably because the distance between the serum cholesterol measurement and the occurrence of the event is becoming too long.

The effect of age on the predictive power of serum cholesterol on CHD was also studied in the Seven Countries Study (32). With the use of 15-year follow-up data of the European cohorts, it was shown that in both northern and southern Europe the odds ratio for serum cholesterol in relation to 5-year CHD mortality decreased with age. In northern Europe the relative risk (odds ratio) for CHD mortality decreased from 4.10 in men aged 40-49 to 1.14 in men aged 60-69. For southern European these odds ratios were 9.77 and 1.04, respectively. These results show clearly that the strength of the association between serum cholesterol and CHD mortality decreases with age.

The association between serum cholesterol and 10-year mortality from CHD in elderly men aged 65-84 at baseline was studied in the Finnish, Dutch, and Italian cohorts of the Seven Countries Study (33). Positive associations were observed in all three countries, but the association reached statistical significance only in the Netherlands. The multivariate risk ratio for the total population was 1.17 (95%CI 1.06-1.29) per 1.00 mmol/l increase in cholesterol level. The multivariate risk ratio in the first five years of follow-up was higher (RR = 1.21 95%CI 1.06-1.38) than that in the second five years (RR = 1.13 95%CI 0.94-1.36). The predictive power in middle-aged men in the Seven Countries Study was 1.25 (95% CI 1.19-1.35) per 1.00 mmol/l increase in cholesterol level (28). These results indicate that serum cholesterol level is still a predictor of CHD risk in elderly men, although the strength of the association diminishes with age.

Relative risk provides information about the strength of the association between a risk factor and a disease. Information about the absolute risk is needed when treatment strategies are implemented for individuals. Absolute risks provide information about the chance of an event for an individual with specified risk factor levels. It is therefore also of great importance to know the absolute risk for CHD at a certain serum cholesterol level.

Figure 4. Twenty-five year coronary heart disease mortality rates in relation to baseline serum total cholesterol quartiles, adjusted for age, smoking, and blood pressure level (28).

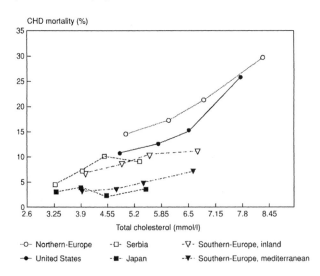

Figure 4 shows the relationship between baseline serum cholesterol levels and 25-year CHD mortality in different populations of the Seven Countries Study. At a serum cholesterol level of 5 mmol/l the 25-year CHD mortality rate is 5 times (15 vs. 3%)

higher in northern Europe than in Mediterranean southern Europe (28). This implies that the absolute risk for CHD mortality based on a certain serum cholesterol level varies greatly among populations; this has large implications for treatment and prevention. The effect of a substantial decrease in serum cholesterol level of individuals through dietary and lifestyle changes or through drugs is much larger in northern Europe than in southern Europe. This also raises questions about the cost-effectiveness of serum cholesterol therapies in different parts of Europe. For instance, the reduction in absolute CHD risk by lowering serum total cholesterol in a high-risk individual from 7 to 5 mmol/l is much larger in northern than in southern Europe. If, in southern Europe, only a small decrease in absolute risk can be obtained by lowering cholesterol, we should question the cost-effectiveness of this therapy.

HDL CHOLESTEROL AND CORONARY HEART DISEASE WITHIN POPULATIONS

Gofman and coworkers first pointed out the importance of different lipoprotein fractions in relation to CHD (2). They isolated lipoprotein fractions by ultracentrifugation, a time-consuming technique that can only be applied in a clinical setting. In an early stage, Anderson and Keys developed a simple method for separating total cholesterol into the atherogenic LDL cholesterol and the protective HDL cholesterol fraction (9). At that time, LDL cholesterol was called ß-lipoprotein cholesterol and HDL cholesterol α-lipoprotein cholesterol. The fractionation of total cholesterol in ß-lipoprotein and α-lipoprotein was done by paper electrophoresis and by cold ethanol precipitation. Keys and coworkers carried out several pilot studies in Finland, Hawaii, and Japan, and found that the Finnish and Japanese differed greatly in ß-cholesterol but very little in α-cholesterol. This suggested to them that α-cholesterol was not important in explaining cross-cultural differences in the occurrence of CHD (13). Since then we learned that just because a risk factor is not important in explaining cross-cultural differences in CHD, it does not mean that this risk factor is unimportant in individual risk (for example, alcohol and fish consumption). A risk factor may not be important in explaining differences in CHD rates among populations, but may very well be important in explaining differences in CHD risks among individuals.

After the discovery of the importance of HDL cholesterol level in the 1950s interest waned because of the small differences in average HDL cholesterol levels among populations. However, a revival in interest in HDL occurred after the landmark publication of Miller and Miller in 1975 (33). Basing findings on metabolic studies, they suggested that HDL is involved in reverse cholesterol transport and that HDL cholesterol may be protective against CHD. Research on HDL cholesterol grew following a publication of the Framingham Heart Study data establishing an inverse relation between the HDL cholesterol level, and individual risk of CHD (5).

HDL cholesterol was measured for the first time in the Seven Countries Study cohorts around 1985 in lipid laboratories in the Netherlands, Finland, and Italy. These laboratories were standardized according to the World Health Organization Lipid Reference Laboratories in Prague, Czech Republic, and Atlanta, Georgia in the U.S. (11). Cholesterol was determined in the HDL lipoprotein fraction after precipitation of apolipoprotein B-containing lipoprotein fractions, using either dextran magnesium chloride, dextran magnesium sulfate or magnesium phosphotungstate.

Table 3. Trend in average HDL cholesterol level (mmol/l) in men aged 65-84 at baseline, in several European cohorts of the Seven Countries Study, in the 1985-1995 period.

Year	1985		1995	
Age (y)	65-84		75-94	
Cohort	N	Mean	N	Mean
East Finland	312	1.22	117	1.09
West Finland	381	1.22	151	1.05
Zutphen	362	1.11	132	1.15
Crevalcore	373	1.31	143	1.18
Montegiorgio	306	1.28	113	1.21
Zrenjanin	148	1.37	50	1.21
Belgrade	198	1.26	123	1.15
Velika Krsna	148	1.31	67	1.36

Average HDL cholesterol levels were highest in elderly men in Italy and Serbia and lowest in elderly men in the Netherlands (11) (Table 3). The average population HDL cholesterol levels decreased in 6 of the 8 cohorts during a follow-up period of 10 years, when average total cholesterol levels also declined. Body Mass Index and cigarette smoking were associated with lower HDL cholesterol, and alcohol consumption with higher levels (11). Changes in body weight and alcohol consumption during the period 1985-1995 were also related to changes in HDL cholesterol level (25), comparable with those observed in controlled experiments. Changes in saturated, monounsaturated and polyunsaturated fatty acids, and dietary cholesterol intake were directly related to changes in HDL cholesterol level. Changes in *trans* fatty acids were inversely related to changes in HDL cholesterol level. Although generally not statistically significant, the strength of the associations among different classes of fatty acids and dietary cholesterol intake in relation to changes in

Figure 5. Ten-year age-adjusted coronary heart disease mortality rates (%) in men aged 65 to 84 years per tertile of baseline HDL cholesterol (32).

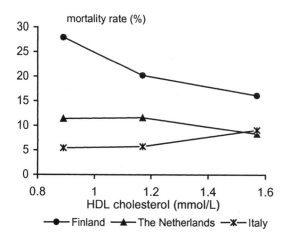

HDL cholesterol levels were comparable to those observed in controlled dietary experiments (20,21).

HDL cholesterol was also studied in relation to 10-year CHD mortality risk in elderly men of cohorts from Finland, The Netherlands, and Italy (34). Different associations were observed in the three countries such that the expected inverse association was found in Finland, but not in the Netherlands or Italy (Fig.5). In Italy, an interaction was noted among HDL cholesterol, Body Mass Index and alcohol consumption. In lean elderly men who drank < 40 g of alcohol daily, an inverse association was noted between HDL cholesterol and CHD mortality. A positive association was observed among elderly overweight men who drank ≥ 40 g of alcohol per day. These results suggest that in thin elderly men with no, or only a moderate, alcohol intake, HDL cholesterol is inversely related to CHD mortality.

COMMENTS

In the Seven Countries Study average population serum cholesterol levels and changes are important determinants of CHD mortality. Within populations serum cholesterol level is an important predictor of CHD mortality in both middle-aged and elderly men.

In a meta analysis, the strength of the relation between serum cholesterol level and CHD incidence was investigated using data of three cross-cultural (ecological) studies including the Seven Countries Study, 10 large cohort studies and 28 randomized controlled trials (34). The reduction in CHD incidence in relation to a 0.6 mmol/l (about 10%) decrease in serum cholesterol level was estimated. For men aged 55-64, the decrease in CHD incidence amounted to 38% in the ecological studies, 27% in the cohort studies and 25% in the randomized trials after 5 years of follow-up. The cohort studies showed that the effect of a 10% decrease in serum cholesterol level on CHD incidence depended on age. The reduction in CHD incidence decreased from 50% at age 40 to 20% at age 70.

The results of the first generation of randomized trials using cholesterol-lowering drugs showed a significant reduction in CHD incidence but were not convincing in relation to all-causes mortality because of the relatively small decrease (about 10%) in serum cholesterol levels. When more effective drugs (statins) became available for serum cholesterol lowering more favorable results were obtained. A meta analysis of five large randomized trials showed a 20% reduction in total cholesterol, 28% reduction in LDL cholesterol and 5% increase in HDL cholesterol level (35). These changes were associated with a 31% reduced risk in major CHD events and 21% in all-causes mortality. The risk reduction was similar for men and women and for middle-aged and elderly persons. We conclude from the results of ecological studies, cohort studies and randomized trials that serum total and LDL cholesterol level are causally related to CHD incidence.

Less evidence is available for the association between serum HDL cholesterol level and CHD incidence. We observed in the FINE Study an inverse association between serum HDL cholesterol level and CHD mortality during 10 years of follow-up in elderly men, especially in thin men with no or moderate alcohol intake. This result is consistent with those of other cohort studies carried out in middle-aged and elderly men (5,36).

The question whether the inverse association between serum HDL cholesterol level and CHD incidence is causal, is difficult to answer. Serum HDL cholesterol levels are inversely associated with serum triglyceride levels. Causality of the inverse association between serum HDL cholesterol level and CHD incidence should therefore preferably be tested in populations with low serum HDL cholesterol, LDL cholesterol and triglyceride levels. The intervention agent should preferably only increase serum HDL cholesterol level in order to establish a protective effect on CHD incidence.

Such a trial was carried out in more than 2,500 men with coronary disease and less than 74 years of age (37). Their serum HDL cholesterol level was 1.0 mmol/l or less, LDL cholesterol level 3.6 mmol/l or less, and triglyceride level 3.4 mmol/l or less. In this trial the effect of 1,200 mg gemfibrozil on CHD incidence during a 5.1 year follow-up was tested. The use of gemfibrozil increased the serum HDL cholesterol level by 6%, lowered the serum triglyceride level by 31%, and did not change LDL cholesterol level. These changes resulted in a reduction in relative risk for CHD incidence of 22%. These findings suggest that the rate of CHD events is reduced by raising serum HDL cholesterol levels and lowering levels of triglycerides without lowering LDL cholesterol levels.

The effect of both an increase in HDL cholesterol level and a decrease in LDL cholesterol level was recently tested in a randomized trial of 160 coronary patients using angiographic and clinical endpoints (38). A lipid modifying therapy of statins in combination with a high dose of niacin was used as intervention. LDL cholesterol levels were lowered by 42% and HDL cholesterol levels increased 26%. Average stenosis progressed by 3.7% in the control group and regressed 0.4% in the statin-niacin group (p<0.001). For clinical cardiovascular events a 60% reduction was observed for the statin–niacin group compared with the predicted 68% reduction in clinical cardiovascular events based on the changes in LDL and HDL cholesterol levels.

We conclude that convincing evidence is in, that serum total and LDL cholesterol level are causally related to CHD incidence and mortality. Evidence is accumulating that the inverse relationship between serum HDL cholesterol level and CHD risk is also causal. Serum LDL cholesterol levels are strongly related to serum total cholesterol levels. Therefore in epidemiologic studies serum total cholesterol level can be measured as a proxy for LDL cholesterol level. Both serum total and HDL cholesterol level should be measured for a proper estimation of CHD risk in individuals.

SUMMARY AND CONCLUSIONS

During the past 35 years the Seven Countries Study has provided insights into the epidemiology of serum cholesterol and its fractions in relation to CHD. First, notable changes occurred in average population serum cholesterol levels in countries with high levels initially (Finland), the high levels decreased, and in those with low levels (Serbia) they increased. Nowadays, the differences in average population serum cholesterol levels in Europe are small. Body weight, and the intake of fatty acids and dietary cholesterol, are important correlates of serum total cholesterol levels in free-living populations. Average population serum total cholesterol levels are an important, but not the only determinant of population differences in CHD mortality rates. Within populations, serum total cholesterol level is an important predictor of CHD, both in middle-aged and older men. However, the strength of the association among individuals diminishes with age. Large differences in absolute risk for CHD

140

mortality at the same serum cholesterol level are, however, observed in different parts of Europe with a high risk in northern Europe and a low risk in southern Europe. Finally, even at older ages, HDL cholesterol level seems to protect from CHD mortality, especially in thin men with no or moderate alcohol intake. Body weight, cigarette smoking, alcohol, fatty acids, and dietary cholesterol are important determinants of individual HDL cholesterol levels

REFERENCES

1. Connor WE. Diet heart research in the first part of the 20th century. Acta Cardiol 1999; 54: 135-149.
2. Gofman JW, Jones HB, Lindgren FT, Lyon TP, Elliott HA, Strisoswer B. Blood lipids and human atherosclerosis. Circulation 1950; 2: 161-178.
3. Brown MS, Kovanen PT, Goldstein JL. Regulation of plasma cholesterol by lipoprotein receptors. Science 1981;212:628-635.
4. Kannel WB, Dawber TR, Kagan A, Revotskie N, Stokes J III. Factors of risk in the development of coronary heart disease. Six-year follow-up experience. The Framingham Study. Ann Intern Med 1961;55:33-50.
5. Gordon T, Castelli WP, Hjortland MC, Kannel WB, Dawber TR. High density lipoprotein as a protective factor against coronary heart disease. Am J Med 1977;62: 707-714.
6. Steinberg D, Parthasarathy S, Carew TE, Khoo JC, Witzum JL. Beyond cholesterol. Modifications of low-density lipoprotein that increase its atherogenicity. N Engl J Med 1989;320:915-924.
7. Abell AA, Levy BB, Brody BB, Kendall FE. A simplified method for the estimation of total cholesterol in serum and demonstration of its specificity. J Biol Chem 1952;195:357-366.
8. Katterman R, Jaworek D, Möller G. Multicentre study of a new enzymatic method of cholesterol determination. J Clin Chem Clin Biochem 1984;22:245-251.
9. Anderson JT, Keys A. Cholesterol in serum and lipoprotein fractions. Its measurement and stability. Clin Chem 1956;2:145-159.
10. Keys A. Adventures of a medical scientist. Sixty years of research in thirteen countries. ISBN 0-9672072-0-7 1999: 1-84.
11. Kromhout D, Nissinen A, Menotti A, Bloemberg B, Pekkanen J, Giampaoli S. Total and HDL cholesterol and their correlates in elderly men in Finland, Italy and the Netherlands. Am J Epidemiol 1990;131:855-863.
12. Keys A. The cholesterol problem. Voeding 1952;13:539-555.
13. Keys A, Aravanis C, Blackburn H, Buzina R, Djordjevic BS, Dontas AS, Fidanza F, Karvonen MJ, Kimura N, Menotti A, Mohacek I, Nedeljkovic S, Puddu V, Punsar S, Taylor HL, Van Buchem FSP. Seven countries. A multivariate analysis of death and coronary heart disease. Cambridge, MA; Harvard University Press, ISBN: 0-674-80237-3, 1980:1-381.
14. Kromhout D, Nedeljkovic SI, Grujic MZ, Ostojic MC, Keys A, Menotti A, Katan MB, Van Oostrom MA, Bloemberg BPM. Changes in major risk factors for cardiovascular diseases during 25 years in the Serbian cohorts of the Seven Countries Study. Int J Epidemiol 1994;23:5-11.
15. Rayner M, Petersen S. Compilers European cardiovascular disease statistics. London: British Heart Foundation, 2000.
16. Kuulasmaa K, Tunstall-Pedoe H, Dobson A, Fortmann S, Sans S, Tolonen H, Evans A, Ferrario M, Tuomilehto J. Estimation of contribution of changes in classic risk factors to trends in coronary-event rates across the WHO MONICA Project populations. Lancet 2000;355:675-687

17. Kromhout D, Keys A, Aravanis C, Buzina R, Fidanza F, Giampaoli S, Jansen A, Menotti A, Nedeljkovic S, Pekkarinen M, Simic BS, Toshima H. Food consumption patterns in the nineteen sixties in Seven Countries. Am J Clin Nutr 1989;49:889-894.

18. Keys A, Anderson JT, Grande F. Serum cholesterol response to changes in the diet IV. Particular fatty acids in the diet. Metabolism 1965;14:776-787.

19. Hegsted DM, McGandy RB, Myers ML, Stare FJ. Quantitative effects of dietary fat on serum cholesterol in men. Am J Clin Nutr 1965;17:281-295

20. Mensink RP, Katan MB. Effect of dietary fatty acids on serum lipids and lipoproteins. A meta-analysis of 27 trials. Atheroscl Tromb 1992;12:911-919

21. Clarke R, Frost C, Collins R, Appleby P, Peto R. Dietary lipids and blood cholesterol: quantitative meta-analysis of metabolic ward studies. BMJ 1997; 314: 112-117.

22. Mensink RP, Katan MB. Effect of dietary trans fatty acids on high-density and low-density lipoprotein levels in healthy subjects. N Engl J Med 1990;323:439-445.

23. Dattilo AM, Kris-Etherton PM. Effects of weight reduction on blood lipids and lipoproteins: a meta-analysis. Am J Clin Nutr 1992;56:320-328.

24. Kromhout D. Body weight, diet and serum cholesterol in 871 middle-aged men during 10 years of follow-up (The Zutphen Study). Am J Clin Nutr 1983;38:591-598.

25. Oomen CM, Ocké MC, Feskens EJM, Kok FJ, Kromhout D. Changes in diet and body weight predict changes in total and high density lipoprotein cholesterol concentrations: A longitudinal study of elderly men. Submitted

26. Keys A. Coronary heart disease in Seven Countries. Circulation 1970;Suppl I:1-211.

27. Menotti A, Blackburn H, Kromhout D, Nissinen A, Fidanza F, Giampaoli S, Buzina R, Mohacek I, Nedeljkovic S, Aravanis C, Toshima H. Changes in population cholesterol levels and coronary heart disease death in Seven Countries. Eur Heart J 1997;18:566-571.

28. Verschuren WMM, Jacobs DR, Bloemberg BPM, Kromhout D, Menotti A, Aravanis C, Blackburn HW, Buzina R, Dontas AS, Fidanza F, Karvonen MJ, Nedeljkovic S, Nissinen A, Toshima H. Serum total cholesterol and long-term coronary heart disease mortality in different cultures. Twenty-five year follow-up of the Seven Countries Study. JAMA 1995;274:131-136.

29. Kromhout D, Bosschieter EB, Drijver M, De Lezenne Coulander C. Serum cholesterol and 25-year incidence of and mortality from myocardial infarction and cancer. The Zutphen Study. Arch Intern Med 1988;148:1051-1055.

30. Pekkanen J, Nissinen A, Punsar S, Karvonen MJ. Short- and long-term association of serum cholesterol with mortality. The 25-year follow-up of the Finnish cohorts of the Seven Countries Study. Am J Epidemiol 1992;135:1251-1258.

31. Mariotti S, Capocaccia R, Farchi G, Menotti A, Verdecchia A, Keys A. Age, period, cohort and geographical area effects on the relationship between risk factors and coronary heart disease mortality. 15-year follow-up of the European cohorts of the Seven Countries Study. J Chron Dis 1986;39:229-242.

32. Houterman A, Verschuren WMM, Giampaoli S, Nissinen A, Feskens EJM, Menotti A, Kromhout D. Total but not high-density lipoprotein cholesterol is consistently associated with coronary heart disease mortality in elderly men in Finland, Italy and the Netherlands. Epidemiol 2000;11:327-332.

33. Miller N, Miller G. Plasma-high-density-lipoprotein concentration and development of ischaemic heart-disease. Lancet 1975;1:16-19.

34. Law MR, Wald NJ, Thompson SG. By how much and how quickly does reduction in serum cholesterol concentration lower risk of ischaemic heart disease? BMJ 1994;308:367-373.

35. La Rosa JC, He J, Vupputuri S. Effect of statins on risk of coronary disease. A meta-analysis of randomized controlled trials. JAMA 1999;282:2340-2346.

36. Gordon DJ, Probstfield JL, Garrison RJ, Neaton JD, Castelli WP, Kroke JD, Jacobs DR Jr, Bangdiwala S, Tyroler HA. High density lipoprotein cholesterol and cardiovascular disease. Four prospective American studies. Circulation 1989;79:8-15.

37. Bloomfield Rubins H, Robins SJ, Collins D, Fye CL, Anderson JW, Elam MB, Faas FH, Linares E, Schaefer EJ, Schectman G, Wilt TJ, Wittes J for the Veterans Affairs High-

density Lipoprotein Cholesterol Intervention Trial Study Group. N Engl J Med 1999;341:410-418.

38. Brown BG, Zhao XQ, Chait A, Fisher LD, Cheung MC, Morse JS, Dowdy AA, Marino EK, Bolson EL, Alaupovic P, Frohlich J, Albers JJ. Simvastatin and niacin, antioxidant vitamins, or the combination for the prevention of coronary disease. N Engl J Med 2001;345:1583-1592.

CHAPTER 3.2

BLOOD PRESSURE AND CARDIOVASCULAR DISEASES IN THE SEVEN COUNTRIES STUDY

Alessandro Menotti

The role of blood pressure, and of high blood pressure, as risk factors for cardiovascular diseases was among the first to be identified in population studies by the Pickering monograph on the distribution of blood pressure in populations (1). Sir George Pickering showed the distribution of blood pressure in the general population to be continuous, roughly normal, and unimodal; therefore, the definition of hypertension was arbitrary. His "enemy and friend," Robert Platt, insisted, however, on the existence of a bimodal distribution of blood pressure, apparently erroneously based on his selection of true hypertensive patients and their relatives on one side and of true non-hypertensives on the other. Later it became clear that Pickering's intuition was correct. Hypertension was simply a quantitative deviation from blood pressure levels associated with lower risk.

At the onset of the Seven Countries Study in the late 1950s, knowledge was needed about the distribution of blood pressure within and among populations, time trends for blood pressure, and its relationship to incidence of and mortality from cardiovascular diseases. It was a logical decision then to measure the blood pressure and to study its relationship to cardiovascular diseases. At that time, treatment of high blood pressure was limited by the few drugs available, most not yet properly tested and most with adverse effects. As a consequence, the proportion of hypertensive subjects treated by drugs was low. Systematic information on treatment of hypertension was collected only at a late stage.

BLOOD PRESSURE LEVELS, PREVALENCE OF HYPERTENSION AND TRENDS

Blood pressure was measured by a standard procedure described in the WHO Cardiovascular Survey Methods Manual (2), with mercury sphygmomanometers located at heart level, on the right arm, in supine position, and taken by trained physicians at the end of the physical examination. Blood pressure was measured twice and systolic, diastolic phase IV and diastolic phase V were recorded. Only even numbers were used as terminal digits. For most analyses the average of two measurements was used. Phase IV diastolic blood pressure was never considered in analysis. Despite training and testing, at entry examination a digit preference for 0 (zero) could be shown in most areas, although to a different extent (3).

The FINE Study used the same methodology with slight differences: sometimes by measuring blood pressure of elderly men in sitting instead of lying position; and taken after 4-5 minutes rest; phase IV was not recorded. In the FINE Study the use of anti-hypertensive drugs was recorded in detail.

Table 1 shows average population levels of systolic and diastolic blood pressure with differences among samples. The distribution did not follow a strictly geographical trend, but altogether higher levels were seen in northern European and North American samples compared to the others. An exception was the high average levels of systolic blood pressure in the rural area of Crevalcore in northern Italy. Mean levels of blood pressure were not elevated in the two Japanese cohorts. Prevalence of hypertension (defined by levels equal to or greater than 160 mmHg for systolic or 95 mmHg for diastolic blood pressure) had a distribution similar to the average levels of blood pressure.

Table 1. Average levels and standard deviation (in parentheses) of blood pressure (BP) and prevalence of hypertension (160 mmHg or more or 95 mmHg or more) at entry examination in the 16 cohorts.

Cohort	Systolic BP (mmHg)	Diastolic BP (mmHg)	Prevalence of hypertension %
U.S. railroad	139.2 (20.8)	86.2 (11.7)	25.9
East Finland	148.4 (20.5)	89.3 (10.8)	37.3
West Finland	139.6 (20.0)	82.1 (10.8)	17.1
Zutphen	144.4 (19.8)	88.8 (12.6)	36.0
Crevalcore	148.0 (21.5)	87.8 (11.2)	33.5
Montegiorgio	137.6 (18.6)	82.2 (10.4)	15.7
Rome railroad	140.4 (18.4)	88.5 (12.6)	32.2
Dalmatia	137.8 (18.2)	82.6 (11.1)	18.9
Slavonia	138.3 (20.9)	82.6 (12.3)	21.6
Zrenjanin	133.6 (19.0)	84.8 (10.6)	17.4
Belgrade	133.9 (18.1)	86.5 (11.0)	18.2
Velika Krsna	131.4 (18.4)	81.8 (10.2)	13.3
Corfu	135.1 (21.2)	82.7 (11.4)	17.8
Crete	137.0 (20.0)	81.6 (11.2)	18.1
Tanushimaru	133.1 (24.4)	73.7 (14.1)	13.8
Ushibuka	136.9 (25.5)	78.3 (13.0)	19.3

Table 2. Mean changes of blood pressure levels in 10 years in the 16 cohorts.

Cohort	Change systolic blood pressure		Change diastolic blood pressure	
	mmHg	%	mmHg	%
U.S. railroad [a]	-2.0	-1.4	-3.1	-3.6
East Finland	+1.0	+0.1	-5.6	-6.2
West Finland	+6.5	+4.7	+1.0	+1.2
Zutphen	+2.6	+1.8	+0.5	+0.6
Crevalcore	+7.1	+4.8	+2.4	+2.8
Montegiorgio	+12.9	+9.3	+7.1	+8.6
Rome railroad	+7.8	+5.5	+0.4	+0.4
Dalmatia	+10.5	+7.6	+4.1	+5.0
Slavonia	+13.7	+9.9	+4.8	+5.8
Zrenjanin	+15.3	+11.4	+4.1	+4.8
Belgrade	+10.7	+8.0	+0.2	+0.2
Velika Krsna	+12.7	+9.7	+2.2	+2.7
Corfu	+13.5	+10.0	+3.9	+4.7
Crete	+0.2	+0.2	-3.8	-4.6
Tanushimaru	+3.7	+2.8	+3.1	+3.1
Ushibuka	+6.2	+4.5	+3.3	+4.2

a = 5 year change

At the time of 5- and 10-year re-examination, blood pressure levels were higher in most cohorts, showing the consequences of aging. The average increase was different

147

among cohorts. A summary of 10-year average changes is reported in Table 2. Here it appears that in North America and northern Europe average levels of blood pressure were stable, only slightly increased or even decreased, while the largest increments were found in southern Europe (except Crete). Reasons for these differential changes cannot be explained by the available data. However, it is known that during those years proper medical control of hypertension started in North America and northern Europe, and later in southern Europe.

Figure 1. Trends of average population systolic blood pressure for 35 years in the cohorts of four countries. The same individuals surviving 35 years are considered. The entry age range was 40-59 years.

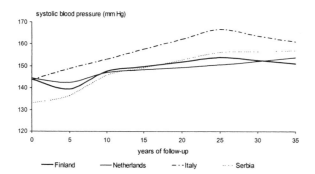

For eight cohorts in four European countries information is available about average systolic blood pressure trends during 35 years (Table 3). A definite increase in systolic blood pressure was seen in the southern European areas, while this was much less evident in Finland and the Netherlands. A similar analysis is reported in Fig. 1 for the four countries involved (Finland, The Netherlands, Italy, and Serbia), where data are given only for men who were still alive at year 35 of the follow-up and therefore deal with the same individuals. Actual measurements are those for years 0, 5, 10, 25, 30 and 35 for the first three countries, and the same except for year 30 for Serbia. The missing values were extrapolated. Figure 1 shows that levels in Finland, The Netherlands, and Italy were similar at entry examination, but later they increased until year 25 when a decline started. Compared to Italy, the increase of blood pressure in Finland and the Netherlands was much less sustained. The average systolic blood pressure in Serbia at year 0 was lower but then continuously increased in the course of 35 years, overtaking the levels of the Dutch cohort between years 15 and 20 and the Finnish cohort around year 25.

Table 4 compares average systolic blood pressure data for men aged 50 in 1960 with data from the Seven Countries Study and in 1985 and 1995 with data from the WHO-MONICA Project (4,5). The table presents pairs of cohorts belonging to roughly similar geographic areas. The general impression is that average systolic blood pressure tends to be stable, or definitely decreasing, in all cultures except in

Table 3. Trends in average systolic blood pressure (mmHg) in men aged 40-59 at baseline in several European cohorts of the Seven Countries Study in the 1960-1995 period.

Year Age (y) Cohort	1960 40-59		1970 50-69		1985 65-84		1995 75-94	
	N	Mean	N	Mean	N	Mean	N	Mean
Eastern Finland	810	148	656	149	318	150	117	149
Western Finland	859	140	720	146	387	157	151	153
Zutphen	876	144	625	147	361	151	132	154
Crevalcore	993	148	799	155	372	167	145	163
Montegiorgio	719	138	606	150	308	166	119	158
Belgrade	540	134	438	145	287	150	140	154
Zrenjanin	517	134	435	149	185	169	55	164
Velika Krsna	511	131	435	144	225	154	74	158

Table 4. Trends in average systolic blood pressure (mmHg) in men aged 50 in the period, 1960-1995 for several European populations

Cohort	1960	1985	1995
North Karelia (SF)	146	144	142
Turku/Loimaa (SF)	138	143	139
Zutphen (NL)	141		
Ghent (B)		127	129
Zrenjanin (S)	130		
Novi sad (S)		135	136
Crevalcore (I)	145		
Friuli (I)		142	140
Montegiorgio (I)	135		
Brianza (I)		137	131

The 1960 data are baseline data from the Seven Countries Study.
The 1985 and 1995 data are from the WHO MONICA Project (4,5).

Serbia, confirming the situations as shown in Table 3 and Fig. 1. The aging effect is found to contrast with the comparison among different generations reaching the same age.

During the first three field examinations, information on the use of anti-hypertensive drugs was collected but not routinely coded. In some areas these drugs were reviewed and reported. For example, in the three Italian areas the proportion of treated hypertensives was 1.2% at entry examination, and most of them used rauwolfia. At examinations for years 5 and 10, the corresponding levels were 9.3% and 12.7%, respectively, and the use of diuretics was the common approach (6).

In the five cohorts of elderly men (ages 65-84) in three countries investigated in the FINE Study in 1985, systematic information was obtained about the use of anti-hypertensive drugs. The prevalence of hypertension (160 mmHg or more for systolic blood pressure, or 95 mmHg or more for diastolic blood pressure, or use of anti-hypertensive drugs) was 33.5 % in Finland, 42.2 % in the Netherlands, and 72.4 % in Italy. The proportion of treated hypertensive patients was 55.7 % in Finland, 28.3 % in the Netherlands, and 45.2 % in Italy, suggesting varying attitudes to the treatment of hypertension. When more recent criteria for hypertension were adopted (i.e. 140 or 90 mmHg or more) the proportion of treated hypertensives dropped to 41.3% in Finland, 16.7 % in the Netherlands, and 36.4 % in Italy.

DETERMINANTS OF BLOOD PRESSURE

Besides drug treatment there has been a long-term interest in the environmental determinants of blood pressure. It is known that overweight people have higher blood pressure than thin people. Salt has been implicated as a determinant of blood pressure since the beginning of the 20th century. Later on it became clear that other minerals such as potassium, calcium, and magnesium could play a role; it was also found that high alcohol consumption increases blood pressure. These determinants were also studied in the Seven Countries Study.

In analyses of the baseline data strong relationships were found between relative body weight, and levels of systolic and diastolic blood pressure, in most cohorts or countries (3). These associations formed the basis for studying the confounding effect of blood pressure on indicators of obesity in their associations with future cardiovascular events.

At the time of the 15th anniversary examination, a subsample of men aged 55-74 in the two Finnish cohorts were studied for 24-hour urinary excretion of sodium and potassium (7). Men in East Finland had lower urine volume (1.64 l in 24 hours) than those in West Finland (1.80 l in 24 hours), but more sodium, corresponding to an estimated intake of 16.0 g/ day and 14.2 g / day, respectively. No difference was found in excretion of potassium between East and West Finland. A slight inverse relationship between sodium excretion and diastolic blood pressure was found (r = -0.22, p<0.05), which is hard to interpret. These results show that the sodium intake in Finland was one of the highest in Europe at the time (1975).

In the Zutphen cohort it was possible to study the relationship of some foods and nutrients to blood pressure, at different field examinations (1960, 1965 and 1970) (8). Potassium intake was inversely related to systolic blood pressure in 1970, and inverse relationships were also found between calcium intake and blood pressure in 1965 and 1970. In all three examinations alcohol intake was directly related to blood pressure levels and its changes also influenced blood pressure levels.

Special attention to the possible determinants of blood pressure was given using the Zutphen data of the FINE Study, at the time of the second examination in 1990 (age range of 70 to 89 years) (9). A cluster analysis was conducted on the average daily intake of selected nutrients, allowing up to four clusters (an alcohol cluster, meat cluster, healthy diet cluster, and refined sugars cluster, called in this way because of characteristic components of the Dutch diet). Systolic and diastolic blood pressure were definitely higher in the alcohol cluster when compared to the others, especially the healthy diet and meat clusters. The prevalence of hypertension was 47% in the alcohol cluster, versus 37% in the healthy diet and meat clusters.

BLOOD PRESSURE AND CARDIOVASCULAR DISEASES FROM A CROSS-CULTURAL PERSPECTIVE

Mean population levels of systolic and diastolic blood pressure were studied against death rates or incidence of CHD during different periods of time and using different starting points (10-12). In a recent unpublished analysis the correlation of population average systolic blood pressure with CHD death rates was strong, but declining by increasing periods of follow-up, although always statistically significant. For example, a correlation coefficient of 0.71 (95% CI 0.31-0.89) found after 5 years of follow-up declined during the next 20 years until reaching the value of 0.58 at year 25 (95% CI 0.09-0.83) (Fig. 2). The association was also observed for baseline levels of systolic blood pressure versus late events, that is, after the 10th anniversary of follow-up. Systolic blood pressure measured in later years (on the 10th anniversary) was associated with CHD death rates to a lesser, and usually not significant, extent compared with baseline measurements.

Figure 2. Cross-cultural association between entry population levels of systolic blood pressure and 25-year age- adjusted death rates from coronary heart disease.

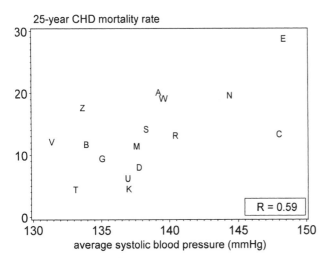

For legend see appendix

The association of population average diastolic blood pressure with CHD death rates was weaker than for systolic blood pressure but it tended to increase for longer follow-up periods. However, when diastolic blood pressure was measured at the 10th year of follow-up, statistically significant associations were no longer found with CHD deaths occurring during the subsequent 5 to 15 years.

In general, it seems that comparing different populations, blood pressure is associated (ecologically) with CHD mortality, but the correlation tends to decline after longer periods of follow-up and when measurements are taken at an older age. However, in multiple regression models of 5, 10, 15, 20 and 25-year CHD death rates, where population average serum cholesterol, smoking habits, body mass index, and physical activity were also included in the model, the association of blood pressure with death rates was never statistically significant (12).

Figure 3. Cross-cultural association between entry average population levels of systolic blood pressure and 25-year age-adjusted death rates from stroke.

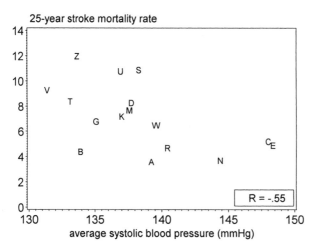

For legend see appendix

The relationship of average population blood pressure to mortality from stroke was preliminarily examined on partial 20-year follow-up data (13) and more systematically after 25 years of follow-up (14). A major limitation of the analyses with stroke as endpoint was the inability to segregate thrombotic from hemorraghic stroke under field conditions. Average entry population levels of systolic blood pressure among cohorts were inversely related to stroke death rates (in the 25-year follow-up data r = -0.55; 95%CI -0.81 and -0.06; p=0.03) (Fig. 3). Within cohorts, as expected, the relationship of blood pressure to stroke was strongly positive, and significant in 14 of the 16 cohorts. Average population levels of serum cholesterol were strongly inversely related to stroke death rates (r = -0.79; 95%CI -0.92 and -0.46; p=0.0003), while the partial correlation coefficient of systolic blood pressure, computed in models including serum cholesterol, was not statistically significant. This suggests that the inverse relationship between blood pressure and stroke mortality, at population level, is reduced when serum cholesterol is taken into account.

Using univariate and multivariate approaches, several potential confounding variable were tested to explain this paradox. Among them, age at death for stroke (average 68.9 ± 7.1 years) was significantly higher than that at death from myocardial infarction and sudden death (average 65.8 ± 7.8 years), suggesting competition between the two endpoints i.e. CHD and stroke deaths. In general, cohorts with medium to low average levels of serum cholesterol were those with lower CHD death rates, higher stroke mortality rates, but also lower average population blood pressure levels. These cohorts had also higher mean age at death for both stroke and CHD. The reverse was true for cohorts having higher average levels of serum cholesterol that had also higher blood pressure levels, higher CHD death rates and lower stroke death rates. The suggestion that part of this relationship could be due to the Japanese cohorts was dismissed when the analysis was re-run after exclusion of the Japanese cohorts. This fits the concept of competing risk between CHD and stroke as well as a possible (direct or indirect) role of low average population cholesterol levels in areas with higher stroke death rates. The occurrence of high CHD death rates prevails when both serum cholesterol and blood pressure levels are high at population level.

BLOOD PRESSURE AND CARDIOVASCULAR DISEASES WITHIN POPULATIONS

The association of individual blood pressure levels with subsequent coronary incidence or mortality was studied by both univariate and multivariate approaches, although the univariate was preferred for the short-term follow-up (up to 10 years) (10,11). There was a consistently positive and significant association of increasing levels of blood pressure (both systolic and diastolic) with increasing rates of CHD incidence (data for the first 5 and 10 years) and mortality (data up to 25 years). Early follow-up data gave the impression that there was no increased risk up to levels of systolic blood pressure above 140 mmHg, but the hypothesis of a threshold could not be confirmed due to the small number of events. More recently, a special analysis on this issue was stimulated by the suggestion that in the Framingham Study there was such a threshold level. (15,16). However, careful analysis of the 25-year relationship between entry blood pressure and all-causes mortality and cardiovascular death confirmed a conventional linear association (17).

The multivariate approach for data dealing with 5 and 10 years of follow-up compelled pooling cohorts into large, supposedly similar, subgroups. This was again due to the small number of events. However, at 5 and 10 years of follow-up, the multivariate coefficients for systolic blood pressure were remarkably similar in northern European cohorts, in the southern European cohorts and in the U.S. cohort. (11, 18) A recent systematic re-analysis of 10-year incidence and mortality data in northern and southern European areas (19) using the multiple logistic function confirmed this finding. For coronary deaths, hard CHD events and any CHD events there were no statistical differences between coefficients of northern and southern European pools. The relative risks (RR) for 20 mmHg difference were as follows: CHD deaths in northern Europe, RR=1.70 (95%CI 1.44-2.01); in southern Europe, RR=1.51 (95%CI 1.29-1.77). The relative risks decreased when the endpoints were more flexible, but were still statistically significant for the softest endpoint of any CHD.

A systematic analysis of the multivariate coefficients of systolic blood pressure in the prediction of CHD death was made in two different publications using the 25-year follow-up data. In the first analysis (20) multivariate proportional hazards coefficients for systolic blood pressure were computed for eight entities (cohort or pool of cohorts in U.S., Finland, The Netherlands, Italy, Croatia, Serbia, Greece, and Japan). Coefficients varied from 0.0094 in Serbia to 0.0218 in Japan, and all of them, except in Serbia and Greece, were statistically significant. The hazard ratio for a difference of 20 mmHg systolic blood pressure ranged from 1.21 in Greece and 1.55 in Japan. A summary of these data, including 95% confidence limits, is given in Table 5. None of the 28 comparisons, made within each possible pair of coefficients, was statistically significant. In this analysis there was no statistically significant correlation between

Table 5. Multivariate coefficients for systolic blood pressure in the eight entities for the prediction of CHD deaths in 25 years. Derived and modified from reference 20.

Country	Coefficients	t-value	Hazard ratio for 20 mmHg	95% CI
United States	0.0149	6.60	1.35	1.23 – 1.47
Finland	0.0186	7.00	1.45	1.30 – 1.61
Netherlands	0.0168	4.89	1.40	1.02 – 1.60
Italy	0.0188	5.35	1.46	1.22 – 1.67
Croatia	0.0111	2.12	1.25	1.02 – 1.53
Serbia	0.0094	1.94	1.21	0.99 – 1.46
Greece	0.0095	1.19	1.21	0.89 – 1.65
Japan	0.0218	3.27	1.55	1.19 – 2.01

Coefficients from the proportional hazards model, adjusted for age, serum cholesterol, and cigarette consumption. Tests between all pairs of coefficients were not statistically significant.

Table 6. Multivariate-adjusted relative risk and 95%CI of death from CHD in 25 years for defined increments in blood pressure before and after adjustment for subject blood pressure variability. Derived and modified from reference 21.

Population	Increment of 10 mmHg in SBP		Increment of 5 mmHg in DBP	
	Unadjusted for within-subject variability	Adjusted for within-subject variability	Unadjusted for within-subject variability	Adjusted for within-subject variability
United States	1.18	1.29	1.16	1.32
	1.13 – 1.23	1.21 – 1.38	1.11 – 1.21	1.23 – 1.41
Northern Europe	1.18	1.30	1.12	1.25
	1.13 – 1.23	1.23 – 1.38	1.07 – 1.16	1.18 – 1.34
Mediterranean	1.23	1.35	1.19	1.38
Southern Europe	1.13 – 1.35	1.19 – 1.52	1.10 – 1.29	1.22 – 1.57
Inland Southern	1.09	1.17	1.06	1.14
Europe	1.03 – 1.16	1.08 – 1.27	1.01 – 1.12	1.06 – 1.24
Serbia	1.23	1.39	1.16	1.34
	1.10 – 1.38	1.20 – 1.61	1.04 – 1.30	1.15 – 1.56
Japan	1.25	1.36	1.18	1.32
	1.10 – 1.42	1.11 – 1.65	1.03 – 1.35	1.07 – 1.63
Total	1.17	1.28	1.13	1.28
	1.14 – 1.20	1.24 – 1.33	1.10 – 1.15	1.23 – 1.33

CI = Confidence Interval   SBP = Systolic Blood Pressure   DBP = Diastolic Blood Pressure

the magnitude of the multivariate coefficients of systolic or diastolic blood pressure, and CHD death rates in 25 years. This means that differences in the size of coefficients (if any) are not associated with differences in CHD incidence and mortality. The best estimate of relative risk (using the eight entities and adjusting for the inverse of variance) for a difference of 20 mmHg of systolic blood pressure was on average 1.38 (95%CI 1.31-1.45).

In the second analysis (21) the 16 cohorts were pooled in six geographic-cultural groups according to similarities in CHD death rates. They were United States, northern Europe, Mediterranean southern Europe, inland southern Europe, Serbia, and Japan. All coefficients for systolic and diastolic blood pressure predicting CHD death in 25 years were statistically significant. Hazards ratios for increments of 10 mmHg for systolic blood pressure and 5 mmHg for diastolic blood pressure were associated with 95% confidence intervals that did not include 1.0 (Table 6). In the same analysis the relative risk for the presence of hypertension (160 or 95 mmHg or more) provided ratios ranging between 1.33 (95% CI 1.01-1.74) (inland southern Europe) and 2.80 (95% CI 1.28-6.11) (Japan). Similar hazard ratios were found for the association between baseline blood pressure and CHD deaths risk in 25 years, which suggests a similar relationship between individual blood pressure and CHD deaths in the various areas. On the other hand, there were large differences between cohorts or groups of cohorts in terms of absolute risk for similar levels of systolic blood pressure as shown in Fig. 4.

Figure 4. Relationship of usual systolic blood pressure with 25-year CHD mortality in six areas. Data adjusted for age, serum cholesterol, cigarette smoking (21).

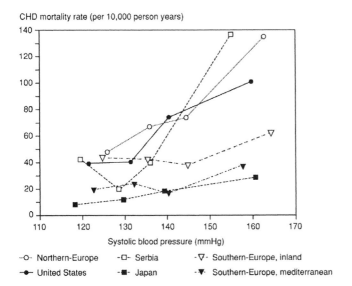

CHD mortality rate (per 10,000 person years)

Systolic blood pressure (mmHg)

··O·· Northern-Europe   -□- Serbia   -∇- Southern-Europe, inland

-●- United States   -■- Japan   -▼- Southern-Europe, mediterranean

The effect of the regression-dilution bias on prediction of events was studied in detail. The specific population adjustment factors for intra-individual variability of blood pressure were estimated, since short-term variation in blood pressure values in individual subjects resulting from measurement bias or random variation may distort the relation between usual blood pressure and mortality. The correction was made through two steps. First, for each subject the usual or average blood pressure during the first 5-year follow-up was estimated from a linear regression model given the values obtained at enrollment and at 5 years of follow-up, taken separately for systolic and diastolic blood pressure. For each subject, the presence or absence of hypertension was also re-assessed according to these estimates. Then the estimates of usual blood pressure and the new hypertension variable were analyzed in Cox models to estimate coefficients for systolic and diastolic blood pressure. To examine the effect of within-person variability in blood pressure on estimated regression coefficients, the adjusted regression coefficients were divided by the unadjusted regression coefficients from the survival analysis to obtain population-specific adjustment factors. The outcome of this process is given by the estimate of the adjustment factor for the coefficients of systolic blood pressure that varied from 1.4 to 1.8 in different areas, and separately for diastolic blood pressure that varied from 1.9 to 2.2. The net effects of using these adjustment factors are given in the right hand column of Table 6, which shows how the multivariate hazard ratios are substantially increased when adjustment is made for within-subject variability, reflecting a greater than expected relationship with the outcome.

Table 7. Proportional hazards model - multivariate coefficients for systolic blood pressure predicting stroke mortality in 25 years for16 cohorts. Derived and modified from reference 22.

Cohort	Coefficient	Hazard ratio per 20 mmHg	95 % CI
U.S. railroad	0.0252	1.66	1.41 – 1.95
East Finland	0.0203	1.50	1.12 – 1.99
West Finland	0.0314	1.87	1.37 – 2.37
Zutphen	0.0113	1.25	0.91 – 1.74
Crevalcore	0.0233	1.60	1.24 – 2.07
Montegiorgio	0.0225	1.58	1.18 – 2.12
Rome Railroad	0.0354	2.03	1.53 – 2.69
Dalmatia	0.0180	1.43	1.04 – 1.96
Slavonia	0.0103	1.23	0.98 – 1.54
Zrenjanin	0.0332	1.94	1.51 – 2.50
Belgrade	0.0118	1.27	0.85 – 1.90
Velika Krsna	0.0255	1.66	1.30 – 2.13
Corfu	0.0356	2.04	1.54 – 2.70
Crete	0.0200	1.49	1.14 – 2.00
Tanushimaru	0.0290	1.79	1.46 – 2.14
Ushibuka	0.0143	1.33	1.10 – 1.61

Coefficients adjusted for age, serum cholesterol, body mass index, cigarette consumption, and physical activity. CI = Confidence Interval

Proportional hazard models were solved, with stroke death in 25 years as endpoint and systolic blood pressure as predictor, where age, physical activity, cigarette smoking, Body Mass Index, and serum cholesterol level were seen as being possible confounding covariates (22). The coefficients for systolic blood pressure were similar among cohorts (Table 7). Out of 120 possible comparisons of these coefficientswithin all pairs of cohorts, only 12 were statistically significant and none of these differences occurred between cohorts of the same country. The magnitude of systolic blood pressure coefficients was unrelated to the stroke death rate of the various cohorts, suggesting that the strength of the association between blood pressure and stroke is independent of the stroke death rate. The pooled estimate of the systolic blood pressure coefficient, weighing for inverse of variance, was 0.0232 with a standard error of 0.0016 and a t-value of 14.60 (relative risk for a difference of 20 mmHg is 1.59; 95%CI 1.49-1.69). The corresponding pooled estimate for diastolic blood pressure was 0.0409, with a standard error of 0.0031 and a t-value of 13.41 (relative risk for a difference of 10 mmHg is 1.50 (95%CI 1.42-1.60).

The overwhelming role of elevated blood pressure in the etiology of cardiovascular diseases was also documented by its predictive value in relation to all-causes mortality according to analyses made in some areas or countries; however, it is not described in this chapter, which deals with cardiovascular diseases (23-25).

BLOOD PRESSURE AND CARDIOVASCULAR DISEASES IN THE ELDERLY

The FINE Study was conducted in five European cohorts, taking as baseline the 25th anniversary follow-up examination, enrolling survivors aged 65 to 84 years. The advantage for obtaining information about anti-hypertensive drugs was counter-balanced by the difficulties in analyzing these data and by the existence of a large proportion of subjects diagnosed with a cardiovascular event. A systematic analysis of the association of blood pressure with 10-year fatal events required that men with a prevalent cardiovascular condition or taking anti-hypertensive drugs be kept separate from those free from both conditions (basically cardiovascular-free and non-hypertensives)(26).

Table 8. Blood pressure, prevalence of cardiovascular diseases, use of anti-hypertensive drugs and 10-year cardiovascular mortality in the three countries of the FINE Study. Derived and modified from reference (26).

Risk factor	Finland		Netherlands		Italy	
Prevalence of CVD or AD	No	Yes	No	Yes	No	Yes
Number	315	350	545	338	292	290
Percentage	47	53	62	38	50	50
	Mean (SD)					
Age (y)	71.5	71.5	71.1	72.1	71.6	72.1
	(5.3)	(5.0)	(5.3)	(5.4)	(4.5)	(4.3)
Systolic BP (mmHg)	152.3	155.5	148.6	155.1	162.8	171.2
	(20.9)	(23.7)	(19.6)	(23.7)	(21.0)	(22.5)
Diastolic BP (mmHg)	86.7	87.2	84.7	86.7	90.4	92.6
	(10.2)	(11.8)	(10.9)	(12.2)	(10.5)	(10.7)
	Percentage					
Hypertension	40.0	47.4	35.0	45.0	61.0	77.6
Anti-hypertensive drugs	-	63.4	-	64.8	-	67.2
Cardiovascular prevalence	-	72.9	-	64.8	-	53.1
	Rate per 1,000 in 10 years					
Cardiovascular mortality	293	674	218	499	222	377

CVD or AD = Cardiovascular diseases or use anti-hypertensive drugs

Table 8 summarizes some of the main findings. The highest elderly population average blood pressure was recorded in Italy, the lowest in the Netherlands. The same applied to the prevalence of hypertensives. On the other hand, the use of anti-hypertensive drugs did not differ between countries (although lower in the Netherlands), while cardiovascular diseases prevalence was much higher in Finland and definitely lower in Italy, with the Netherlands in between. Cardiovascular mortality among cardiovascular- and anti-hypertensive drug- free elderly men was definitely lower than among men with cardiovascular conditions or taking anti-hypertensive drugs, this being true in the three countries.

Multivariate analyses (not reported here in detail) were run to study the associations of systolic, diastolic, and pulse pressure with cardiovascular mortality in the sub-groups of subjects free from cardiovascular disease and not taking anti-hypertensive drugs (26). In none of the three countries or the pooled countries, did blood pressure, either systolic or diastolic, show an association with cardiovascular diseases. However, in the pooled analysis pulse pressure was significantly associated with cardiovascular mortality. These results suggest that in this age range the role of blood pressure in predicting cardiovascular events is a minor one, compared to that in younger people.

CHANGES IN BLOOD PRESSURE AND SUBSEQUENT CHANGES IN CARDIOVASCULAR RISK

The expectation from observational longitudinal studies is that changes in blood pressure over time, whatever the reason, are associated with a different risk for cardiovascular events. The risk could supposedly be reduced or increased depending upon the direction of changes in blood pressure levels. The overall changes recorded during the first 10 years within each country or cohort, already described in Table 2, tend to hide the fact that sub-groups of men had variable amounts of changes in their blood pressure in different directions. Two different methodological types of analysis were run to look at blood pressure changes related to cardiovascular events during 10 years, and dealing with different sets of data and different endpoints.

The first analysis was done on changes of systolic blood pressure recorded during the first 10 years of follow-up in cohorts of six countries (Finland with 2 cohorts, The Netherlands with 1 cohort, Italy with 3 cohorts, Serbia with 2 cohorts, Greece with 2 cohorts, and Japan with 2 cohorts) in relation to all cardiovascular deaths occurring during the subsequent 10 years (27). Initially using a relatively simple procedure, we stratified subjects in four age–specific (quinquennia) quartiles of entry systolic blood pressure (SBP). The changes observed during the first 10 years of follow-up (Delta-SBP, computed through a geometrical procedure) were divided into two classes of relative change defined by levels located above (relative increase) versus below (relative decrease) the median. The relative risk for increasing vs. decreasing Delta-SBP was estimated in each quartile. A summary Mantel-Haenszel relative risk was also calculated (Table 9). In the majority of cells describing the six countries and the four quartiles, the relative risk of increasing versus decreasing systolic blood pressure was greater than 1 with only 3 exceptions in 24 cells. The relative risk in the six cells of the summary Mantel-Haenszel were all greater than 1, and 6 cells in two countries showed statistically significant relative risks.

Table 9. Relative risk of increasing versus decreasing delta-systolic blood pressure in age-specific quartiles of entry systolic blood pressure. Derived and modified from reference (27).

Entry quartile of SBP	Finland	Netherlands	Italy	Serbia	Greece	Japan
1	0.84	2.77	1.49*	1.57	1.20	2.80
2	1.27	1.84	1.28	2.78*	1.58	2.82
3	1.45	1.45	1.78*	1.58	1.79	1.52
4	0.93	1.04	1.30	2.14*	1.74	0.94
MH	1.12	1.67	1.50*	2.15*	1.64	1.47

The risk bound to relative changes of systolic blood pressure in 10 years is related to the cardiovascular deaths occurring during the next 10 years. MH = Mantel-Haenszel summary statistic. * = P < 0.05

A multivariate analysis dealing with the same material, and using the Cox model, produced coefficients for baseline systolic blood pressure alone and then in the presence of Delta-SBP. In both cases, five possible confounding covariates were considered and the endpoint was cardiovascular death in the 10 years following the observed blood pressure changes. In each of the six country groupings, the coefficients of Delta-SBP were statistically significant; this was also true for baseline systolic blood pressure. All models showed a significant improvement in chi-square when the Delta-SBP variable was added. This suggests that changes in systolic blood pressure during the first 10-years of follow-up are directly related to risk for cardiovascular deaths in the following 10 years, while the entry levels of systolic blood pressure retain their strong predictive value.

The second type of analysis was carried out in relation to stroke mortality in all the 16 cohorts (22). Change in blood pressure during the first 10 years of follow-up (five years for the U.S. railroad cohort) was analyzed to predict stroke mortality occurring between years 10 and 25. A general linear model was solved with stroke mortality as endpoint. The average of the available blood pressures at years 0, 5, and 10 was used as baseline, and changes in 10 years (five years for the U.S. railroad cohort) were expressed as differences in blood pressure at year 10 minus pressure at year 0. Further covariates were age at baseline, the interaction term of blood pressure with its changes and the dummy variables for cohorts when data were pooled. Separate analyses were made for continuous systolic and diastolic blood pressure variables. Models were used to compute rates adjusted by age, cohort, average blood pressure, changes in blood pressure, and interaction of average with changes in blood pressure. Similar models were made with baseline blood pressure and changes expressed in 4 and 3 classes, respectively. Categories of 10-year change in systolic blood pressure were 0 or decrease, 1 to 19 mmHg increase and 20 or more mmHg increase. Those for diastolic blood pressure were 0 or decrease, 1 to 9 mmHg increase and 10 or more mmHg increase. Models were run for all populations and for geographic pools of North American and northern European cohorts (low stroke mortality), pools of southern European cohorts (intermediate stroke mortality), and Japan (high stroke mortality).

For all cohorts combined, when continuous blood pressure terms were used, there was a significant interaction between blood pressure levels and blood pressure change (for systolic p=0.017 and for diastolic blood pressure p=0.029). The predominant feature was a clear increase in stroke death rate with greater average systolic and diastolic blood pressure. The effect of change in blood pressure, holding average levels fixed, was smaller and varied depending on average level. Change in systolic blood pressure in the second intermediate class (140 to 159 mmHg) and in the highest class (≥160 mmHg) was accompanied by an increased stroke mortality risk. In the first intermediate systolic class (125 to 139 mmHg), changes in the first 10 years did not relate to stroke mortality in the next 15 years. In contrast, in the lowest class of average systolic blood pressure (< 125 mmHg) an increase in blood pressure levels of the first 10 years was associated with a slight decreased mortality risk. This decreased risk is basically restricted to those whose blood pressure increase is moderate and does not reach hypertensive levels. The regression analysis dealing with categories of blood pressure showed that in those with the highest average blood pressure level (≥160 mmHg), late mortality from stroke was lower among those with the largest declines in blood pressure during the first 10 years. Similar conclusions were obtained when using diastolic instead of systolic blood pressure.

In general, a moderate increase of blood pressure, either systolic or diastolic, was associated with reduced risk when it occurred at low levels of usual blood pressure (< 125 mmHg for systolic and < 80 mmHg for diastolic). That stroke mortality risk was increased when blood pressure increased from a low level into the hypertensive range cannot be excluded, but this phenomenon rarely occurred. In the intermediate levels of usual blood pressure little or no effect could be attributed to blood pressure change. In contrast, changes in blood pressure starting from higher usual levels (≥ 140 mmHg for systolic or ≥ 90 mmHg for diastolic) were associated with an excess risk when blood pressure increased. This was most convincingly shown for systolic blood pressure in southern Europe. This might, however, simply be a reflection of a larger error bound to smaller numbers in Japan. However, for cohorts in North America and northern Europe (in countries where anti-hypertensive treatment started to be common in the late 1960s), it could be supposed that possible protection occurred through anti-hypertensive treatment, which may have started after the higher blood pressure levels were detected in the survey prior to the 10-year follow-up. Unfortunately, detailed information on anti-hypertensive treatment was not available in the early phases of the Seven Countries Study.

COMMENTS

Inter-cohort differences in average blood pressure levels were not large, although higher levels, with some exceptions, were found in northern Europe and North America compared to other locations. Detailed analyses on the relationship of diet with blood pressure were not conducted. However, the results obtained in some specific analyses were in accord with those of the recent DASH trials. These trials showed that using a diet rich in fruit and vegetables, low-fat dairy products and low in salt was able to reduce blood pressure (28,29). In general, the DASH diet is similar to that of the Seven Countries' Mediterranean areas.

The Seven Countries Study was first to show in cross-cultural analyses a relationship between average population blood pressure and CHD mortality rates, although this was true only in the univariate approach. The univariate association of blood pressure with CHD death was somewhat stronger than that found in an early ecological analysis of the WHO-MONICA Project, where the correlation coefficients between the proportion of subjects with high blood pressure and CHD death rates ranged between 0.30 and 0.39, depending upon gender and adjustment for other factors (30). However, these MONICA data refer to entry levels in the population samples and the subsequent 3-year mortality data in the registration area (not in the population samples).

The population inverse relationship between average systolic blood pressure level and stroke mortality rates could partially be explained by the association between average population serum cholesterol and blood pressure levels that created competition between the occurrence of stroke and CHD, the latter occurring more frequently than stroke when both factors were high. On the other hand, the findings of the ecological analysis of the MONICA Project provided correlation coefficients between the proportion of subjects with high blood pressure, and mortality rates from stroke, ranging from 0.35 to 0.49, depending on gender and the adjustment for other factors (30). Reasons for these different relationships are unclear and were not investigated. We can suppose that different combinations of cohorts might have influenced this outcome. Moreover it should be taken into account that the Seven Countries Study used a true longitudinal approach while in the MONICA Project blood pressure levels were derived from sub-samples of the population and stroke mortality rates from data of registrations in the several regions. This may also produce different results.

As for other major risk factors, the multivariate coefficients of blood pressure predicting CHD or stroke events in individuals were substantially similar among cohorts, or entities or groups of cohorts, suggesting a universal law determining the strength of the association between blood pressure levels and cardiovascular events. On the other hand, major differences in incidence and mortality exist (absolute risk) for the same levels of blood pressure due to unmeasured or unknown factors.

The positive and strong relationship between blood pressure levels and subsequent CHD and stroke events at the individual level has been shown in many studies all over the world, at least when middle-aged persons were involved. The MRFIT observational follow-up data (31) of some 300,000 middle-aged men found entry blood pressure related to subsequent CHD mortality; a large meta analysis involving many studies run all over the world found a clear-cut positive and strong relationship between habitual (prolonged) levels of diastolic blood pressure, and subsequent coronary, and stroke deaths (32). Results from the Seven Countries Study were basically confirmatory and some of its data contributed to another meta analysis where among almost 445,000 subjects based on diastolic blood pressure showed a strong positive relationship with the occurrence of stroke deaths (33).

Systolic and diastolic blood pressure measured in advanced ages, as in the FINE Study, were not associated with excess risk of cardiovascular deaths. However, the interference of prevalent cardiovascular conditions, anti-hypertensive treatment, and small numbers prevented us from drawing a firm conclusion. In contrast, pulse pressure was significantly associated with cardiovascular death as shown, more convincingly, in other studies (34-36).

Changes in blood pressure levels over time were associated with a differential risk for stroke and cardiovascular death using different analytical techniques. Unfortunately, the explanation for those different trends can only be hypothesized, since firm documentation on changes in blood pressure due to drug treatment is lacking.

The overwhelming role of high blood pressure as determinant of cardiovascular diseases found in the Seven Countries Study was confirmed not only by the meta analysis dealing with observational data as mentioned above (32) but also by the results of pooled data of intervention trials (37). The latter provided convincing evidence for a causal role of blood pressure in the occurrence of cardiovascular diseases and on the possible benefits from proper intervention.

SUMMARY AND CONCLUSIONS

The distribution of blood pressure levels among the 16 cohorts showed differences of lesser magnitude compared with other risk factors such as serum cholesterol. Higher levels were typical in northern Europe and in northern Italy. The association of average population blood pressure levels with CHD was direct and statistically significant (at least on a univariate basis), while it was inverse with stroke. This paradox could partially be explained by the association between average population serum cholesterol and blood pressure creating competition between the occurrence of stroke and CHD.

In middle-aged men blood pressure at the individual level was a universal predictor of CHD and stroke mortality. Multivariate coefficients and relative risk were similar across cohorts and cultures, although for the same levels of blood pressure, the absolute risks of cardiovascular events were different. The relationship of blood pressure with CHD events became more marked after having taken into account regression-dilution bias.

Increasing levels of average blood pressure due to aging in 10 years were larger in southern Europe (and even more in 35 years in Serbia and Italy) than in northern Europe. Analyses relating changes of blood pressure in 10 years at the individual level with cardiovascular mortality risk during the subsequent years showed reduced risk (at levels of 140 mmHg systolic or 90 mmHg diastolic or higher) for those exhibiting a decline or, little increase, compared to those who had a definite increase in blood pressure.

REFERENCES

1. Pickering G. The nature of essential hypertension. London, J & A Churchill ltd, 1961: 1-149.
2. Rose G, Blackburn H. Cardiovascular Survey Methods. Geneva, World Health Organization . 1968:1-188.
3. Keys A, Blackburn HW, Van Buchem FSP, Buzina R, Djordjevic BS, Dontas AS, Fidanza F, Karvonen MJ, Kimura N, Lekos D, Monti M, Puddu V, Taylor HL. Epidemiological studies related to coronary heart disease: characterstics of men aged 40-59 in seven countries. Acta Med Scand 1967; Suppl 460: 1-392.
4. Rayner M.Petersen S. Compilers European cardiovascular disease statistics. London: British Heart Foundation, 2000:1-132.
5. Kuulasma K, Tunstall-Pedoe H, Dobson A, Fortmann S, Sans S, Tolonen H. Evans A, Ferrario M, Tuomilehto J. Estimation of contribution of changes in classic risk factors to trends in coronary-event rates across the WHO MONICA Project populations. Lancet 2000;355:675-687.

6. Menotti A, Lanti M, Puddu PE. Epidemiologia delle malattie cardiovascolari. Insegnamenti dalle aree Italiane del Seven Countries Study. Roma, Cardioricerca Ed. 1999.
7. Karvonen MJ, Punsar S. Sodium excretion and blood pressure of West and East Finns. Acta Med Scand 1977; 202: 501-507
8. Kromhout D, Bosschieter EB, de Lezenne Coulander C. Potassium, calcium, alcohol intake and blood pressure: the Zutphen Study. Am J Clin Nutr 1985; 41: 1299-1304.
9. Huijbregts PPCW, Feskens EJM, Kromhout D. Dietary patterns and cardivoascuilar risk factors in elderly men. The Zutphen Elderly Study. Int J Epidemiol 1995; 24: 313-320.
10. Keys A (Ed). Coronary heart disease in seven countries. Circulation 1970;41 Suppl 1:1-211.
11. Keys A, Aravanis C, Blackburn H, Buzina R, Djordjevic BS, Dontas AS, Fidanza F, Karvonen MJ, Kimura N, Menotti A, Mohacek I, Nedeljkovic S, Puddu V, Punsar S, Taylor HL, Van Buchem FSP. Seven countries. A multivariate analysis of death and coronary heart disease. Cambridge, MA; Harvard University Press, ISBN: 0-674-80237-3, 1980:1-381.
12. Menotti A, Keys A, Kromhout D, Blackburn H, Aravanis C, Bloemberg B, Buzina R, Dontas A, Fidanza F, Giampaoli S, Karvonen M, Lanti M, Pekkanen J, Punsar S, Seccareccia F, Toshima H. Inter-cohort differences in coronary heart disease mortality in the 25-year follow-up of the Seven Countries Study. Eur J Epidemiol 1993; 9: 527-536
13. Menotti A, Keys A, Blackburn H, Aravanis C, Dontas A, Fidanza F, Giampaoli S, Karvonen M, Kromhout D, Nedeljkovic S, Nissinen A, Pekkanen J, Punsar S, Seccareccia F, Toshima H. Twenty-year mortality and prediction of stroke in twelve cohorts of the Seven Countries Study. Int J Epidemiol 1990; 19: 309-315.
14. Menotti A, Blackburn H, Kromhout D, Nissinen A, Karvonen M, Aravanis C, Dontas A, Fidanza F, Giampaoli S. The inverse relation of average population blood pressure and stroke mortality rates in the Seven Countries Study: a paradox. Eur J Epidemiol 1997; 13: 379-386.
15. Port S, Demer L, Jennerich R, Walter D, Garfinkel A. Systolic blood pressure and mortality. Lancet 2000; 355: 175-180.
16. Port S, Garfinkel A, Boyle N. There is non-linear relationship between mortality and blood pressure. Eur Heart J 2000; 21: 1635-1638.
17. Van den Hoogen P, Seidell J, Nagelkerke N, Menotti A, Kromhout D. Relation between blood pressure and mortality: is there a threshold? Eur Heart J 2001;22:2132-2133
18. Keys A, Aravanis C, Blackburn H, Van Buchem FSP, Buzina R, Djordjevic BS, Fidanza F, Karvonen M, Menotti A, Puddu V, Taylor HL. Probability of middle-aged men developing coronary heart disease in five years. Circulation 1972; 45: 815-828.
19. Menotti A, Lanti M, Puddu PE, Kromhout D. Coronary heart disease incidence in northern and southern European populations: a reanalysis of the Seven Countries Study for a European coronary risk chart. Heart 2000; 84: 238-244.
20. Menotti A, Keys A, Blackburn H, Kromhout D, Karvonen M, Nissinen A, Pekkanen J, Punsar S, Fidanza F, Giampaoli S, Seccareccia F, Buzina R, Mohacek I, Nedeljkovic S, Aravanis C, Dontas A, Toshima H, Lanti M. Comparison of multivariate predictive power of major risk factors for coronary heart disease in different countries: results from eight nations of the Seven Countries Study, 25-year follow-up. J Cardiov Risk 1996; 3: 69-75.
21. Van den Hoogen PCW, Feskens EJM, Nagelkerke NJD, Menotti A, Nissinen A, Kromhout D. The relation between blood pressure and mortality due to coronary heart disease among men in different parts of the world. N Engl J Med 2000: 342: 1-8.
22. Menotti A, Jacobs DR, Blackburn H, Kromhout D, Nissinen A, Nedeljkovic S, Buzina R, Mohacek I, Seccareccia F, Giampaoli S, Dontas S, Aravanis C, Toshima H. Twenty-five-year prediction of stroke deaths in the Seven Countries Study. The role of blood pressure and its changes. Stroke 1996; 27: 381-387.
23. Menotti A, Keys A, Kromhout D, Nissinen A, Blackburn H, Fidanza F, Giampaoli S, Karvonen M, Pekkanen J, Punsar S, Seccareccia F. All cause mortality and its

determinants in middle-aged men in Finland, the Netherlands and Italy in a 25-year follow-up. J Epidemiol Comm Hlth 1991; 45: 125-130.

24. Dontas AS, Menotti A, Aravanis C. Ioannidis P, Seccareccia F. Comparative total mortality in 25 years in Italian and Greek middle aged rural men. J Epidemiol Comm Hlth 1998; 52: 638-644.

25. Menotti A, Blackburn H, Kromhout D, Nissinen A, Adachi H, Lanti M, for the Seven Countries Study Research Group. Cardiovascular risk factors as determinants of 25-year all-cause mortality in the Seven Countries Study . Eur J Epidemiol, 2001 (in press).

26. Van den Hoogen PCW, Seidell JC, Feskens EJM, Nissinen A, Menotti A, Kromhout D. Systolic, diastolic and pulse pressure and 10-year cardiovascular mortality among elderly men in Finland, Italy and the Netherlands. Submitted, 2001.

27. Menotti A, Keys A, Blackburn H, Karvonen M, Punsar S, Nissinen A, Pekkanen J, Kromhout D, Giampaoli S, Seccareccia F, Fidanza F, Nedeljkovic S, Aravanis C, Dontas A, Toshima H. Blood pressure changes as predictors of future mortality in the Seven Countries Study. J Hum Hypertension 1991; 5: 137-144.

28. Appel LJ, Moore TJ, Obarzanek E, Vollmer WM, Svetkey LP, Sacks FM, Bray GA, Vogt TM, Cutler JA, Windhauser MM, Lin PH, Karanja N. A clinical trial of the effect of dietary patterns on blood pressure. DASH Collaborative Research Group. N Engl J Med 1997; 336: 1117-1124.

29. Sacks FM, Svetkey LP, Vollmer WM, Appel LJ, Bray GA, Harsha D, Obarzanek E, Conlin PR, Miller ER 3rd, Simons-Morton DG, Karanja N, Lin PH, DASH-Sodium Collaborative Research Group. Effects on blood pressure of reduced dietary sodium and the Dietary Approaches to Stop Hypertension (DASH) diet. DASH-Sodium Collaborative Research Group. N Engl J Med 2001; 344: 3-10.

30. World Health Organization MONICA Project. Ecological analysis of the association between mortality and major risk factors of cardiovascular disease. Int J Epidemiol 1994; 23: 505-516.

31. Martin MJ, Hulley SB, Browner WS, Kuller LH, Wentworth D. Serum cholesterol, blood pressure and mortality: implications from a cohort of 361,662 men. Lancet 1986;2:933-936.

32. MacMahon S, Peto R, Cutler J, Collins R, Sorlie P, Neaton J, Abbott R, Goodwin J, Dyer A, Stamler J. Blood pressure, stroke and coronary heart disease. Part 1, prolonged differences in blood pressure: prospective observational studies corrected for the regression dilution bias. Lancet 1990; 334: 765-774.

33. Prospective Studies Collaboration. Cholesterol, diastolic blood pressure and stroke: 13,000 strokes in 450,000 people in 45 prospective cohorts. Lancet 1995; 346: 1647-1452.

34. Glynn RJ, Chae CUC, Guralnik JM, Taylor JO, Hennekens CH. Pulse pressure and mortality in older people. Arch Intern Med 2000; 160: 2765-2772.

35. Franklin SS, Khan SA, Wong ND, Larson MD, Levy D. Is pulse pressure useful in predicting risk of coronary heart disease ? Circulation 1999; 100: 354-360.

36. Blacher J, Staessen JA, Girerd X, Gasowski J, Thijs L, Liu L, Wang JG, Tagard RH, Safar ME. Pulse pressure not mean pressure determines cardiovascular risk in older hypertensive patients. Arch Intern Med 2000; 160: 1085-1089.

37. Collins R, Peto R, MacMahon S, Hebert P, Fiebach NH, Eberlein KA, Goodwin J, Qizilbash N, Taylor JO, Hennekens CH. Blood pressure, stroke and coronary heart disease. Part 2, Short-term reductions in blood pressure: overview of randomized drug trials in their epidemiological context. Lancet 1990; 335: 827-838.

CHAPTER 3.3

BODY FATNESS, CORONARY HEART DISEASE AND ALL-CAUSES MORTALITY IN THE SEVEN COUNTRIES STUDY

Daan Kromhout

Body weight can be divided into fat mass and fat-free mass (e.g. muscle and bone). Overweight can therefore be due to either an increase in fat mass, an increase in fat-free mass, or an increase in both. In relation to risk of CHD and chronic diseases, in general, it is necessary to differentiate between overweight due to an increase in fat mass and that due to an increase in fat-free mass. Fat mass and fat-fee mass are, however, difficult to measure. Time-consuming methods (e.g. underwater weighing or dilution techniques such as doubly-labelled water) are needed to measure these compartments of the body. For this reason there was a need to develop a simple, easy-to-measure index of relative weight representing body fatness. As early as the 19th century the Belgian mathematician, Quetelet, proposed body weight/height^2 as an index of body build. Keys and coworkers showed that this index is relatively independent of height, and correlates well with different measures of body fatness (1). Nowadays, the Quetelet Index or Body Mass Index (BMI in the American literature) is the most commonly used indicator of body fatness.

Recent research shows that the BMI is neither completely independent of height nor perfectly correlated to body fatness (2). It is therefore better to find a more direct measure of body fatness. The subscapular skinfold thickness is such a measure. In the Seven Countries Study both the triceps and the subscapular skinfold thickness were measured. The subscapular skinfold thickness is more strongly related to CHD risk than the triceps skinfold thickness (3), and reflects subcutaneous truncal fat. Recent research has shown that truncal subcutaneous and intra-abdominal fat, measured as waist circumference, is not only related to CHD and all-causes mortality, but also to quality of life (4).

In this chapter we describe the trends in body fatness in a 35-year period using the two indicators, BMI and subscapular skinfold thickness. At the population level indicators of body fatness have been studied in relation to both physical activity and dietary determinants and long-term risk of CHD and all-causes mortality. Physical activity and dietary determinants of these indicators of body fatness are also studied at the individual level. In prospective analyses linking indicators of body fatness to mortality risk, the emphasis will be on BMI as an indicator of body fatness, as the subscapular skinfold thickness has not yet been analyzed in relation to long-term mortality risk. Finally, weight changes in relation to subsequent mortality risk will be described.

TRENDS IN INDICATORS OF BODY FATNESS IN THE 35-YEAR PERIOD

In the Seven Countries Study height, weight, and subscapular and triceps skinfold thickness were measured in a standardized way (5). Height and weight are relatively easy to standardize, but triceps and subscapular skinfold thickness are much more difficult to measure. The protocol required skinfold thickness to be measured in duplicate on the right side of the body. Calipers exerting a constant pressure were used. The triceps skinfold thickness was measured on the upper arm, halfway between the tip of the acromial process and the tip of the elbow. The subscapular skinfold thickness was measured just below the tip of the scapula.

In the baseline survey the average BMI of the 16 cohorts varied from 21.8 kg/m^2 in men from Tanushimaru to 26.6 kg/m^2 in men from Rome. Information on long-term trends in BMI is only available for eight European cohorts. Between 1960 and 1985, average BMI increased in six of the European cohorts (Table 1). The largest increase was observed in men from Finland. The average BMI of men from

166

Table 1. Trends in average BMI (kg/m²) in men aged 40-59 at baseline in several European cohorts of the Seven Countries Study in the period 1960-1995.

| Year | 1960 | | 1970 | | 1985 | | 1995 | |
| Age (y) | 40-59 | | 50-69 | | 65-84 | | 75-94 | |
Cohort	N	Mean	N	Mean	N	Mean	N	Mean
East Finland	797	23.3	631	24.4	306	25.3	116	25.5
West Finland	836	24.1	697	25.1	375	26.0	148	26.0
Zutphen	876	24.0	618	25.1	361	25.4	129	25.5
Crevalcore	978	25.7	753	26.6	359	25.8	129	26.3
Montegiorgio	715	24.4	570	25.4	291	26.0	109	26.0
Belgrade	540	26.2	433	26.5	265	26.1	139	25.8
Zrenjanin	517	25.1	433	26.3	159	26.5	49	26.1
Velika Krsna	510	22.1	437	22.3	201	23.3	71	23.7

Table 2. Trends in average BMI (kg/m²) in men aged 50 in the period of 1960-1995 in several European populations (6,7,8).

Cohort	1960	1985	1995
North Karelia (SF)	23.0	26.9	27.5
Turku/Loimaa(SF)	23.7	26.9	27.1
Zutphen (NL)	24.0		
Ghent (B)		26.1	26.4
Zrenjanin (S)	24.7		
Novi Sad (S)		26.7	27.3
Crevacore (I)	25.6		
Friuli (I)		26.6	26.9
Montegiorgio (I)	23.9		
Brianza (I)		25.7	26.4

The 1960 data are the baseline data from the Seven Countries Study.
The 1985 and 1995 data are data from the WHO MONICA Project.

Crevalcore, and Belgrade did not change much during the 25-year follow-up period. Between 1985 and 1995, the average BMI remained stable in the elderly men examined.

The trends described in Table 1 are confounded by aging. A comparison of European men with an average age of 50 years examined in 1960 in the Seven Countries Study, and in 1985 and 1995 in the WHO-MONICA Project, showed a continuous increase in average BMI during this 35-year period (7,8) (Table 2). This average increase varied between 1.3 in Italian men and 4.5 kg/m² in men from East Finland, an average increase in weight from 4 to 13.5 kg. The 10-year average increase in BMI was larger between 1960 and 1985 than that between 1985 and 1995.

Figure 1: Average population subscapular skinfold thickness in 16 cohorts around 1960.

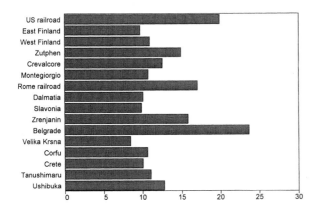

average subscapular skinfold thickness (mm)

Table 3. Trends in average subscapular skinfold thickness (mm) in men aged 40-59 at baseline in several European cohorts of the Seven Countries Study in the period of 1960-1985.

Year	1960		1970		1985	
Age (y)	40-59		50-69		65-84	
Cohort	N	Mean	N	Mean	N	Mean
East Finland	813	9.7	643	11.1		
West Finland	859	10.9	709	13.0		
Zutphen	876	14.9	618	14.3	361	18.7
Crevalcore	989	12.5	741	16.5	356	19.4
Montegiorgio	715	10.7	563	14.7	292	19.0
Belgrade	540	23.7	430	23.2	264	17.8
Zrenjanin	517	15.9	427	15.1	150	15.2
Velika Krsna	510	8.4	431	13.0	197	8.1

This increase in average body weight is accompanied by a substantial increase in the prevalence of obesity in middle-aged European men.

Large differences were observed for the average subscapular skinfold thickness in the baseline survey (Fig.1). The lowest quantity of average subcutaneous fat was found in men from Velika Krsna (8.4 mm) and the highest in Belgrade professors (23.7 mm). Information on long-term trends in subscapular skinfold thickness is only available for eight European cohorts.

The average subscapular skinfold thickness increased between 1960 and 1970 in 5 of the 8 European cohorts (Table 3). The exceptions were the men from Zutphen and the Serbian cohorts in Belgrade and Zrenjanin. Between 1970 and 1985 the average subscapular skinfold thickness increased in the Zutphen, and Italian cohorts in

Crevalcore and Montegiorgio, remained stable in Zrenjanin, and decreased in the Serbian cohorts, Belgrade and Velika Krsna.

We conclude that the average BMI increased continuously in middle-aged men between 1960 and 1995. In aging cohorts of originally middle-aged men, the average BMI generally increased between 1960 and 1985, but remained stable in elderly men between 1985 and 1995. The trends were less consistent in average subscapular skinfold thickness. In most cohorts an increase in average subscapular skinfold thickness was observed between 1960 and 1970, and different trends were found in the following 15 years.

PHYSICAL ACTIVITY AND DIETARY DETERMINANTS OF BODY FATNESS IN POPULATIONS

The development of obesity is the consequence of a chronic and sustained energy imbalance when energy intake exceeds energy expenditure. Therefore it is necessary to take both sides of the energy equation simultaneously into account. Both energy imbalance and maintenance of obesity are thought to be facilitated by energy-dense diets and sedentary lifestyles (9).

When there is an energy balance, the average provision of energy from the diet is a good index of the total energy expenditure of the groups under study. Of total energy intake, about 10% is used for diet-induced energy expenditure. The remaining 90% is used for basal metabolism and physical activity. Both basal metabolism and the energy costs of body movements are related to body mass. Therefore when groups of men were compared, total energy intake, expressed as energy per unit body weight, was used as an indicator of physical activity (10).

Using baseline data from 14 of the 16 cohorts, Keys showed that the average sum of two skinfold thicknesses at the population level is strongly inversely associated ($r =$ -0.75) with total energy intake per kg body weight (10). A similar association was obtained for the relationship between average energy from physical activity per kg body weight and average sum of two skinfold thicknesses (10). These results suggest that at the population level energy intake per kg body weight may be used as an indicator of physical activity.

Energy intake per kg body weight is however not a perfect indicator of physcial activity. Energy intake may be underestimated especially in populations with a high prevalence of obesity. Obese people tend to underreport their energy intake. It is therefore better to have an indenpendent indicator of physical activity. Besides physical activity energy-density is an other determinant of body fatness. We re-analyzed the relationships between physical activity , energy-density and body fatness at the population level using the baseline data of the Seven Countries Study cohorts.

At the beginning of the Seven Countries Study in the period of 1958-1964, differences in energy expenditure in middle-aged men were largely due to differences in job-related physical activity. The men were therefore classified according to their job-related habitual physical activity pattern (5). Class 1 men were 13 of the 12,763 men who were bedridden and did not have job-related physical activity. Class 2 men were sedentary and engaged in little physical activity. Class 3 men were moderately active during a substantial part of the day, and Class 4 men performed hard physical labor. For each cohort the percentage of men in each class was determined and multiplied by either 1, 2, 3, or 4 for each activity class, added up for the four classes and divided by 100. This average population physical activity index was multiplied by

1000 to get values on the order of magnitude comparable to energy expenditure expressed in kcal. The average energy, fat, and fiber intake of the cohorts was determined chemically in food composites representing the average food intake of each cohort (11).

The physical activity index for the average population varied from 2,006 in Belgrade professors to 3,982 in farmers in Velika Krsna. Average-population energy intake varied from 2,251 kcal per day in American railroad employees to 3,609 kcal per day in farmers in Slavonia. The correlation between the average-population physical activity index and energy intake was 0.45 (p< 0.10). This low correlation coefficient indicates substantial measurement error in both physical activity and energy intake. Dietary fat intake varied from 33 g per day in farmers from Tanushimaru to 179 g per day in farmers from Slavonia. Fishermen in Ushibuka consumed 21 g of fiber per day compared with 57 g/day in farmers from Corfu .

Figure 2. Relationship between average population Physical Activity Index and subscapular skinfold thickness in men aged 40-59 around 1960 (11).

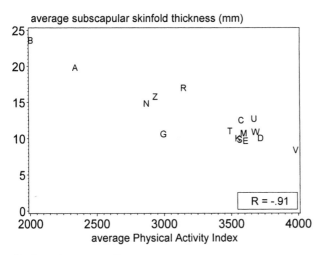

For legend see appendix

The average-population physical activity index was significantly inversely related to average-population BMI. This association remained after multivariate analyses. However, average-population fat and dietary fiber intake were not related to average-population BMI. Average population physical activity index was inversely related to average population subscapular skinfold thickness (Fig. 2). Population dietary fiber was inversely related to average population subscapular skinfold thickness (Fig. 3), but dietary fat was not related. Multivariate analyses showed that average-population physical activity index, and dietary fiber intake, collectively explained 90% of the variance in average-population subscapular skinfold thickness.

The results of these analyses show that average population physical activity index was strongly inversely related with average-population subscapular skinfold thickness. Besides physical activity, dietary fiber intake was also inversely related to average population subscapular skinfold thickness. The associations of physical activity and

Figure 3. Relationship between average population dietary fiber intake and subscapular skinfold thickness in men aged 40-59 around 1960 (11).

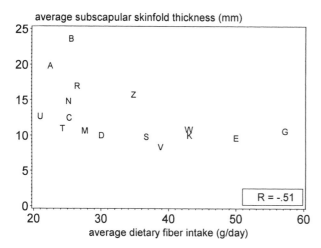

For legend see appendix

dietary fiber with BMI were weaker and in case of dietary fiber even non-existent. This suggests that physical activity and dietary fiber are stronger determinants of body fatness than of overweight. The results also imply that in these populations physical activity is the strongest determinant of body fatness.

PHYSICAL ACTIVITY AND DIETARY DETERMINANTS OF BODY FATNESS IN INDIVIDUALS

In the 1980s the determinants of BMI and skinfold thickness were studied at the individual level in the Zutphen Study (12,13). Data used for these analyses were collected in 1960 and 1965. In 1960 information was collected on height, weight, triceps, and subscapular skinfold thickness and diet. In 1965 the same information was collected but also information on energy expenditure and smoking. Dietary data were collected by the cross-check dietary history method that provides information on the *usual* food intake of the participant. Energy expenditure was measured by the questionnaire developed for studies in occupational medicine. Information was collected on the usual energy expenditure for five working days and two weekend days. Both the time spent on the activity and its intensity were estimated.

The 1960 data of the Zutphen Study showed that overweight and obese men consumed on average 300 to 400 kcal per day less than lean men (12). This was due to a lower intake of all macro nutrients except alcohol. Energy intake per kg body weight was strongly inversely related to BMI and skinfold ticknesses. The 1965 data of the Zutphen Study confirmed the inverse relation between energy intake per kg body weight, and the different indicators of body fatness (13). These results suggest that physical activity may be a determinant of body fatness in individuals.

171

In 1965 physical activity was not only indirectly measured by dividing energy intake by body weight but also directly from total energy expenditure (13). Basic

Table 4. Standardized regression coefficients for energy expenditure on working- and weekend days, and other determinants of body fatness for 525 men aged 45-64 from Zutphen (13).

Determinants	Subscapular skinfold		Body Mass Index	
	UV	MV	UV	MV
Energy intake – expenditure	-0.38	-0.40	-0.47	-0.49
Energy expenditure on working days	-0.23	-0.24	-0.15	-0.15
Energy expenditure on weekend days	-0.17	-0.12[**]	-0.20	-0.20
Smoking	-0.20	-0.14	-0.19	-0.12[**]
R^2		0.26		0.31

UV = Univariate analysis   MV = Multivariate analysis
Multivariate model: indicator of body fatness = energy expenditure on working days + expenditure on weekend days + (energy intake - expenditure) + smoking
[**] $p \leq 0.01$. All other standardized regression coefficients $p < 0.001$

metabolic rate was subtracted from total energy expenditure in order to obtain physical activity and divided by body weight. This was done because the energy costs of different types of activities are directly related to body weight. Physical activity per kg body weight was inversely associated with indicators of body fatness in both uni- and multivariate analyses (Table 4) Energy expenditure on working days and weekend days, and smoking were independently inversely associated with BMI and subscapular skinfold thickness (Table 4).

The effect of other thermogenic stimuli on indicators of body fatness was also studied (13). Coffee and tea contain caffeine that increases thermogenesis. Coffee but not tea was consistently inversely related to indicators of body fatness. After multivariate analyses, only the effect of smoking on body fatness remained, probably due to the strong correlations between smoking and coffee. These results support a thermogenic effect of smoking on different indicators of body fatness but not of coffee and tea.

We conclude physical activity to be an important determinant of body fatness. The difference between energy intake and energy expenditure was, in contrast to expectation, inversely related to different indicators of body fatness. This was probably due to under-reporting of food consumption in obese men and a thermogenic effect of smoking in lean men. Smoking was consistently inversely related with indicators of body fatness.

BODY FATNESS, CORONARY HEART DISEASE, AND ALL-CAUSES MORTALITY FROM A CROSS-CULTURAL PERSPECTIVE

The ecological relationships between population levels of indicators of body fatness and population rates of CHD and all-causes mortality rates were studied for the 16 cohorts. Population average BMI at baseline tended to be inversely associated with

10-year mortality rates from CHD (r = -0.37) (6). This non-significant inverse correlation was due to the cohort of East Finland. This cohort consisted of men characterized by a high level of job-related physical activity. Most of the men in this cohort were lumberjacks and farmers. Excluding this cohort would suggest a positive association between the average BMI at baseline and 10-year population CHD mortality rates.

Figure 4. Relationship between entry average population Body Mass Index and 25-year-adjusted mortality rates from coronary heart disease.

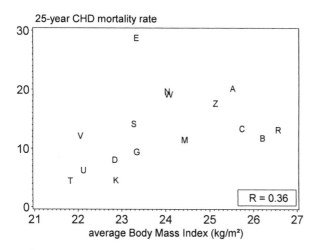

For legend see appendix

This association could be studied in more detail using 25-year mortality data. A non-significant positive association (r = 0.36) was observed between average baseline BMI and 25-year CHD mortality rates (Fig.4). This association became statistically significant (r = 0.56, p <0.05) after exclusion of the cohort from East Finland. These results are suggestive for a positive association between BMI and CHD mortality at the population level. Average-population subscapular skinfold thickness was not related to either 25-year population mortality rates from CHD (r = -0.37) or all-causes (r = 0.16). Neither was average population BMI related to 25-year population mortality rates from all-causes.

We conclude that at the population level consistent relationships between different indicators of body fatness and long-term mortality from CHD and all-causes were not observed.

BODY FATNESS, CORONARY HEART DISEASE, AND ALL-CAUSES MORTALITY IN INDIVIDUALS

For the first 10 years of follow-up associations between skinfold thickness, CHD incidence, and all-causes mortality were investigated (6,16). Using 5- and 10-year follow-up data, the sum of two skinfold thicknesses, triceps and subscapular, was, with the exception of the Zutphen cohort, not related to CHD incidence and mortality. The 5-year follow-up data indicated a relationship between the sum of skinfold thicknesses and the "soft" diagnosis of CHD in the U.S. and southern Europe (16), but this was not found using 10-year follow-up data (6). Neither were clear associations observed for the relation between the sum of skinfold thicknesses, and 10-year all-causes mortality (6). There was even a tendency to an inverse relation in the cohorts from Finland, Croatia, Serbia, Italy, Greece, and Japan. Similar relationships were observed between BMI, and the 5- and 10-year morbidity and mortality data (6,14).

Keys found no consistent associations between BMI at entry and 25-year mortality from all-causes in the 16 cohorts (15). We analyzed the relationships between BMI and 25-year all-causes mortality in the 13 European cohorts stratified by smoking status. These results showed that in both non-smokers and smokers a U-shaped relationship is seen between BMI and all-causes mortality (Fig. 5). The lowest mortality rates were observed in non-smokers with a BMI of 22.5-25 kg/m^2, and in smokers with a BMI of 20-30 kg/m^2. In all BMI classes the mortality rate from all-causes was higher in smokers compared with non-smokers. This difference was larger at low BMI levels (< 20 kg/m^2) compared with high BMI levels (>27.5 kg/m^2).

Figure 5. 25-year all-causes mortality by level of Body Mass Index at baseline in European cohorts.

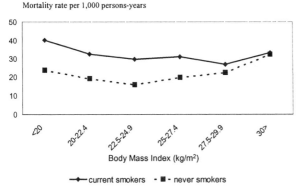

Mortality during the first 5 years of follow-up was excluded. Adjustments were made for age and cohort.

In the European cohorts also the relationship between underweight and overweight was studied in relation to 15-year all-causes mortality in men aged 40-59, and 50-69 years (16). BMI was defined according to the guidelines of WHO (17). Underweight was defined as a BMI of less than 18.5 kg/m^2, the reference category as 18.5-25.0 kg/m^2, grade I overweight as 25.1-30.0 and Grade II overweight (also called severe overweight or obesity) as more than 30. The data were stratified by smoking status (Table 5). The hazard ratio for underweight was 2.1 (95%CI: 1.5-2.8) for men aged 40-59, and 1.7 (95%CI: 1.3-2.2) for men aged 50-69. Grade I overweight was not related to increased mortality. Among never-smokers the hazard ratio for grade II overweight was 1.8 (95%CI:1.2-2.8) for men aged 40-59, and 1.4 (95%CI: 1.0-1.9) for men aged 50-69. Grade II overweight was not related to increased mortality among current smokers.

Table 5. Hazard ratios (95% Confidence Intervals) of 15-year all-causes mortality[a] among European men by category of Body Mass Index[b] (16).

Follow-up period	Body Mass Index (kg/m^2)			
Smoking category	<18.5	18.5-24.9	25.0-29.9	≥30.0
1960-1975				
Never smokers	2.1 (0.8-5.7)	1.0	1.3 (0.9-1.7)	1.8 (1.2-2.8)
Ex-smokers	2.0 (0.5-8.2)	1.0	1.0 (0.7-1.3)	1.3 (0.8-2.1)
Current smokers	2.1 (1.5-2.8)	1.0	0.9 (0.8-1.1)	1.0 (0.7-1.4)
1970-1985				
Never smokers	2.3 (1.0-5.3)	1.0	1.0 (0.8-1.2)	1.4 (1.0-1.9)
Ex-smokers	2.5 (1.3-4.8)	1.0	1.1 (0.9-1.4)	1.4 (1.0-1.8)
Current smokers	1.5 (1.1-2.1)	1.0	1.0 (0.9-1.1)	1.0 (0.8-1.3)

a = Mortality during the first five years of follow-up was excluded.

b = Adjustments were made for age and cohort

These results show that a BMI at the tails of the distribution either underweight or severely overweight is associated with excess mortality (16). For underweight this association was present in never- and ex-smokers, and current smokers. The association between underweight and all-causes mortality declined when the follow-up period was extended from 15 to 25 years. This may be due to confounding by subclinical disease in the early years of follow-up, although the first five years of follow-up were excluded. There was no information available about whether weight loss was intentional or unintentional. The increased mortality among the men with a low BMI is therefore difficult to interpret.

Never-smokers with severe overweight had an increased risk of all-causes mortality (16). This association was not influenced by the length of the follow-up period. Severely overweight ex-smokers also had an increased mortality risk, which tended to increase with extension of the follow-up period. After 25 years they approached the relative risk of never-smokers. Severe overweight was not related to increased mortality in current smokers. This is probably due to the high absolute risk of smokers compared with never-smokers. Smoking is such a dominant risk factor for increased mortality that overweight adds no detectable additional risk to the already increased absolute risk of mortality among smokers.

Data on BMI collected in men aged 65-84 years around 1985 have been analyzed in relation to 5- and 10-year all-causes mortality data (18,19). The 5-year mortality data showed a parabolic relation with BMI (18). In the 10-year data an inverse relationship was noted (19). However, when mortality during the first five years of follow-up was excluded, BMI was not related to all-causes mortality. This was done to exclude deaths that could be associated with weight loss. These results suggest that in healthy elderly men, BMI is not related to 10-year all-causes mortality.

In summary, the results of the Seven Countries Study show that in middle-aged men different indicators of body fatness are not consistently associated with 10-year mortality from CHD, and all-causes. However, detailed analyses using longer follow-up periods showed that the tails of the BMI distribution were associated with increased mortality. Underweight (BMI < 18.5 kg/m^2) was associated with an increased relative risk for all-causes mortality. Obesity (BMI > 30 kg/m^2) was related to increased mortality in never-and ex-smokers, but not in current smokers. In men aged 65-84, BMI was not related to all-causes mortality.

WEIGHT CHANGES AND MORTALITY

Changes in body weight were analyzed in relation to CHD and all-causes mortality in the European cohorts (20). This could be done because information on body weight was collected at baseline and after 5 and 10 years of follow-up. Changes in body weight were related to 15-year mortality data. To minimize the effect of confounding by weight loss due to subclinical disease, deaths in the first five years were excluded in the main analyses.

Four categories of weight patterns were defined as follows:
- Men with a change in body weight between +2 or –2 kg during the first and third examination were called "constant".
- Men who gained more than 2 kg fell into the category "increasing",
- Men who lost more than 2 kg were categorized as "decreasing ".
- Men were defined as "fluctuating" when their weight at the second examination differed more than 2 kg with their weight at examination 1 or 3.

The average weight of men with constant weight was 66.4 kg; their BMI was 23.4 kg/m^2 at examination 3. Men with increasing weight put on an average of 7 kg, and their weight and BMI were 76.3 kg and 26.6 kg/m^2, respectively. Men with decreasing weight lost on average 5.1 kg, and their weight and BMI were 64.4 kg and 22.5 kg/m^2, respectively. Men with fluctuating weight lost on average 0.7 kg, and their average weight and BMI were 73.4 kg and 25.5 kg/m^2, respectively.

For comparing men with decreasing weight to those with constant weight, the hazard ratio for 15-year CHD mortality was 1.19 (95%CI:0.91-1.56) and 1.33 (95%CI:1.15-1.54) for all-causes mortality. For fluctuating weight these hazard ratios were 1.47 (95%CI:1.13-1.91) for CHD mortality, and 1.21 (95%CI:1.03-1.41) for all-causes mortality. The least increased risks relative to constant weight were observed for increasing weight: 1.18 (95%CI:0.94-1.48) for CHD mortality and 1.05 (95%CI:0.92-1.20) for all-causes mortality.

These analyses showed that middle-aged men who kept a constant weight had the lowest CHD and all-causes mortality risk. An average gain of 7 kg was associated with a non-significant 18% increase in coronary, and a 5% increase in all-causes mortality. The highest relative risks were observed for middle-aged men with decreasing and fluctuating body weight. Especially striking was the 47% higher relative risk for CHD mortality among men with fluctuating weight.

COMMENTS

In the Seven Countries Study body fatness was quantified by measuring BMI and the thickness of triceps and subscapular skinfolds. In most of the analyses BMI was used as indicator of body fatness. The long-term trends in average BMI in eight European cohorts were more consistent than those in subscapular skinfold thickness. This may be due to measurement error. Measurement of skinfold thicknesses is much more difficult than that of height and weight. In spite of all efforts to standardize the measurement of skinfold thicknesses, errors occurred because during the course of the long follow-up period change in staff took place.

Interesting changes in average BMI were seen in eight European cohorts during the 35 year follow-up period. Between 1960 and 1985 average BMI increased in six of the eight cohorts. The two cohorts with stable average BMI were Crevalcore and Belgrade. These cohorts had in 1960 the highest average BMI of about 26 kg/m². The average BMI in the other cohorts were 1-4 units lower. These cohorts, with the exception of Velika Krsna, increased their average BMI till about 26 kg/m² between 1960 and 1985. In Velika Krsna the average BMI increased from 22 to 24 kg/m².

These results suggest that the average BMI remained stable in cohorts with a high average BMI at baseline. The average BMI in the other cohorts increased. The largest increase was observed in the cohorts of East and West Finland in which the average BMI increased by 2 units. Also a comparison of middle-aged men examined in 1960 and 1985, showed that the largest increase in average BMI took place in men from Finland (Table 2). This was probably due to a large decrease in physical activity.

Between 1969 and 1989 the average energy intake decreased in Finnish cohorts by about 5 MJ (Chapter 2.1, Table 8). This was much larger than the average decreases of 1.8-3.5 MJ observed in the Dutch and rural Italian cohorts during the same period (Chapter 2.1, Tables 10 and 12). Similar results were found in comparing the average energy intake of middle-aged men examined about 25 years apart (see chapter 2.1, Table 6). The Finnish men had a very high average energy intake in 1960 of about 16 MJ because of their energy-demanding jobs as lumberjacks and farmers. Because of increasing mechanization they decreased their physical activity very much as indicated by energy intake during the course of the follow-up.

Around 1985 the age of the cohorts varied between 65 and 84 years. During the next 10 years of follow-up the average BMI of the survivors remained stable. Comparison of cross-sectional samples of men aged 35-64 in the WHO-MONICA Project showed an increase in average BMI in most centers between 1979-1989 and 1989-1996 (21). A comparison of the results for middle-aged men examined in the Seven Countries Study around 1960 and in the MONICA Project around 1985 and 1995 (Table 2) showed that the 10-year increase in average BMI was larger in the period 1960-1985 than in the period 1985-1995. These results suggest that in middle-aged men the largest increase in the prevalence of obesity in European countries occurred between 1960 and 1985, but this increase continued at a slower rate thereafter.

Because of the increasing epidemic of obesity it is of great importance to identify the determinants of body fatness. The results of the Seven Countries Study showed that physical activity was the strongest determinant of BMI and skinfold thickness both at the population and at the individual level. These associations were found for proxy variables such as energy intake divided by body weight as for direct measures of physical activity (quantifying job-related physical activity during the baseline survey and later on by estimating both job- and leisure time related physical activity).

The difference between energy intake and energy expenditure is hypothesized to be positively associated with different indicators of body fatness. Contrary to expectation, this difference was strongly inversely related to these indicators (13).

This relationship was found in both obese and lean men. In obese men this association may be due to under-reporting of food consumption. This hypothesis was supported by an analysis in non-smoking men that showed a difference in average energy intake and total energy expenditure of + 60 kcal per day in lean men (BMI < 25 kg/m^2), and –252 kcal per day in overweight men (BMI > 27 kg/m^2) (13). An overview of studies comparing self-reported energy intake with simultaneously objectively measured energy expenditure by doubly labeled water showed an underestimation of reported energy intake (22). The under-reporting was related to body fatness and was much higher in obese persons. These results show that a valid estimate of energy intake cannot be obtained in overweight and obese men.

The inverse relation between the difference in energy intake and energy expenditure and indicators of body fatness in lean men may be due to the influence of smoking. This hypothesis is supported by the positive relationship between smoking and the difference between energy intake and energy expenditure observed in lean men. The energy intake of lean men who smoked was 322 kcal per day higher than their energy expenditure (13). This difference amounted to only 60 kcal per day for lean non-smokers. These results suggest that a thermogenic effect of 262 kcal per day can be ascribed to smoking. A study in a metabolic chamber showed that in lean men smoking 24 cigarettes for a period of 24 hours, energy expenditure was increased 215 kcal compared with not smoking (23). This difference was independent of energy intake and physical activity.

Besides physical activity and smoking, diet is also a determinant of body fatness. Energy-dense diets that are high in fat and low in carbohydrate, promote obesity. Therefore dietary fat and the dietary fat-carbohydrate ratio have been suggested as determinants of body fatness (24,25). We explored this concept by studying dietary fat and dietary fiber in relation to body fatness. We chose dietary fiber instead of carbohydrate because a high fiber intake leads to "bulky" diets which limit spontaneous intake of energy (26).

We found that at the population level dietary fat was not associated with BMI and subscapular skinfold thickness (11). Average dietary fiber intake was however inversely related with average population subscapular skinfold thickness. This association was independent of physical activity. A similar association was also observed in individuals (26). These results suggest that besides physical activity and smoking, dietary fiber also could play a role in the etiology of obesity.

We observed differences in average BMI between cohorts but these differences were even larger when subscapular skinfold thickness values were compared. However, these differences in indicators of body fatness were not consistently correlated with differences in population rates of CHD and all-causes mortality. These results suggest that average population levels of BMI and subscapular skinfold thickness do not contribute to population differences in CHD and all-causes mortality.

During the first 10-years of follow-up of the Seven Countries Study consistent relationships between BMI and the sum of triceps and subscapular skinfold thickness and different CHD endpoints were not observed. After 10-years of follow-up the emphasis in studying associations between indicators of body fatness and endpoints was on all-causes mortality.

We found a U-shaped relationship between BMI and 25-year mortality from all-causes in both smokers and non-smokers. As expected the absolute mortality risk was higher in smokers than in non-smokers. Underweight (BMI <18.5 kg/m^2) was associated with excess mortality in never-, ex- and current smokers. Severe overweight (BMI >30 kg/m^2) was associated with an increased risk of all-causes mortality in non-smokers and ex-smokers but not in current smokers.

Besides body weight, weight changes may also influence mortality risk. Changes in weight during 10 years of follow-up were related to 15-year mortality from CHD and all-causes. Men with constant weight had the lowest risk. A non-significant increase in mortality was observed for men with increasing weight. Men with decreasing weight had the highest mortality from all-causes. The highest relative risk for CHD mortality was observed for men with fluctuating weight. Similar results were observed in several other cohort studies (27).

We conclude that in middle-aged men the lowest risk for all-causes mortality is observed in never-smokers with a BMI of 22.5-24.9 kg/m^2. If these men keep their weight constant they have the lowest risk. An increase in body weight is associated with a non-significant increase in CHD and all-causes mortality. The largest increase in risk is found for men with decreasing and fluctuating weight.

In the FINE Study of men aged 65-84 BMI was not related to 10-year all-causes mortality (19). In the Rotterdam Study among never smokers only the highest category of BMI (BMI > 30 kg/m^2) was related to increased mortality (28). The proportion of mortality attributable to a large waist circumference (an indicator of abdominal fatness) among never smokers was three- fold the proportion attributable to a high BMI. Such associations were not seen in ex- and current smokers. These results suggest that among never smoking elderly men, waist circumference may be more important than BMI.

SUMMARY AND CONCLUSIONS

In the Seven Countries Study BMI and skinfold thickness were used as indicators of body fatness. In middle-aged men at baseline differences in average BMI between cohorts were relatively small. In six of the eight European cohorts, a strong increase in average BMI was observed between 1960 and 1985, but BMI remained stable in elderly men between 1985 and 1995. At baseline, a threefold difference in average subscapular skinfold thickness was found among the 16 cohorts. Between 1960 and 1985 inconsistent trends were observed in average subscapular skinfold thickness in different European countries. At the population level, physical activity was the most important determinant of subscapular skinfold thickness. Population average dietary fiber intake was also inversely associated with average subscapular skinfold thickness. Population average body fatness indicators were not related to long-term risk of mortality from CHD and all-causes. At the individual level, physical activity and smoking were consistently inversely associated with indicators of body fatness. Indicators of body fatness were not consistently related to 10-year incidence of and mortality from CHD, and all-causes. However, underweight (BMI < 18.5 kg/m^2), and obesity (BMI > 30 kg/m^2), among never- and ex-smokers were compared to the reference BMI of 18.5-25 kg/m^2 and were associated with an increased all-causes mortality. Weight change was related to CHD and all-causes mortality. Men with constant weight had the lowest risk. The highest relative risk for CHD mortality was observed for men with fluctuating weight, and for all-causes for men who lost weight.

REFERENCES

1. Keys A, Fidanza F, Karvonen MJ, Kimura N, Taylor HL. Indices of relative weight and obesity. J Chron Dis 1972;25:329-343.
2. Han TS, Seidell JC, Curral JEP, Morrison CE, Deurenberg P, Lean MEJ. The influence of height on waist circumference as an index of adiposity in adults. Int J Obesity 1997;21:83-89.
3. Donahue RP, Abbott RD, Bloom E, Reed DM, Yano K. Central obesity and coronary heart disease in men. Lancet 1987;1:821-824.
4. Lean ME, Han TS, Seidell JC. Impairment of health and quality of life in people with large waist circumference. Lancet. 1998;351:853-856.
5. Keys A, Aravanis C, Blackburn HW, Van Buchem FSP, Buzina R, Djordjevic BS. Dontas AS, Fidanza F, Karvonen MJ, Kimura N, Lekos D, Monti M, Puddu V, Taylor HL. Epidemiological studies related to coronary heart disease: characteristics of men aged 40-59 in seven countries. Acta Med Scand 1967;460 Suppl:24-27.
6. Keys A. Seven Countries: a multivariate analysis of death and coronary heart disease. Cambridge, MA: Harvard University Press, 1980:161-195.
7. Rayner M, Petersen S. Compilers European cardiovascular disease statistics. London: British Heart Foundation, 2000:1-132.
8. Kuulasmaa K, Tunstall-Pedoe H, Dobson A, Fortmann S, Sans S, Tolonen H, Evans A, Ferrario M, Tuomilehto JL. Estimation of contribution of changes in classic risk factors to trends in coronary-event rates across the WHO MONICA Project populations. Lancet 2000;355:675-687.
9. World Health Organization. Obesity: preventing and managing the global epidemic. Geneva: World Health Organization, 1998.
10. Keys A (Ed). Coronary heart disease in seven countries. Circulation 1970;41 Suppl I:175-183.
11. Kromhout D, Bloemberg B, Seidell JC, Nissinen A, Menotti A, for the Seven Countries Study Group. Physical activity and dietary fiber determine population body fat levels. The Seven Countries Study. Int J Obesity 2001;25:301-306.
12. Kromhout D. Energy and macronutrient intake in lean and obese middle-aged men (The Zutphen Study). Am J Clin Nutr 1983;37:295-299.
13. Kromhout D, Saris WHM, Horst CH. Energy intake, energy expenditure, and smoking in relation to body fatness: the Zutphen Study. Am J Clin Nutr 1988;47:668-674.
14. Keys A, Aravanis C, Blackburn H, Van Buchem FSP, Buzina R, Djordjevic BS, Fidanza F, Karvonen MJ, Menotti A, Puddu V, Taylor HL. Coronary heart disease: Overweight and obesity as risk factors. Ann Intern Med 1972;77:15-27.
15. Keys A. Longevity and body size of men in middle age: Twenty-five-year survival in the Seven Countries Study. CVD Prevention 2000;3:4-10.
16. Visscher TLS, Seidell JC, Menotti A, Blackburn H, Nissinen A, Feskens EJM, Kromhout D. Underweight and overweight in relation to mortality among men aged 40-59 and 50-69 years. Am J Epidemiol 2000;151:660-666.
17. World Health Organisation Expert Committee. Physical status: The use and interpretation of anthropometry. WHO technical report series 854. Geneva, Switzerland. World Health Organisation, 1995.
18. Menotti A, Kromhout D, Nissinen A, Giampaoli S, Seccareccia F, Feskens E, Pekkanen J, Tervahanta M. Short term all-cause mortality and its determinants in elderly populations in Finland, The Netherlands and Italy. The FINE-study. Prev Med 1996;25(3):319-327.
19. Menotti A, Mulder I, Nissinen A, Feskens E, Giampaoli S, Kromhout D. Cardiovascular risk factors and 10-year all-cause mortality in elderly European male populations. (the FINE study). Eur Heart J 2001;22:573-579.
20. Peters EThJ, Seidell JC, Menotti A, Aravanis C, Dontas A, Fidanza F, Karvonen M, Nedeljkovic S, Nissinen A, Buzina R, Bloemberg B, Kromhout D. Changes in body weight

in relation to mortality in 6,441 European middle-aged men: the Seven Countries Study. Int J Obesity 1995;19:862-868.

21. Molarius A, Seidell JC, Sans S, Tuomilehto J, Kuulasmaa K. Educational level, relative body weight, and changes in their association over 10 years: an international perspective from the WHO-MONICA Project. Am J Publ Health 2000;90:1260-1268.

22. Trabulski J, Schoeller DA. Evaluation of dietary assessment instruments against doubly labeled water, a biomarker of habitual energy intake. Am J Physiol Endocrinol Metab 2001;281:E891-E899.

23. Hofstetter A, Schutz Y, Jéquier E, Wahren J. Increased 24-hour energy expenditure in cigarette smokers. N Engl J Med 1986;314:79-82.

24. Bray GA, Popkin BM. Dietary fat intake does effect obesity! Am J Clin Nutr 1998;68:1157-1173.

25. Saris WHM, Astrup A, Prentice AM, Zunft HJF, Formiguera X, Verboeket- van de Venne WPHG, Raben A, Poppitt SD, Seppelt B, Johnston S, Vasilaras TH, Keogh GF. Randomized controlled trial of changes in dietary carbohydrate fat ratio and simple versus complex carbohydrates on body weight and blood lipids: the CARMEN study. Int J Obesity 2000;24:1310-1318.

26. Rolls BJ, Bell EA, Castellanos VH, Chow M, Pelkman CL, Thorwart ML. Energy density but not fat content of foods affected energy intake in lean and obese women. Am J Clin Nutr 1999;69:863-871.

27. Lissner L, Brownell KD. Weight cycling, mortality and cardiovascular disease: A review of epidemiologic findings. In: Obesity. Björntorp P, Brodoff BN (Eds). J.B. Lippincott Company, Philadelphia, 1992:653-661.

28. Visscher TLS, Seidell JC, Molarius A, Kuip A van der, Hofman A, Witteman JCM. A comparison of Body Mass Index, waist-hip ratio and waist circumference as predictors of all-cause mortality among elderly: The Rotterdam Study. Int J Obes Relat Metab Disorders 2001;25:1730-1735.

CHAPTER 3.4

TYPE 2 DIABETES, GLUCOSE TOLERANCE AND CARDIOVASCULAR DISEASES IN THE SEVEN COUNTRIES STUDY

Daan Kromhout, Edith Feskens

The prevalence and incidence of type 2 diabetes (formerly called non-insulin-dependent diabetes) are increasing worldwide. The WHO predicts that the number of diabetic patients will increase from 143 million in 1997 to about 300 million in 2025 (1). A major determinant of diabetes is obesity and large increases in the prevalence of obesity were observed in the developed countries during the last decades of the 20th century and in developing countries more recently. Worldwide more than 250 million people are estimated to be obese (2). Another important determinant of diabetes is physical inactivity. There is now evidence from ecological, cross-sectional, and cohort studies that physical activity is inversely related to risk of type 2 diabetes (3).

Diet has always been viewed as a major determinant of diabetes. In an ancient Hindu document from 400 BC the diabetic syndrome was described to include "honey-like urine" (4). It took, however, till 1776 before it was demonstrated that the sweet substance in the urine of diabetic patients was glucose. A major event in the history of diabetes was the discovery of the hormone insulin in 1921, when Banting and Best produced the first insulin preparation for treatment of diabetic patients.

Carbohydrates influence ß-cell activity and have therefore been suspected to influence glucose tolerance and diabetes. Himsworth suggested in 1935 that insulin sensitivity increased with a high-carbohydrate diet and this became the basis of a standard recommendation regarding dietary preparation for the oral glucose tolerance test (5). He also suggested that not only the energy density of carbohydrates but also dietary fat might play a role in the etiology of diabetes (6).

The diet traditionally prescribed for diabetic patients was low in carbohydrate and high in fat (7) and contained a large amount of saturated fat, thus promoting the occurrence of CHD. Currently, a diet low in saturated fat and high in fiber-rich carbohydrates is recommended for the prevention and amelioration of both diabetes and CHD (7).

There is also a genetic basis for diabetes; a family history of diabetes occurs more frequently in diabetic than in non-diabetic women (8). It is not clear whether type 1 (insulin-dependent) and type 2 diabetes have the same genetic basis. There is quite some evidence suggesting that type 2 diabetes results from an interaction among genetic, dietary, and lifestyle factors (9).

This chapter summarizes the findings of the Seven Countries Study on type 2 diabetes and glucose tolerance. We will describe trends in prevalence of diabetes over 35 years, including the relationships among body fatness, physical activity and diabetes from a cross-cultural perspective. Also described are the relationships among body fatness, lifestyle, dietary and genetic determinants of glucose tolerance and diabetes at the individual level. Finally, the relationship between diabetes and the risk of cardiovascular and all-causes mortality will be outlined.

TRENDS IN THE PREVALENCE OF DIABETES OVER A 35-YEAR PERIOD

In the Seven Countries Study, information about prevalence of diabetes had been collected since the baseline survey in 1958-1964. The diagnosis was based on a typical history of diabetes under treatment. During follow-up the cumulative prevalence was calculated, which means that a man who was diagnosed as a diabetic stayed a prevalent case during the whole follow-up period. The prevalence of diabetes varied at baseline between 0% in Japan and 2.1% in Belgrade. Ten years later the cumulative prevalence was found between 0% in Japan and 12.8% in Belgrade (Fig. 1).

Figure 1. The prevalence of diabetes in 16 cohorts around 1960 and 1970.

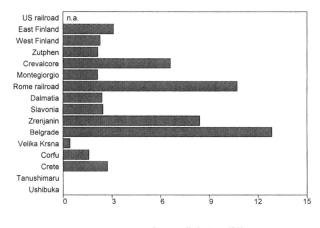

prevalence diabetes (%)

n.a. = not available

Table 1. Age-adjusted cumulative prevalence of clinical diabetes (%) in men aged 40-59 at baseline among several European cohorts of the Seven Countries Study in the period 1960-1995.

Year	1960		1970		1985		1995	
Age (y)	40-59		50-69		65-84		75-94	
Cohort	N	%	N	%	N	%	N	%
East Finland	817	0.8	656	3.1	316	14.1	119	7.0
West Finland	860	0.2	720	2.3	387	8.4	150	14.1
Zutphen	878	0.9	627	2.1	361	7.5	146	15.4
Crevalcore	993	0.9	799	6.6	373	12.4	146	11.4
Montegiorgio	719	0.5	606	2.1	309	11.7	121	11.3
Zrenjanin	517	0.3	436	8.4	180	8.2	54	11.8
Belgrade	538	2.1	436	12.8	286	20.2	139	28.8
Velika Krsna	511	0.2	437	0.4	227	1.2	74	0.5

For eight European cohorts information on the prevalence of diabetes was collected repeatedly between 1960 and 1995. Table 1 provides information about the cumulative prevalence of diabetes during a follow-up period of 35 years. With a few exceptions, a continuous increase in the prevalence of diabetes was observed in these aging cohorts between 1960 and 1995.The largest increase was observed in the Belgrade cohort: 2.1% in 1960 to 28.8% in 1995. In contrast, the prevalence of diabetes in the Serbian cohort of Velika Krsna varied only between 0.2 and 1.2% during this 35-year period. Another remarkable feature was the 50% reduction in prevalence of diabetes in the cohort from East Finland between 1985 and 1995. This is probably due to the high all-causes mortality rate of this cohort, so only relatively healthy men with a low prevalence of diabetes survive.

185

Information on glucose tolerance was collected only in the Dutch and Finnish cohorts. In 1970 a glucose tolerance test was carried out in the Zutphen cohort using a glucose load of 50 g. A blood sample was obtained from the subjects after an overnight fast. Repeated blood samples were taken by venipuncture 30, 60, 120, and 150 minutes after oral glucose. In 1990 the oral glucose tolerance test was repeated using a glucose load of 75 g, with fasting; 60- and 120-minute glucose values determined. In 1970, glucose was measured using o-toludine reagent and in 1990 with the hexokinase method.

In Finland, oral glucose tolerance tests were carried out in 1984 and 1989. A 75-g glucose load was used and fasting and 2-hour post-load glucose values were determined. In 1984 the participants were requested to fast for at least 4 hours before examination. Between 08.00 and 16.30, fasting and 2-hour post-load capillary blood samples were collected. A refractometric method was used for glucose determination. In 1989 the subjects were asked to fast at least 12 hours; the test took place between 08.00 and 12.00. Blood glucose was measured from venous blood samples using a glucose dehydrogenase method. Because of differences in methodology only the 1989 results on glucose tolerance collected in Finland and the 1990 results from Zutphen are comparable. A similar methodology was also used in the Cremona Study from Italy (10) carried out outside the context of the Seven Countries Study. This makes it possible to compare the prevalence of diabetes in elderly men in northern and southern Europe.

The 1985 WHO criteria were used to define the prevalence of diabetes based on an oral glucose tolerance test (10). This includes known diabetes or diabetes defined as a fasting glucose level ≥ 7.8 mmol/l or by a 2-hour postload glucose level ≥ 11.1 mmol/l in venous blood or plasma. Impaired glucose tolerance was defined as 2-hour post-load blood glucose between 7.8 and 11.1 mmol/l. A study in which five repeated tolerance tests were carried out in 237 elderly subjects from the Netherlands showed that the reliability coefficient for the area under the curve for glucose tolerance (r = 0.81) was similar to that for serum total cholesterol (r = 0.80) (11).

The prevalence of diabetes in men aged 50-70 in Zutphen in 1970 was about 4% (Table 2). Twenty years later the prevalence of diabetes in this cohort of elderly men had increased to about 15%. Around 1990, glucose tolerance tests using a similar methodology were also carried out in the cohorts from Finland, and in elderly men

Table 2. Average Body Mass Index (BMI) and prevalence of diabetes in three European populations of elderly men (10,12,13)

Cohort	Year survey	No.	Age (y)	BMI (kg/m²)	Prevalence of DM (%)[a] Known	WHO[b]
Zutphen	1970	437	50-70	25.1	4.3	4.3[c]
Zutphen	1990	485	69-90	25.5	8.0	15.4
Finland	1989	411	69-89	26.4	13.9	21.9
Cremona[d]	1990/91	334	69-88	26.7	7.2	20.1

a = Diabetes mellitus
b = WHO criteria: known diabetes or diabetes defined by 2-hour glucose (≥ 11.1 mmol/l)
c = Based on a glucose tolerance test using a glucose load of 50 g in euglycemic men only
d = Cohort study outside the Seven Countries Study

aged 69-88 from Cremona (Italy). The results of these studies showed that about 1 in 5 elderly men in Finland and Italy, and 1 in 7 in Zutphen had diabetes conforming to WHO criteria. In Finland about 35% of these men were newly diagnosed, in Zutphen almost 50%, and in Italy about 65%. This shows that in elderly men about one-half of the men who have diabetes are unaware of their disease. We conclude that clinically diagnosed diabetes is a common disorder in European elderly men. In addition, a large proportion of the men with diabetes is not detected.

BODY FATNESS AND THE PREVALENCE OF DIABETES FROM A CROSS-CULTURAL PERSPECTIVE.

The ecological relationships between indicators of body fatness and diabetes risk were studied using data on Body Mass Index (BMI), subscapular skinfold thickness and information on the prevalence of diabetes. Average population values were calculated for BMI and subscapular skinfold thickness from data collected in 1960, and related to the prevalence of diabetes 10 years later.

Figure 2. Relationship between average population Body Mass Index in 1960 and cumulative prevalence of diabetes in 1970.

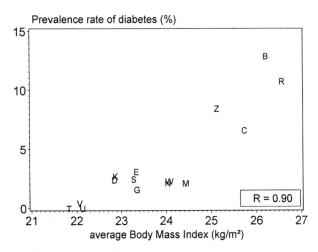

For legend see appendix

Both average population BMI and subscapular skinfold thickness in 1960 were strongly related to diabetes prevalence in 1970. These correlations were 0.90 (p< 0.001) for BMI (Fig. 2) and 0.85 (p< 0.001) for subscapular skinfold thickness. These results suggest that at an average population BMI below 25 kg/m^2 the prevalence of diabetes is low: 3% or less (Fig.2). Above this cut-off point, the relationship between average population BMI and the prevalence of diabetes increases in a graded manner. Average population BMI between 26 and 27 kg/m^2 in men aged 40-59 is associated with a more than 10% prevalence of diabetes 10 years later. These results show the importance of keeping average population BMI below 25 kg/m^2 for prevention of type 2 diabetes.

Figure 3. Relationship between average population physical activity in 1960 and cumulative prevalence of diabetes in 1970.

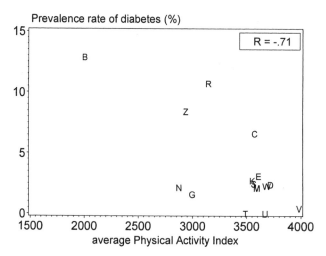

For legend see appendix

Average population physical activity in 1960 was inversely associated with 10-year prevalence of diabetes (r = -0.71, p< 0.01) (Fig. 3). Also average population dietary fiber intake in 1960 was inversely related to 10-years prevalence of diabetes (r = -0.23), but this association was not statistically significant. Multivariate analysis showed that both average population BMI and average population physical activity were significantly associated with the 10-year prevalence of diabetes. BMI and physical inactivity are apparently the strongest determinants of diabetes prevalence in a population.

BODY FATNESS, PHYSICAL ACTIVITY AND SMOKING AS RISK FACTORS FOR GLUCOSE TOLERANCE AND DIABETES IN INDIVIDUALS

The relationship between indicators of body fatness and glucose tolerance was investigated in Dutch and Finnish cohorts (12,13). In the Zutphen cohort of men aged 50-70, BMI was strongly associated with fasting, the 60-minute glucose level, and the area under the glucose curve (13). In multivariate analyses, also taking subscapular skinfold thickness into account, these associations were no longer statistically significant. In the Finnish cohorts of men aged 65-84 in 1984, fasting and 120 minute glucose were not related to BMI (12). Changes in BMI were, however, associated with changes in fasting and 120 minute glucose values for 5 years of follow-up (12). BMI at baseline was strongly correlated with glucose intolerance or diabetes 5 years later. The risk ratio for persons with a BMI $\geq$ 27 kg/m^2, compared to non-obese persons, was 2.25 (95%CI 1.06-4.80). However, BMI did not have an impact on the development of overt diabetes among men with glucose intolerance.

The associations between BMI, insulin and glucose tolerance were studied prospectively in the Dutch and Finnish cohorts (14). At the 30-year follow-up fasting insulin levels were strongly related to glucose tolerance. Among men with hyperinsulinaemia (fasting insulin $\geq$ 9.2 mU/l) BMI was already high 30 years before the current insulin measurements. Similar results were obtained for the relation between BMI and glucose tolerance. Insulin and glucose tolerance were both associated with blood pressure. The strongest association was observed for glucose tolerance and blood pressure. It may therefore be questioned whether insulin is the underlying metabolic risk factor for both abnormal glucose tolerance and hypertension.

Subscapular skinfold thickness is, in contrast to BMI, a direct measure of body fatness. In the Zutphen Study subscapular skinfold thickness was strongly correlated with fasting, 60 and 120 minutes glucose values, and with the area under the glucose curve (13). These associations remained after multivariate analyses. Subscapular skinfold thickness measured in 1960 was also independently related to the 25-year incidence of diabetes (15) (Table 3).

Evidence for a protective effect of physical activity on glucose tolerance was obtained in the Zutphen Elderly Study (16). Information on different types of activity was collected with a validated questionnaire designed for retired men. Men taking physical activity 30 minutes per day or more had a lower prevalence of glucose intolerance (OR = 0.32, 95%CI 0.18-0.57). Analyses using different types of physical activity showed that especially cycling and gardening, but not walking, were "protective." Repeatedly collected physical activity data in 1985 and 1990 showed that the lowest risk for glucose intolerance was found in men who were physically active for at least 30 minutes per day in both years (RR = 0.41, 95%CI 0.23-0.76). Physical activity was also inversely related with serum insulin levels during the glucose tolerance test (17).

Table 3. Adjusted hazard ratios of 25-year diabetes incidence for selected risk factors in 841 men initially free of diabetes (15).

Risk factor	All men N = 841		CVD free men N = 343	
	HR	95%CI	HR	95%CI
Subscapular skinfold (>18 vs <10 mm)	3.2	1.7-6.1	3.9	1.5-10.1
Cigarette use (> 20 vs 0 cig/d)	3.3	1.4-7.9	3.9	1.0-14.3
Alcohol intake (≥ 10 vs 0 g/d)	1.1	0.6-2.3	2.5	0.9-7.4

CVD = Cardiovascular diseases   HR = Hazard ratio   CI= Confidence Interval

The relationship between cigarette smoking and the incidence of diabetes was investigated using 25-year follow-up data of the Zutphen Study (15). Heavy cigarette smoking (>20 cigarettes/day) was strongly associated with 25-year diabetes incidence (Table 3). This association was stronger in men who remained free from cardiovascular diseases. Alcohol consumption in 1960 was not associated with 25-year diabetes incidence. This may be explained by the relatively low prevalence (43%) of drinkers in 1960 in this population.

We can conclude that subscapular skinfold thickness, physical activity, and heavy cigarette smoking are independent predictors of glucose intolerance and/or diabetes. The associations between subscapular skinfold thickness and glucose intolerance or diabetes, were stronger than those for BMI.

DIET, GLUCOSE TOLERANCE, HYPERINSULINEMIA AND DIABETES

The classic diet of diabetic patients was low in carbohydrate and high in fat, especially saturated fat (7). This type of diet promotes the occurrence of CHD, therefore nowadays a diet low in saturated fat and high in fiber-rich carbohydrates is advocated (7). It is therefore of interest to know about the current diet of diabetic patients.

The diet of elderly men from Finland, The Netherlands, and Italy with non-insulin-dependent diabetes was compared with that of non-diabetic men (18). These men were 70-90 years old in 1990, and about 8-9% had a history of diabetes. Generally, the differences in the diet between diabetic and non-diabetic men in the three countries were small. The most characteristic difference in the diet of diabetic men was the low consumption of added sugar. In addition, diabetic men consumed more fruit in the Netherlands and Italy, and more vegetables in Italy. The Dutch diabetics also had a higher consumption of milk (products), cheese, meat (products), and a lower consumption of alcoholic beverages. These differences were reflected in a lower intake of carbohydrates by Finnish and Dutch diabetics, and a higher intake of protein and dietary fiber by Dutch and Italian diabetics. The Dutch diabetics also had a lower alcohol intake than the non-diabetics. It was concluded that the diet of the diabetic men from Finland, The Netherlands, and Italy resembled more the diet of non-diabetic men from the respective countries than the diet of diabetic men from other countries. In the diet of Italian diabetic men, the proportion of saturated fat and carbohydrates was nearest the recommended levels.

The cross-sectional relationship between diet and glucose tolerance was investigated using data of the Zutphen cohort collected in 1970 in 394 men aged 50-70. For the association between diet and hyperinsulinemia, data collected in 1990 in 389 men aged 70-89 were used.

The intake of saturated fat and dietary cholesterol was positively associated with the fasting glucose level (19). These associations were no longer statistically significant when both variables were simultaneously entered into the multivariate model. Saturated fatty acid intake was not related to postload glucose levels but was, however, positively associated with the area under the insulin curve and with fasting C peptide in both uni- and multivariate analyses (17). These results suggest that saturated fatty acid intake is more strongly related to indicators of insulin resistance and hyperinsulinemia than to glucose intolerance.

The intake of mono- and disaccharides, and of the soluble fiber, pectin, was inversely associated with postload glucose level in both uni- and multivariate analyses (19). In 1970 consumption of sugar products was inversely related to both fasting glucose and area under the glucose curve (19). An inverse relationship between sugar products and fasting glucose was also observed using the 1990 data of the Zutphen Elderly Study (20). Such associations were not observed for total dietary fiber. However, total dietary fiber was inversely associated with the area under the insulin curve (Fig. 4) and fasting C peptide after both uni- and multivariate analyses (17). These results provide evidence that sugar products and the water-soluble fraction of dietary fiber, pectin, are inversely related with postload glucose level, and total dietary fiber with postload insulin level and fasting C-peptide. Total dietary fiber is also inversely associated with insulin sensitivity and beta cell mass (16).

190

Figure 4. Insulin levels (mean and standard deviation) during an oral glucose tolerance test in 389 men aged 70-89 years by quartiles of dietary fiber intake (17).

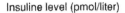

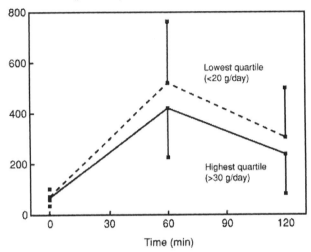

Time (min)

PROSPECTIVE ANALYSES ON DIET, GLUCOSE TOLERANCE AND DIABETES

In the Finnish and Dutch cohorts of the Seven Countries Study dietary data using the cross-check dietary history method were collected around 1970 and 1990 (21). These data were used to study prospectively the associations between diet, glucose intolerance and diabetes. Between 1971 and 1975 an epidemiological study was carried out in elderly persons in Rotterdam, The Netherlands (22). In this study dietary data were collected in 1971 using the cross-check dietary history method. Between 1971 and 1975 glucose tolerance tests were carried out yearly. These unique data could be used to study diet in relation to 4-year incidence of glucose intolerance.

In prospective analyses of the Zutphen data no associations was found between dietary data collected in 1960 and 25-year incidence of clinical diabetes (15). In the Finnish and Dutch cohorts of the Seven Countries Study the relationships between dietary variables assessed around 1970, changes in diet between 1970 and 1990, and impaired glucose tolerance, and newly established diabetes in 1990 were investigated (21). An increase in the consumption of vegetables and legumes, potatoes and fish during the 20-year follow-up was inversely related to the 2-hours postload glucose level in 1990. An independent inverse association was observed for vitamin C in 1970 and the dietary fiber intake in 1970 was also inversely associated, but this latter association did not reach statistical significance.

In the elderly study from Rotterdam the consumption of legumes was inversely related to the incidence of glucose intolerance (22). An inverse relationship was also observed between fish consumption and the incidence of glucose intolerance (23). Pastries, a rich source of *trans* fatty acids, were positively associated with the incidence of glucose intolerance (22).

Currently there is a great interest in the effect of the glycemic index on the occurrence of type 2 diabetes and CHD (24). The glycemic index refers to the increase in blood glucose concentration in the three hours after consumption of a test meal containing 50 g of available carbohydrate. The index is calculated as a percentage increase in blood glucose concentration produced by a reference food, typically white bread, with equivalent carbohydrate content. Although foods with a high fiber content generally have a low glycemic index, the two concepts are independent. Foods with a low glycemic index and high fiber content typically raise post-prandial blood glucose concentrations less than foods that have the same fiber content but higher glycemic index values.

A possible protective effect of a low glycemic index and high fiber content of the diet was shown in relation to the risk of non-insulin dependent diabetes in the Nurses Health and the Health Professionals Follow-up Studies (25,26). The strongest effects were observed in the nurses. In comparing the highest with the lowest quintile of dietary glycemic load, the relative risk was found to be 1.47 (95%CI 1.16-1.86). For cereal fiber the relative risk for the extreme quintiles was 0.72 (95%CI 0.58-0.90). The combination of high glycemic load and low cereal fiber intake further increases the risk of diabetes (RR= 2.50, 95%CI 1.14-5.51). In the Nurses Health Study a lower glycemic load was also associated with a reduced risk of CHD (27).

The relationships among dietary glycemic index, hyperinsulinemia, hyperglycemia, dyslipidemia, and CHD risk were also investigated in elderly men from Zutphen (20). Cross-sectional analyses using the 1990 data showed no associations among the dietary glycemic index and fasting glucose and insulin, and blood lipids. A high glycemic index in 1985 was compared with a low index and was not associated with CHD incidence during the 10 years of follow-up (RR= 1.11, 95%CI 0.66-1.87).

These different results may be due to differences in age and gender since the Zutphen population consisted of elderly men. The glycemic index was a stronger predictor of HDL cholesterol concentrations in women than men (28). Also the food pattern determining the glycemic index may have differed substantially in the different study populations. On the other hand, the variation in dietary glycemic index in the Zutphen Elderly Study was similar to that in the American and British studies (25-28). Lack of variation is therefore unlikely to be an explanation for the differences in results, because the expected inverse relationship between dietary fiber and indicators of insulin resistance and hyperinsulinemia was also observed in the Zutphen Elderly Study (17).

The results from the reported cross-sectional and prospective studies carried out in the Seven Countries Study suggest that saturated and *trans* fatty acid rich foods may promote insulin resistance and glucose intolerance. The consumption of fish and plantfoods, especially legumes, a rich source of dietary fiber, may be protective against insulin resistance and glucose intolerance. We did not observe effects of the glycemic index on hyperinsulinemia, hyperglycemia, dyslipidemia, and CHD.

DIETARY AND LIFESTYLE INTERVENTIONS ON GLUCOSE TOLERANCE AND DIABETES

The observational data from the Finnish and Dutch cohorts of the Seven Countries Study suggest that saturated fatty acids promote insulin resistance and hyperinsulinemia and are positively associated with the 2-hour postload glucose level.

Recently a controlled dietary intervention study was carried out in 162 healthy volunteers (29) to study the effect of saturated fat on insulin sensitivity (29). A reduction in saturated fat from 17.6 to 9.6 percent of energy reduced insulin sensitivity by 10%, but sensitivity did not change on the monounsaturated fatty acid diet. These results suggest that a low saturated fat diet has a favorable effect on insulin sensitivity.

There is strong observational evidence for a protective effect of water-soluble and total dietary fiber on glucose intolerance and indicators of insulin resistance and hyperinsulinemia (17,19,20). These results were confirmed in a controlled dietary experiment among 13 patients with type 2 diabetes (30). For six weeks, patients got either 24 g (8 g soluble and 16 g insoluble) or 50 g (25 g soluble and 25 g insoluble) of fiber using unfortified foods. The high-fiber diet lowered the area under the curve for 24-hour plasma glucose and insulin concentrations by 10 and 12%, respectively. The high-fiber diet also lowered plasma cholesterol concentrations by 6.7%, and triglyceride concentrations by 10.2%. These results confirm that a high-fiber diet containing both soluble and insoluble fiber improves glycemic control, decreases hyperinsulinemia, and lowers plasma lipid concentrations in diabetic patients.

The hypothesis that weight loss, increase in physical activity, decrease in saturated fat, and increase in dietary fiber intake may improve glucose tolerance and reduce the incidence of diabetes was tested experimentally in a controlled intervention study carried out in middle-aged subjects with impaired glucose tolerance (31). These persons were advised to reduce their weight by 5% or more, to increase physical activity to at least 30 minutes per day, to decrease their saturated fat intake to less than 10 percent of energy, and to increase dietary fiber intake to at least 15g/1000 kcal. These goals were realized by 43, 86, 26 and 25%, respectively, of the experimental group compared with 13, 71, 11 and 12%, respectively, in the control group. The net loss in body weight by the end of the second year differed by 2.7 kg (p< 0.001) between the experimental and the control group. The cumulative incidence of diabetes after 4 years was 11% in the experimental group (95% CI 6-15%), and 23% (95%CI 17-29%) in the control group. These results show that type 2 diabetes can be prevented by changes in lifestyle and diet of high-risk persons

We conclude that body fatness and physical activity are the most important determinants of type 2 diabetes both in populations and individuals. Observational and controlled intervention studies showed that in individuals, besides body fatness and physical activity, a low intake of saturated fat and a high intake of dietary fiber improve glycemic control and insulin sensitivity.

GENETIC SUSCEPTIBILITY, GLUCOSE INTOLERANCE AND NON-INSULIN-DEPENDENT DIABETES

The influence of a family history on glucose tolerance was investigated in the Zutphen Elderly Study (32). Based on a history of diabetes and a glucose tolerance test, 14.5% of the men aged 70-90 were diabetic. In diabetic men a family history of diabetes occurred more often (22.1%) than in men with normal glucose tolerance (6.8%). The odds ratio for a history of diabetes in diabetic men compared with men with normal glucose tolerance was 3.9 (95%CI 1.9-7.9). These results support an effect of genetic susceptibility on the occurrence of type 2 diabetes.

Both type 1 and 2 diabetes are multifactorial diseases with a strong genetic basis (33). Progress in identifying genes involved in type 2 diabetes has been slow. For type

1 diabetes the major genetic susceptibility has been shown to be explainable by associations with HLA genes located on chromosome 6. Using HLA haplotype data from the Finnish childhood study, 37 haplotypes were identified that explained genetic susceptibility in 84% of the probands. Another 20 haplotypes were identified later for type 1 diabetes. These 57 haplotypes were then used to study the genetic basis of type 2 diabetes in 131 elderly men from the Finnish cohorts.

Diabetes-associated haplotypes were present in 94% (85/90) of the diabetic men, in 79% (27/34) of men with glucose intolerance and in only 13% (3/23) of non-diabetic men. Mean fasting blood glucose was significantly higher in men with diabetes-associated haplotypes than in men with no diabetes-associated haplotypes (6.1 vs. 5.5 mmol/l, p = 0.037). The difference in a 2-hour post-challenge glucose concentration was much larger between these two groups (10.4 vs. 6.4 mmol/l, p< 0.001). These results suggest that HLA haplotypes are a common genetic determinant of both type 1 and 2 diabetes.

The predictive power for diabetes-associated HLA haplotypes to detect abnormal glucose tolerance was 97% (30). This may provide possibilities to identify high-risk persons based on specific HLA haplotypes. Because it has been shown in a controlled intervention study that weight reduction, in combination with increased physical activity, decreased intake of saturated fat, and increased intake of dietary fiber, reduced the risk of diabetes incidence by 58%, an effective preventive program through lifestyle and dietary changes can be offered to high-risk persons (31).

FASTING INSULIN, GLUCOSE TOLERANCE, TYPE 2 DIABETES, AND THE RISK OF CARDIOVASCULAR DISEASES

Macrovascular diseases (cardiovascular diseases) are major complications of type 2 diabetes. The relationships between fasting insulin, glucose tolerance, diabetes, and cardiovascular diseases were investigated in the Dutch and the Finnish cohorts of the Seven Countries Study.

The relationship between fasting serum insulin level and the prevalence of CHD could be studied in elderly men in Zutphen examined in 1990 (34). This association was studied in 390 non-diabetic men aged 70-89. Men in the highest quartile of the fasting insulin distribution had a significantly higher prevalence of CHD compared with men with lower fasting insulin levels. This result was independent of potential confounding variables as well as possible intermediates (Odds Ratio 2.43, 95% CI 1.33-4.47).

The relationship between glucose tolerance and cardiovascular mortality was investigated in 400 euglycemic men from Zutphen in 1970 (35) (Table 4). After adjustment for other cardiovascular risk factors, glucose intolerance was significantly associated with 15-year risk for fatal and non-fatal CHD. The relationship with cerebrovascular disease incidence did not reach statistical significance (RR = 1.90, 95%CI 0.88-4.10). Peripheral arterial disease incidence was not related to glucose tolerance. In a prospective study among 202 elderly persons, in which repeated glucose tolerance tests were carried out in the period 1971-1975, it was shown that average area under the glucose curve was related to 12-year mortality from CHD (36). The relative risk for the highest versus the lowest tertile was 3.10 (95%CI 1.11-8.67). These results suggest that glucose tolerance is related to fatal and non-fatal CHD risk.

In the Zutphen cohort, 46 cases of non-insulin-dependent diabetes developed be-ween 1960 and 1985 (35) (Table 4). The median age of these men at the time of *Table*

194

4. Adjusted risk ratios for cardiovascular diseases to glucose tolerance and clinically diagnosed diabetes (35)

Incidence of disease	Glucose tolerance[a] and 15-year CVD[b]		Diabetes and 25-year CVD[b]	
	HR	95%CI	HR	95%CI
Fatal coronary heart	2.27	1.03-5.01	2.21	0.97-5.04
Coronary heart	1.59	1.02-2.46	1.33	0.70-2.51
Cerebrovascular	1.90	0.88-4.10	1.95	0.87-4.37
Peripheral arterial	0.83	0.41-1.71	2.84	0.97-8.35

a = above vs below median   HR = Hazard ratio
b = cardiovascular diseases   CI = Confidence interval

diagnosis was 61. Compared with 230 matched controls who did not have diabetes, the relative risks were 2.21 (95%CI 0.97- 5.04) for fatal CHD, 1.95 (95%CI 0.87-4.37) for cerebrovascular disease incidence, and 2.84 (95%CI 0.97-8.35) for peripheral arterial disease. The relative 5-year mortality risk from cardiovascular diseases in Finnish men with diabetes, aged 65-84 diabetes was 1.55 (95%CI 0.84-2.85) (37). These results suggest that the risk for cardiovascular disease incidence and mortality among diabetic men is higher compared with controls. The relative strength of this association seems to decrease with age.

The relationship between the prevalence of diabetes and all-causes mortality has also been investigated in the Seven Countries Study (38,39). The adjusted relative risk for all-causes mortality during 15 years of follow-up of diabetic men aged 50-69 was 1.24 (95%CI 0.69-2.22) in Finland, 1.43 (95%CI 0.52-3.94) in the Netherlands, and 1.78 (95%CI 1.28-1.48) in Italy (38). In diabetics of ages 65-84 from these countries, who were followed for 10 years, these relative risks were 1.41 (95%CI 1.02-1.96) for Finland, 1.40 (95%CI 0.96-2.04) for the Netherlands and 1.49 (95%CI 1.03-2.14) for Italy (39). Generally, these relative risks for all-causes mortality were of the same order of magnitude as those for the prevalence of different cardiovascular diseases (38,39). These results suggest that the prevalence of diabetes is an important determinant of all-causes mortality. From 50-69 years onwards, the risk for all-causes mortality is about 40% higher compared to non-diabetic persons.

The associations among glucose intolerance, clinical diabetes, cardiovascular and all-causes mortality were also analyzed in the DECODE Study (40). This study combines the results of 10 prospective European cohort studies including the Finnish and Dutch cohorts of the Seven Countries Study. In total more than 15,000 men and 7,000 women aged 30 to 89 underwent a glucose tolerance test and were followed for a median of 8.8 years. For known diabetic men risk ratios of about 2 were found for CHD, stroke and all-causes mortality. Generally lower risk ratios were found for men with impaired glucose tolerance and newly diagnosed diabetes.

We conclude that both glucose intolerance and diabetes are associated with CHD, stroke and all-causes mortality. The strength of the associations increased with the severity of glucose intolerance.

SUMMARY AND CONCLUSIONS

Data from cohorts of the Seven Countries Study show that in men aged 40-59 in 1960 the cumulative prevalence of diabetes varied between 0% in Japan and 2.1% in Belgrade. Thirty-five years later the prevalence of diabetes in eight Europea cohorts varied between 0.5% in Velika Krsna and 28.8% in Belgrade. In 1990 a glucose tolerance test was carried out in Finland and the Netherlands. According to WHO criteria, the prevalence of diabetes in elderly men aged 69-90 was 22% in Finland and 15% in the Netherlands, and in about half of these men, it was newly diagnosed. BMI and physical inactivity were the most important associations of diabetes at the population level. Results from the Zutphen Study showed that subscapular skinfold thickness, physical inactivity, and heavy smoking are independent predictors of glucose intolerance and/or diabetes at the individual level. Studies on diet and glucose tolerance carried out in the Zutphen cohort showed that intake of sugar products is inversely related to fasting glucose level. Water- soluble and total dietary fiber were inversely related with different indicators of glucose intolerance and insulin resistance. Studies on the genetic basis of type 2 diabetes in the Finnish cohorts showed the HLA haplotypes to be a major genetic determinant of glucose intolerance and diabetes. Results from the Zutphen Study provided evidence that glucose intolerance and diabetes are related to mortality from CHD and cerebrovascular disease incidence. In the Seven Countries Study diabetes is a strong determinant of all-causes mortality.

REFERENCES

1. World Health Organization. Life in the 21st century. A vision for all. World Health Report, Geneva, Switzerland, WHO, 1998
2. Seidell JC. Obesity, insulin resistance and diabetes- a worldwide epidemic. Br J Nutr 2000;83:S5-8
3. Manson JE, Spelsberg A. Primary prevention of non-insulin dependent diabetes mellitus. Am J Prev Med 1994;10:172-184
4. Krall LP, Levine R, Barnet DM. The history of diabetes. In: Joslin's diabetes mellitus. Kahn CR, Weir GC (Eds), Pennsylvania. Lea&Febiger, 1994
5. Himsworth HP. The dieting factor determining the glucose tolerance and sensitivity to insulin in healthy men. Clin Sci 1935;2:67-94
6. Himsworth HP. Diet and the incidence of diabetes mellitus. Clin Sci 1935;2:117-148.
7. Blades M. Morgan JB, Dickerson JW. Dietary advice in the management of diabetes mellitus- history and current practice. J R Soc Hlth 1997;117:143-150.
8. Morris RD, Rimm DL, Hartz AJ, Kalkhoff RK, Rimm AA. Obesity and heredity in the etiology of non-insulin dependent diabetes mellitus in 32,662 adult white women. Am J Epidemiol 1989;130:112-121
9. Barsch GS, Faroogi IS, O'Rahilly S. Genetics of body weight regulation. Nature 2000;404:644-651.
10. DECODE Study Group on behalf of the European Diabetes Epidemiology Study Group. Will new diagnostic criteria for diabetes mellitus change phenotype of patients with diabetes? Reanalyses of European epidemiological data. BMJ 1998;317:371-375.
11. Feskens EJM, Bowles CH, Kromhout D. Intra- and interindividual variability of glucose tolerance in an elderly population. J Clin Epidemiol 1991;44:947-953.
12. Stengård JH, Pekkanen J, Tuomilehto J, Kivinen P, Kaarsalo E, Tamminen M, Nissinen A, Karvonen MJ. Changes in glucose tolerance among elderly Finnish men during a five-year follow-up: The Finnish cohorts of the Seven Countries Study. Diab Metab 1993;19:121-129.

13. Feskens EJM, Kromhout D. Effects of body fat and its developments over a ten-year period on glucose tolerance in euglycemic men: The Zutphen Study. Int J Epidemiol 1989;18:368-373.

14. Feskens EJM, Tuomilehto J, Stengård JH, Pekkanen J, Nissinen A, Kromhout D. Hypertension and overweight are associated with hyperinsulinaemia and glucose tolerance: a longitudinal study of the Finnish and Dutch cohorts of the Seven Countries Study. Diabetologia 1995;38:839-847.

15. Feskens EJM, Kromhout D. Cardiovascular risk factors and the 25-year incidence of diabetes mellitus in middle-aged men. Am J Epidemiol 1989;130:1101-1108.

16. Dam RM van, Schuit AJ, Feskens EJM, Seidell JC, Kromhout D. Physcial activity and glucose tolerance in elderly men. The Zutphen Study. Med Sci Sports Exerc. Accepted.

17. Feskens EJM, Loeber JG, Kromhout D. Diet and physical activity as determinants of hyperinsulinemia: The Zutphen Elderly Study. Am J Epidemiol 1994;140:350-360.

18. Virtanen SM, Feskens EJM, Räsänen L, Fidanza F, Tuomilehto J, Giampaoli S, Nissinen A, Kromhout D. Comparison of diets of diabetic and non-diabetic elderly men in Finland, The Netherlands and Italy. Eur J Clin Nutr 2000; 54:181-186.

19. Feskens EJM, Kromhout D. Habitual dietary intake and glucose tolerance in euglycemic men: the Zutphen Study. Int J Epidemiol 1990;19:953-959.

20. Dam RM van, Visscher AWJ, Feskens EJM, Verhoef P, Kromhout D. Dietary glycemic index in relation to metabolic risk factors and incidence of coronary heart disease: the Zutphen Elderly Study. Eur J Clin Nutr 2000; 54:726-731.

21. Feskens EJM, Virtanen SM, Räsänen L, Tuomilehto J, Stengård J, Pekkanen J, Nissinen A, Kromhout D. Dietary factors determinating diabetes and impaired glucose tolerance. A 20-year follow-up of the Finnish and Dutch cohorts of the Seven Countries Study. Diabetes Care 1995;18:1104-1112.

22. Feskens EJM, Bowles CH, Kromhout D. Carbohydrate intake and body mass index in relation to the risk of glucose intolerance in an elderly population. Am J Clin Nutr 1991;54:136-140.

23. Feskens EJM, Bowles CH, Kromhout D. Inverse association between fish intake and risk of glucose intolerance in normoglycemic elderly men and women. Diabetes Care 1991;14:935-941

24. Rendell M. Dietary treatment of diabetes mellitus. N Engl J Med 2000;342:1440-1441.

25. Salmeron J, Manson JE, Stampfer MJ, Colditz GA, Wing AL, Willett WC. Dietary fiber, glycemic load and risk of non-insulin dependent diabetes. JAMA 1997;277:472-477.

26. Salmeron J, Ascherio A, Rimm EB, Colditz GA, Spiegelman D, Jenkins DJ, Stampfer MJ, Wing AL, Willett WC. Dietary fiber, glycemic load and risk of non-insulin dependent diabetes mellitus in men. Diabetes Care 1997;20:545-550.

27. Liu S, Willett WC, Stampfer MJ, Hu FB, Sampson L, Hennekens CH, Manson JE. A prospective study of dietary glycemic load, carbohydrate intake and risk of coronary heart disease in U.S. women. Am J Clin Nutr 2000;71:1455-1461.

28. Frost G, Leeds AA, Doré CJ, Madeiros S, Brading S, Dornhorst A. Glycaemic index as a determinant of serum HDL-cholesterol concentration. Lancet 1999;353:1045-1048.

29. Vessley B, Uusitupa M, Hermansen K, Ricardi G, Rivellese AA, Tapsell LC, Nalsen C, Berglund L, Louheranta A, Rasmussen BM, Calvert CD, Maffetone A, Pedersen E, Gustafsson IB, Storlien LH. Substituting dietary saturated fat for monounsaturated fat impairs insulin sensitivity in healthy men and women: the KANWU Study. Diabetologia 2001;44:312-319.

30. Chandala M, Garg A, Lutjohann D, Von Bergmann K, Grundy S, Brinkley LJ. Beneficial effects of high dietary fiber intake in patients with type 2 diabetes mellitus. N Engl J Med 2000;342:1392-1398.

31. Tuomilehto J, Lindström J, Eriksson JG Valle TT, Hamalainen H, Ilanne-Parikka P, Keinanen-Kiukaanniemi S, Laakso M, Louheranta A, Rastas M, Salminen V, Uusitupa M. Finnish Diabetes Prevention Study Group. Prevention of type 2 diabetes mellitus by changes in lifestyle among subjects with impaired glucose tolerance. N Engl J Med 2001;344:1343-1350.

32. Boer JMA, Feskens EJM, Kromhout D. Characteristics of non-insulin-dependent diabetes mellitus in elderly men: Effect modification by family history. Int J Epidemiol 1996;25:394-402.

33. Tuomilehto-Wolf E, Tuomilehto J, Hitman GA, Nissinen A, Stengård J, Pekkanen J, Kivinen P, Kaarsalo E, Karvonen MJ. Genetic susceptibility to non-insulin dependent diabetes mellitus and glucose intolerance are located in HLA region. BMJ 1993;307:155-159.

34. Feskens EJM, Kromhout D. Hyperinsulinaemia, risk factors and coronary heart disease. The Zutphen Elderly Study. Arterioscler Thromb 1994;14:1641-1647.

35. Feskens EJM, Kromhout D. Glucose tolerance and risk of cardiovascular diseases: the Zutphen Study. J Clin Epidemiol 1992;45:1327-1334.

36. Feskens EJM, Bowles CH, Kromhout D. Glucose tolerance and ischaemic heart disease mortality in an elderly population: impact of repeated measurements. Ann Epidemiol 1993;3:336-342.

37. Stengård JH, Tuomilehto J, Pekkanen J, Kivinen P, Kaarsalo E, Nissinen A, Karvonen MJ. Diabetes mellitus, impaired glucose tolerance and mortality among elderly men: The Finnish cohorts of the Seven Countries Study. Diabetologia 1992;35:760-765.

38. Menotti A, Blackburn H, Seccareccia F, Kromhout D, Nissinen A, Aravanis C, Giampaoli S, Mohacek I, Nedeljkovic S, Toshima H. The relation of chronic diseases to all-cause mortality risk. The Seven Countries Study. Ann Med 1997;29:135-141.

39. Menotti A, Mulder I, Nissinen A, Giampaoli S, Feskens EJM, Kromhout D. Prevalence of morbidity and co-morbidity in elderly male populations and their impact on 10-year all-cause mortality. The FINE Study. J Clin Epidemiol 2001;54:680-686

40. The DECODE Study Group, on behalf of the European Diabetes Epidemiology Group. Glucose tolerance and cardiovascular mortality. Comparison of fasting and 2-hour diagnostic criteria. Arch Intern Med 2001;161:397-404.

CHAPTER 3.5

ELECTROCARDIOGRAPHIC PREDICTORS OF CORONARY HEART DISEASE IN THE SEVEN COUNTRIES STUDY

Alessandro Menotti, Henry Blackburn

The electrocardiogram (ECG) displays information about the heart, whether there has been a heart attack or the muscle lacks oxygen, whether conduction of the heart beat is disturbed or its rate or rhythm altered. It is useful as a rapid indicator of the diagnosis and is easy, painless and inexpensive to record. Also used to monitor severely ill patients, the record made in healthy people at rest or undergoing an exercise test helps predict risk of future coronary disease.

The electrocardiograph was invented by Willem Einthoven in Leiden, the Netherlands, around 1900, when he displayed the deflections representing differences in electrical potential between the arms and legs, amplifying the tiny current passing through the body with each heart beat. Now data are recorded from the chest wall and the limbs and displayed on paper or TV screens. Tracings are interpreted by physicians or technicians and, in digital form, are analyzed automatically with computers.

The ECG was recorded in the Seven Countries Study from the outset in 1958 to identify such characteristics relevant to cardiovascular diseases as myocardial infarction, hypertrophy, arrhythmia and conduction defects. ECG findings were also used as predictors of future events, independent of the medical history and the physical examination. The advantage was a quantitative record that could be preserved, capable to characterize an individual objectively in central blinded coding.

The development of a coding system, known as the Minnesota Code (1,2), was the consequence of the need for a quantitative procedure to measure characteristics and severity of the ECG findings and to classify them following precise criteria and rules. The Minnesota Code was based on careful review of validated criteria at the time. Its procedure was to obtain uniform, precise and reproducible codes within and among observers, as required for population studies. The Minnesota Code provides a quantitative description of major relevant findings such as large Q waves, ST and T deviations, conduction defects and arrhythmias. The Minnesota Code and procedure diminishes observer disagreement and is widely used in population studies.

ECG tracings were systematically recorded at rest and after exercise at baseline and 5- and 10- year follow-up examinations. Resting ECGs were also taken at regular intervals in the cohorts of the FINE Study in elderly men of three countries. ECG findings, in the absence of clinical diagnoses of coronary disease of any type, were used to test their predictive power for CHD events.

ECG RECORDING AND CODING

The ECG coding followed strict rules as published in the WHO Cardiovascular Survey Methods Manual (2). Records were taken using 2- or 3-channel ink-jet machines, in 12 standard leads, following protocol for the preparation of skin, positioning of electrodes, number of beats to be recorded in each group of leads, their sequence and the freedom from baseline artifacts. The paper speed was 25 mm per second and the calibration 10 mm per mV. The simple field exercise test, after exclusion of subjects with clinical contra-indications, was based on a single-step test (step of 30 cm, 60 ascents and 60 descents in 3 minutes) or a bicycle ergometer at 150 W for 3 minutes. The post-exercise record was taken starting about 30 seconds after the end of exercise.

All records were centrally coded at the Laboratory of Physiological Hygiene, University of Minnesota, by a team led by Henry Blackburn, following standard rules and quality control. The up-dated version of the Code published in 1968 was used (2).

200

The same edition was used to code the records collected at 5- and 10-year examinations. For the FINE Study (3), the same rules were followed, but the post-exercise ECG was not taken. Readings were made separately in each country by different coders who were under quality control of the WHO ECG Reference Center in Budapest, Hungary.

The ECG findings contributed to the diagnosis of coronary events together with other clinical data in the criteria for prevalence and incidence of CHD presented in chapter 1.4. However, the majority of analyses reported here refer to prevalence of ECG findings in the population samples, mainly of "silent" findings, that is, those found in the absence of clinical symptoms and signs of cardiovascular diseases. These "silent" findings were employed here for prediction of future fatal and non-fatal events, mainly coronary or cardiovascular diseases. For analyses reported here, the following Minnesota Code (MC) items were considered without attributing a precise diagnostic meaning, rather using them as descriptive findings:

- Q-QS findings (MC 1.1-3) as possible indicators of myocardial infarction (QQS);
- left axis deviation (MC 2.1) (LAD);
- ST depression (MC 4.1-4) and/or negative or flat T waves (MC 5.1-3) as possible indicators of myocardial damage or ischemia (STT);
- high R waves in left ventricular leads (MC 3.1 and 3.3) as possible indicators of left ventricular hypertrophy (MC 3.3 corresponding to Sokolow criteria) (HRW);
- a pool of arrhythmias (MC 8.1-8.6 or 8.9 or 6.1-2 or 6.4 or 6.8) corresponding to frequent atrial or ventricular premature beats, ventricular tachycardia, atrial flutter or fibrillation, supraventricular tachycardia, idioventricular rhythm, A-V nodal rhythm, arrhythmias not mentioned above, atrioventricular block of 2nd or 3rd degree, Wolff-Parkinson-White pattern or the presence of an artificial pacemaker (ARR);
- bundle branch block (MC 7.1-2, 7.4) corresponding to complete left and right bundle branch block and intra-ventricular block (BLO).

On some occasions, combinations were used and are described. ECG findings for epidemiological studies are used differently than in clinical settings; mainly considered as objective indicators of existing disease or precursors of future clinical disease.

PREVALENCE OF ECG FINDINGS AT ENTRY AND AFTER 25 YEARS.

Table 1 presents rates for selected ECG findings for three large geographic – cultural groups at the baseline survey. Rates are shown separately for men with and without cardiovascular diseases at entry examination, as classified by clinical criteria. (In Japan, the use of non-standardized clinical diagnoses made it impossible to segregate the rare men with cardiovascular diseases at entry). Prevalence of ECG findings is higher in men with cardiovascular diseases than in those free from those diseases. Prevalence of ECG findings among CVD-free men is higher than the prevalence of clinical cardiovascular conditions.

The most common post-exercise findings among men with a "normal" resting ECG (Table 2) were similar in North American, northern European and the southern European men, while in Japan their prevalence was only about half. The similarity between Northern and Southern Europe might be explained by the fact that men with cardiovascular diseases (and thus with an abnormal resting ECG) were removed from the denominator.

Information on the prevalence of ECG findings in older men, aged 65 to 84 years, was collected in the three European countries participating in the FINE Study (3). In this analysis special combinations of ECG findings were considered beyond the basic Minne-

Table 1. Prevalence rates per 1,000 of major ECG findings in men with and without clinically prevalent cardiovascular diseases at entry. Reconstructed from reference 3.

ECG findings	NA and NE CVD absent N=4560	NA and NE CVD present N=549	southern Europe CVD absent N=6308	southern Europe CVD present N=305	Japan CVD absent N=992	Japan CVD present N=0
QQS	24	131	21	72	12	-
STT	42	248	38	193	35	-
LAD	33	47	40	66	13	-
HRW	70	128	60	151	96	-
ARR	15	49	14	79	11	-
BLO	13	40	10	20	9	-
ANY	175	441	160	390	167	-

NA = North America NE = northern Europe
CVD = cardiovascular diseases STT = MC 4.1, 4.2, 4.3, 5.1, 5.2, or 5.3;
MC= Minnesota Code LAD = Left axis deviation MC 2.1;
QQS = MC 1.1, 1.2, or 1.3; HRW = High R wave in left ventricular leads MC 3.1
ARR = Arrhythmias, any of the following MC: 8.1, 8.2, 8.3, 8.4, 8.5, 8.6, 8.9, 8.0, 6.1, 6.2, 6.4 corresponding to frequent atrial or ventricular premature beats, ventricular tachycardia, atrial flutter or fibrillation, supraventricular tachycardia, idioventricular rhythm, A-V nodal rhythm, arrhythmias not mentioned above, atrioventricular block of 2nd or 3rd degree, and Wolff-Parkinson-White pattern.
BLO= Bundle branch blocks MC 7.1-2 or 7.4, corresponding to complete left and right bundle branch block and intra-ventricular block.

Table 2. Prevalence of post-exercise ECG findings per 1000 in subjects free from cardiovascular diseases and having normal resting ECG at entry. Reconstructed from reference 3.

ECG finding	NA and NE N = 3478	SE N = 4830	Japan N = 726
ST segment, severe depression MC 11.1	4	4	0
ST segment, upward sloping, MC 11.1-4	33	37	5
T-wave, negative or flat MC 12.1-3	12	11	23
STT MC 11.1-3 or 12.1-3	24	21	23
Frequent premature beats, MC 15.1	11	11	0
Overall prevalence of post-exercise findings	52	54	26

NA=North America NE= northern Europe SE= southern Europe MC = Minnesota Code

sota Code items. In particular an operational definition of definite myocardial infarction was based on the presence of large Q waves or smaller Q waves accompanied by negative T waves; the definition of possible myocardial infarction was based in the presence of smaller Q waves and negative T waves; the definition of left ventricular hypertrophy was based on the presence of high R waves in the left ventricular leads or the Sokolow criteria accompanied by ST-T findings.

Table 3. Prevalence rates of ECG findings per 1,000 in men aged 65-84 years with and without heart disease (HD) at entry examination in the FINE Study. Reconstructed from reference 4.

| ECG finding | Prevalent heart disease rates per 1,000 | | | | | |
| | Finland | | The Netherlands | | Italy | |
	Without HD	With HD	Without HD	With HD	Without HD	With HD
N at risk	505	181	713	167	567	115
QQS	95	254	66	365	46	191
STT	261	530	257	503	136	252
LAD	121	99	139	114	132	96
HRW	139	215	128	126	192	209
ARR	119	188	95	186	42	130
BLO	65	116	80	126	72	87
ANY	551	757	529	802	508	626
Definite MI	20	116	27	198	12	78
Possible MI	18	105	20	72	21	35
Left VH	63	193	58	102	27	61

HD = prevalence of myocardial infarction, angina pectoris or heart failure.
MC = Minnesota Code
QQS = QQS MC 1.1-3   LAD = Left axis deviation MC 2.1
STT codes = STR-T MC 4.1-3 and 5.1-3   HRW = High R waves MC 3.1 or 3.3
ARR = arrhythmias MC 8.1-8.6 or 8.9 or 6.1-2 or 6 4 or 6.8, corresponding to frequent atrial or ventricular premature beats, ventricular tachycardia, atrial flutter or fibrillation, supraventricular tachycardia, idioventricular rhythm, A-V nodal rhythm, arrhythmias not mentioned above, atrioventricular block of 2nd or 3rd degree, Wolff-Parkinson-White pattern or the presence of an artificial pacemaker.
BLO = Bundle branch blocks MC 7.1-2 or 7.4
Definite myocardial infarction = MC 1.1 or (1.2 + 5.1 or 5.2)
Possible myocardial infarction = MC 1.3 + (1.5 or 5.2)
Left ventricular hypertrophy = MC 3.1 or 3.3 + 4.1-3 or 5.1-3

The older age range explains why the prevalence of selected ECG findings is high (Table 3) – greater than 50% among men free from clinically diagnosed heart disease, and 63 to 80 % among men with diagnosed heart disease. Higher levels were seen in Finland, intermediate in the Netherlands, and lower in Italy. The Dutch group had the highest prevalence of ECG findings among men with heart disease. In all groups the most common conditions were ST-T codes; composite ECG findings were rather common, such as Q waves plus negative T waves, and "left ventricular hypertrophy."

PREDICTION OF CORONARY EVENTS AS A FUNCTION OF ECG FINDINGS

"Major" ECG findings (large Q waves, negative T waves and atrial fibrillation) at the entry examination (ignoring the presence or absence of clinically diagnosed cardiovascular conditions) were associated with 5-year CHD deaths after adjustment for

Table 4. Major resting ECG findings at entry examination and 5-year CHD deaths. Reconstructed and modified from reference (3).

ECG code	Ratio Observed / Expected cases	P-value Fisher's exact test
Large Q waves, MC 1.1	15.25	< 0.001
Small Q waves+negative T waves, MC 1.2 + 5.1-2	6.54	0.108
Negative T waves, MC 5.3	9.82	< 0.001
Left bundle branch block, MC 7.1	3.40	0.214
Right bundle branch block, MC 7.2	0	0.594
Intraventicular block, MC 7.4	0	0.594
Atrial fibrillation, MC 8.3	12.90	< 0.001

MC = Minnesota Code

six risk factors (4) (Table 4). The small numbers involved, even after pooling all cohorts, probably explains the lack of association for the other listed ECG codes. The association of "minor" ECG findings with any-CHD incident events among cardiovascular disease-free men is seen for left axis deviation (in the European pool only), for minor T wave code 5.3, for 1st degree atrio-ventricular block and for the presence of frequent premature beats (data not reported in detail).

Table 5. Post-exercise ECG findings at entry examination and 5-year any-CHD incidence in CHD-free men at entry of all cohorts except the Japanese ones. Reconstructed and modified from reference 3.

ECG code	Observed Ratio / Expected[a] cases	Chi square
"Ischemic" ST depression, MC 11.1-11.3	1.82	16.39*
Junctional ST depression, MC 11.4	1.24	0.41
Negative T waves, MC 12.1 – 12-3	1.35	1.60
Premature beats, MC 15.1	1.59	3.65*

a = Observed and expected cases were matched, with adjustment for age, sum of two skinfolds, systolic blood pressure, serum cholesterol, smoking habits and physical activity.
MC = Minnesota Code   * = p < 0.05

Post-exercise ECG findings were studied as possible predictors of any-CHD event among CHD-free men at entry (Table 5). "Ischemic" ST depression and frequent premature beats post-exercise were associated with excess risk for a CHD event.

In men free of clinically diagnosed cardiovascular diseases at baseline (Table 1), ECG findings were related to 25-year CHD deaths. Three major geographic–cultural areas were considered, and six groups of ECG findings were tested, adjustments were made by the Cox proportional hazards model using age, systolic blood pressure, serum cholesterol, smoking habits and Body Mass Index as confounders. The results differed

Table 6. Twenty-five year CHD death rates (per 1,000) in men free of cardiovascular diseases in three geographical pools to ECG findings.

ECG findings		NA and NE N=4560	SE N=6308	Japan N=992
No findings	N at risk	3761	5301	166
	Death rate	182	102	52
QQS	N at risk	111	131	12
	Death rate	270	176	0
	Crude RR	1.41	1.60	-
	Adjusted HR	1.45	1.39	-
	95%CI	1.00 – 2.11	0.91 - 2.13	
LAD	N at risk	152	251	13
	Death rate	243	175	77
	Crude RR	1.27	1.61	1.45
	Adjusted HR	1.22	1.51	3.78
	95%CI	0.87 – 1.71	1.11 - 2.06	0.50 - 28.28
STT	N at risk	191	239	35
	Death rate	330	205	86
	Crude RR	1.76	1.90	1.65
	Adjusted HR	1.59	1.51	2.43
	95%CI	1.22 – 2.06	1.12 - 2.06	0.73 - 8.00
HRW	N at risk	317	381	95
	Death rate	218	160	53
	Crude RR	1.14	1.48	0.98
	Adjusted HR	0.94	1.32	1.
	95%CI	0.73 – 1.22	1.00 - 1.73	0.40 - 2.60
ARR	N at risk	67	88	11
	Death rate	209	205	182
	Crude RR	1.08	1.86	3.50
	Adjusted HR	0.91	2.35	1.59
	95%CI	0.52 – 1.57	1.45 - 3.82	0.21 – 12.25
BLO	N at risk	58	61	9
	Death rate	310	180	0
	Crude RR	1.61	1.62	-
	Adjusted HR	1.82	1.60	-
	95%CI	1.13 – 2.96	0.88 - 2.92	

NA=North America   NE= northern Europe   SE= southern Europe
Crude rates for men with no ECG findings are reported as reference. Adjustments were made for five major risk factors.
RR = Relative risk   HR = Hazard ratio   CI = Confidence interval
For legend ECG findings see table 1

Table 7. Ten-year CHD mortality among heart disease-free men as a function of silent ECG findings at entry conventionally defined as absent-marginal, minor and major (see text for definitions) (4).

ECG findings	Finland	Netherlands	Italy	Pool
Absent or marginal				
N at risk	220	360	360	940
N deaths	19	21	18	58
Rate per 1000	86	58	50	62
Minor				
N at risk	232	286	179	697
N deaths	37	27	18	82
Rate per 1000	160	94	101	118
Crude RR	1.86	1.62	2.02	1.90
Adjusted HR	1.93	1.69	1.60	1.79
95%CI	1.09 –3.40	0.95 – 3.01	0.80 – 3.22	1.26 – 2.53
Major				
N at risk	53	67	28	148
N deaths	12	12	3	27
Rate per 1000	226	179	107	182
Crude HR	2.63	3.09	2.14	2.93
Adjusted HR	3.24	3.57	1.96	3.12
95%CI	1.52 – 6.91	1.70 – 7.50	0.44 – 8.64	1.92 – 5.06

RR = Relative risk   HR = Hazard ratios   CI = Confidence intervals,
Adjustments were made for age, systolic blood pressure, serum cholesterol, Body Mass Index, smoking habits and cohorts.
Marginal or no findings = all codes not mentioned below
Minor findings = lesser Q waves (MC 1.2 or 1.3) or left axis deviation (MC 2.1), or ST-T pattern (MC 4.2-4 or 5.2-3); or WPW syndrome (MC 6.4); or right bundle branch blocks (MC 7.2-3); or frequent premature beats (MC 8.1)
Major findings = severe Q waves (MC 1.1); or severe ST-T pattern (MC 4.1 or 5.1); or left or intraventricular block (MC 7.1 or 7.4); or atrial fibrillation (MC 8.3); or pacemaker (MC 6.8)
Note AV blocks of 2nd and 3rd degree and severe arrhythmias were not mentioned here because they were never found.

somewhat by area, since Q-QS findings, ST-T findings, and blocks were significantly predictive of CHD deaths in North America and northern European areas. Left axis deviation, ST-T findings, high R waves and arrhythmia were predictive in Southern Europe, while the small numbers involved likely prevented the Japanese data reaching statistical significance. Multivariate coefficients in northern European and American areas were not significantly different from those for southern Europe (Table 6).

The presence of "clinically meaningful" ECG findings (data not reported in detail) was strongly associated with risk of sudden coronary death, CHD death and any cardiovascular deaths in the next 25 years. This was the case for major Q waves and ST-T codes, but not for "left ventricular hypertrophy" codes. Similar analyses were duplicated, segregating the outcome of the first 5 years from that of the subsequent 20 years. In general, the association of single resting ECG findings was much stronger for the short-term than for distant events.

Another analysis was made on post-exercise ECG findings to predict 25-year CHD deaths (details not reported). Severe ST depression (code 11.1), all types of ST depression (code 11.1-4) and the pool of ST depression (codes 11.1-3) with negative T wave (codes 12.1-3) were highly predictive of CHD deaths in both the North American and northern European and in the southern European cohorts, whereas negative T waves alone (codes 12.1-3) did so only in the North American and northern European areas. The hazard ratios for the two major geographic–cultural areas were not statistically different. No findings related to Japanese areas were statistically significant.

An analysis among men participating in the FINE Study (3) focused on the aggregation of silent ECG findings of different severity for the prediction of 10-year CHD deaths (Table 7). Compared with subjects with no or "marginal" ECG findings, crude death rates were higher among those with minor findings and much higher among those carrying major ECG findings. Although the rates of different ECG findings were higher in Finland, intermediate in the Netherlands and lower in Italy, the relative risks, both crude and adjusted for six covariates, were similar among entities, confirming the pattern of all the predictors of CHD events. The adjusted hazards ratios were statistically significant for minor findings in Finland, and in the three countries pooled. This also applied to major findings in Finland, the Netherlands and all the pooled countries, except Italy. This analysis was complemented by the computation of indices of predictivity. Sensitivity (compared with those free from ECG findings) was only 0.50 for minor ECG findings and 0.61 for major; the corresponding specificity was 0.61 and 0.92 respectively.

SPECIAL ANALYSES

In some areas and for specific follow-up periods and endpoints, special analyses were conducted based on ECG measurements independent of the Minnesota Code rules and coding system.

In the Dutch cohort of Zutphen five different analyses were performed. A Cardiac Infarction Injury Score was developed to measure the presence and the probability of a previous myocardial infarction. A high score was associated, in the next 5 years of follow-up, with excess risk of angina pectoris, myocardial infarction and CHD deaths, with significant relative risks of 2.2, 2.4 and 5.8 respectively (5).

Compared with a corrected QTc interval of less than 385 msec, a QTc interval of 420 msec or more was associated with a relative risk of 3.3 (95% CI 1.0-11.8) for 5-year CHD death, independent of age and other major risk factors (6). The presence of a prolonged corrected QTc was associated with insulin resistance syndrome (7).

The high voltage of T waves $\geq$ 1.5 mV was associated with a lower CHD incidence and mortality risk compared with a T wave voltage of 0.05-0.15 mV. A slight elevation of the ST segment was "protective" compared with the presence of an isoelectric ST. ST depression had a relative risk of 2.2 (95% CI 1.4-3.4) for CHD deaths, compared with the absence of ST depression (8).

Low heart rate variability based on a 20-second resting ECG and defined by the standard deviation of RR interval duration (i.e. < 20 msec), was associated, at least in middle aged men, with excess all-causes mortality and a relative risk of 1.9 (95% CI 1.3-2.7), while the same was true for elderly men, but only marginally (9).

In the pool of two rural Italian areas and for an average follow-up period of 22 years, an indicator of left ventricular hypertrophy, made by the 12 lead QRS voltage sum, was predictive of sudden coronary death, whereas ST-T findings did so only for non-sudden coronary deaths (10).

COMMENTS

At the baseline survey silent ECG findings were fairly common in the general population, occurring in 17% of men who had no symptoms, signs, or clinical diagnosis of cardiovascular diseases. Codable ECG findings were observed in about 40% of cases with clinical cardiovascular disease. However, the majority of ECG findings in the population were found in men free from cardiovascular diseases. This means that a simple resting ECG may reveal a large number of ECG findings that cannot be classified as "normal" because they carry a risk for the development of future fatal or non-fatal clinically defined coronary events. Most of these ECG findings would be classified, nowadays, as possible "silent" forms of CHD.

The prevalence of ECG findings was much higher in the baseline survey of the FINE Study, in which men aged 65-84 years in three European countries were examined. More than half of those free from heart disease had codable ECG findings, compared to about 70% among those with clinically diagnosed heart disease. Among these men a definite myocardial infarction, by FINE criteria, was found in 12 to 20 per 1000 of men without, and among 78 to 198 per 1000 of men with, a diagnosis of cardiovascular disease.

Most of the analyses on ECG findings dealt with the predictive power of ECG findings in CHD- or cardiovascular disease-free subjects; so-called "silent" findings. About 6% of 25-year CHD deaths in originally middle-aged men could be attributed to ECG findings. In heart disease-free elderly men the highest rate of CHD mortality occurred among men with minor ECG findings. Most of the clinically silent major ECG findings were associated with excess CHD mortality.

We consider a most relevant finding to be the similarity in multivariate hazards ratios among men from different cultures and populations characterized by different levels of absolute CHD risk. This finding resembles conclusions reached in analyses dealing with traditional risk factors and confirms and clarifies the independent predictive importance of the resting and post-exercise ECG.

The Seven Countries Study data, extending over a long period of follow-up, confirm the short- and long-term predictive power of ECG findings, as relatively recently reported in several other studies on resting ECG findings (11-26). In most of the literature, prediction was usually studied for particular ECG findings, most often the risk of "left ventricular hypertrophy" (LVH), defined variously. Few studies here separated the clinically latent cases from the overt ones (already manifesting disease). Nevertheless, our findings are largely in agreement with the relevant prior reports, that is, those that had substantial follow-up among healthy populations and where statistical adjustment was attempted for ascertaining the influence of other risk characteristics. The exception is the finding of little independent predictive importance for ECG-LVH. All these conclusions are confirmed in a comprehensive recent review of CVD prediction in population studies (27).

Similar statements can be made considering part of the vast literature on the post-exercise ECG (28-36). If relative risk and predictive power in the Seven Countries Study was frequently lower than that in other studies, this may be due to the light exercise performed by the Seven Countries Study men 40 years ago compared with standard graded tread-mill or bicycle testing today.

This approach to the electrocardiogram in populations dates back more than 40 years with publication of the Minnesota Code, then devised to compare whole populations by objective measures relevant to ischaemic heart disease yet free of the bias of different clinical customs and terms. The Minnesota Codes were arranged to reflect magnitude of Q, ST, T, and R waves, arrhythmias and blocks, used diagnostically in the clinic, but without giving them disease labels. For epidemiologic comparisons, general validity, objectivity, and repeatability over-ride precise diagnostic accuracy for every individual.

Clearly, however, diagnostic criteria have progressed over the last 40 years and more objective and automated ECG measurements are now possible. But the classifications remain relevant to disease and the opportunity was presented here for predictive analyses through the prolonged follow-up available among entire populations of working middle-aged men in different cultures. Therein lies the strength of this study, showing the universality of ECG prediction in cultures at different overall risk. The limitations are equally clear: from the present more sophisticated diagnoses of coronary disease, as well as from changes over the decades in the nature and severity of coronary disease – and thus changes of the meaning inherent in ECG findings.

SUMMARY AND CONCLUSIONS

Among culturally diverse, representative population samples of middle-aged men followed for 25 years, about 17% showed, at the ages 40-59, clinically silent major or minor resting ECG findings, codable by the Minnesota Code. At the ages of 65-84, more than 50% had these findings. This forms a likely indication that the prevalence of "silent" CHD is very common among middle-aged and elderly men in the western world. Another important finding is that across large geographic-cultural areas the relative risk for a CHD event as a function of silent ECG findings is roughly the same. Despite limitations in comparability of study design, the relative risks reported for common major ECG findings in the literature are comparable to those found among Seven Countries Study areas, which differ greatly in absolute CHD risk. This suggests that the ECG is a universal predictor of *relative risk* for CHD events, similar in strength to, and independent of, the classical cardiovascular disease risk factors. This long-term, population-based international study confirms that clinically silent ECG findings, found casually in systematic surveys, contain predictive information for the individual and add to the profile of risk based on traditional risk factors and thus may help in planning preventive interventions.

REFERENCES

1. Blackburn H, Keys A, Simonson E, Rautaharju P, Punsar S. The electrocardiogram in population studies: a classification system. Circulation 1960;21:1160-1175.
2. Rose G, Blackburn H. Cardiovascular Survey Methods. World Health Organization, Geneva, 1968:1-188.
3. Keys A (Ed). Coronary heart disease in seven countries. Circulation 1970; 41 Suppl 1: 1-211.
4. Menotti A, Mulder I, Kromhout D, Nissinen A, Feskens EJM, Giampaoli S. The association of silent electrocardiographic findings with coronary deaths among elderly men in three European countries. The FINE study. Acta Cardiol 2001; 56: 27-36.

209

4. Dekker J, Schouten EG, Kromhout D, Klootwijk P, Pool J. The Cardiac Infarction Injury Score and coronary heart disease in middle-aged and elderly men: the Zutphen Study. J Clin Epidemiol 1995; 48: 833-840.

6. Dekker J, Schouten EG, Klootwijk P, Pool J, Kromhout D. Association between QT interval and coronary heart disease in middle-aged and elderly men. The Zutphen Study. Circulation 1994; 90: 770-785.

7. Dekker J, Feskens EJ, Schouten EG, Klootwijk P, Pool J, Kromhout D. QTc duration is associated with levels of insulin and glucose intolerance. The Zutphen Elderly Study. Diabetes 1996; 45: 376-380.

8. Dekker J, Schouten EG, Klootwijk P, Pool J, Kromhout D. ST segment and T wave characteristics as indicators of coronary heart disease risk: the Zutphen Study. J Am Coll Cardiol 1995; 25: 1321-1326.

9. Dekker J, Schouten EG, Klootwijk P, Pool J, Swenne CA, Kromhout D. Heart rate variability from short electrocardiographic recordings predicts mortality from all causes in middle-aged and elderly men. The Zutphen Study. Am J Epidemiol 1997; 145: 899-908.

10. Lanti M, Puddu PE, Menotti A. Voltage criteria of left ventricular hypertrophy in sudden and non-sudden coronary artery disease mortality: the Italian section of the Seven Countries Study. Am J Cardiol 1990; 15 : 1181-1185.

11. Rabkin SW, Mathewson FAL, Tate RB. The electrocardiogram in apparently healthy men and the risk of sudden death. Br Heart J 1982;47:546-552.

12. Cullen K, Stenhouse NS, Wearne KL, Cumpston GN. Electrocardiograms and 13-year cardiovascular mortality in the Busselton Study. Br Heart J 1982;47:209-212.

13. Cedres BL, Liu K, Stamler J, Dyer AR, Stamler R, Berkson DM, Paul O, Lepper M, Lindberg HA, Marquardt J, Stevens E, Schoenberger JA, Shekelle RB, Collette P, Garside D. Independent contribution of electrocardiographic abnormalities to risk of death from coronary heart disease, cardiovascular disease and all causes. Findings of three Chicago epidemiologic studies. Circulation 1982;65:146-153.

14. Brand FN, Abbott RD, Kannel WB, Wolf PA. Characteristics and prognosis of lone atrial fibrillation. 30-year follow-up in the Framingham Study. JAMA 1985;254:3449-3453.

15. Liao Y, Liu K, Dyer A, Schoenberger JA, Shekelle RB, Colette P, Stamler J. Major and minor electrocardiographic abnormalities and risk of death from coronary heart disease, cardiovascular diseases and all causes in men and women. J Am Coll Cardiol 1988;12:1494-1500.

16 Levy D, Labib SB, Anderson KM, Christiansen JC, Kannel WB, Castelli WP. Determinants of sensitivity and specificity of electrocardiographic criteria for left ventricular hypertrophy. Circulation 1990;81:1144-1146.

17. Wolf PA, Abbott RD, Kannel WB. Atrial fibrillation as an independent risk factor for stroke: the Framingham Study. Stroke 1991;22:983-988.

18. Kannel WB, Cobb J. Left ventricular hypertrophy and mortality. Results from the Framingham Study. Cardiology 1992;81:291-298.

19. Furberg CD, Manolio T, Psaty BM, Bild DE, Borhani NO, Newman A, Tabatznik B, Rautaharju PM. Major electrocardiographic abnormalities in persons aged 65 years and older (the Cardiovascular Health Study). Cardiovascular Health Study Collaborative Research Group. Am J Cardiol 1992; 69: 1329-1335

20. Sutherland SE, Gazes PC, Keil JE, Gilbert GE, Knapp RG. Electrocardiographic abnormalities and 30-year mortality among white and black men of the Charleston Heart Study. Circulation 1993;88:2685-2692.

21. De Bacquer D, Martins-Pereira LS, De Backer G, De Henauw S, Kornitzer M. The predictive value of electrocardiographic abnormalities for total and cardiovascular disease mortality in men and women. Eur Heart J 1994;15:1604-1610.

22. Iacovino JR. Mortality analysis of complete right and left bundle branch block in a selected community population. J Insur Med 1997; 29: 91-99.

23. Greenland P, Xie X, Liao Y, Daviglus M, Walsh M, Stamler J. Isolated nonspecific resting ECG ST and/or T abnormalities predict 22-year risk of cardiovascular death in men and

women: the Chicago Heart Association Detection Project in Industry [abstract]. Can J Cardiol 1997;13 Suppl B:372.

24. Menotti A, Seccareccia F and the RIFLE Research Group. Electrocardiographic Minnesota Code findings predicting short term mortality in asymptomatic subjects. The Italian RIFLE Pooling Project (Risk Factors and Life Expectancy) G Ital Cardiol 1997;27:40-49.

25. De Bruyne MC, Mosterd A, Hoes AW, Kors JA, Kruijssen DA, Van Bemmel JH, Hofman A, Grobbee DE. Prevalence, determinants, and misclassification of myocardial infarction in the elderly. Epidemiol 1997; 8: 495-500.

26. De Bacquer D, De Backer G, Kornitzer M, Myny K, Doyen Z, Blackburn H. Prognostic value of ischemic electrocardiographic findings for cardiovascular mortality in men and women. J Am Coll Cardiol 1999;33:1491-1498.

27. Ashley, EA, Raxwal VK, Froelicher VF. The prevalence and prognostic significance of electrocardiographic abnormalities. Probl Cardiol 2000;21:1-72.

28. Wilhelmsen L, Bjure J, Ekstrom-Jodal, B, Aurell M, Grimby G, Scardsudd K, Tibblin G, Wedel H. Nine years' follow-up of a maximal exercise test in random population sample of middle-aged men. Cardiology 1981; 68 Suppl 2: 1-8.

29. Bruce RA, Hossack KF, DeRouen TA, Hofer V. Enhanced risk assessment for primary coronary heart disease events by maximal exercise testing: 10 years' experience of Seattle Heart Watch. J Am Coll Cardiol 1983; 2: 565-573.

30. Rautaharju PM, Prineas RJ, Eifler WJ, Furberg CD, Neaton JD, Crow RS, Stamler J, Cutler JA for the MRFIT Research Group. Prognostic value of exercise electrocardiogram in men at high risk of future coronary heart disease: Multiple Risk Factor Intervention Trial experience. J Am Coll Cardiol 1986; 8: 1- 10

31. Bruce RA, Fisher LD. Exercise-enhanced assessment of risk factors for coronary heart disease in healthy men. J Electrocardiography 1987; 20 Suppl: 162-166.

32. Rautaharju PM, Neaton JD. Electrocardiographic abnormalities and coronary heart disease mortality among hypertensive men in the Multiple Risk Factor Intervention Trial. Clin Invest Med 1987; 10: 606-615.

33. Ekelund LG, Suchindran CM, McMahon RP, Heiss G, Leon AS, Romhilt DW, Rubenstein CL, Probstfield JL, Ruwitch JF. Coronary heart disease morbidity and mortality in hypercholesterolemic men predicted from an exercise test: the Lipid Research Clinics Coronary Primary Prevention Trial. J Am Coll Cardiol 1989; 14: 556-563.

34. Siscovick DS, Ekelund LG, Johnson JL, Troung Y, Adler A. Sensitivity of exercise electrocardiography for acute cardiac events during moderate and strenuous physical activity. The Lipid Research Clinics Coronary Primary Prevention Trial. Arch Intern Med 1991; 151: 325-330.

35. Pedersen F, Sandoe E, Laekerborg A. Prevalence and significance of an abnormal exercise ECG in asymptomatic males. Outcome of thallium myocardial scintigraphy. Eur Heart J 1991; 12: 766-769.

36. Fleg JL. Prevalence and prognostic significance of exercise-induced silent myocardial ischemia in apparently healthy subjects. Am J Cardiol 1992; 69: 14B-18B.

CHAPTER 3.6

MULTIVARIATE ANALYSIS OF MAJOR RISK FACTORS AND CORONARY HEART DISEASE RISK IN THE SEVEN COUNTRIES STUDY

Alessandro Menotti

Multivariate analytical techniques in the Seven Countries Study were first made using cross- classifications compacted by the Mantel-Haenszel method (1). This used multiple cells in a cross- classification to take into account several risk factors simultaneously (each subdivided into a few classes) in relation to an outcome variable, such as mortality from CHD. Observed and expected cases were computed for a summary chi-square with one degree of freedom. Variances were calculated of the number of cases (events) in specified classes from sums of the expected and observed cases. However, cross-classification of risk factors became increasingly difficult with a greater number of risk factors, so a new approach was needed in multivariate analysis.

The Framingham Study led in development of the multiple logistic function for predicting morbid or fatal events. A milestone first paper on this technique was published in 1967 (2), and other relevant reports came later (3,4). The multiple logistic function has the advantage of treating the dependent variable (the event) as a probability. Mathematically speaking, the multiple logistic function represents the extension to many risk factors of the computation of odds ratios derived from simple 2 x 2 contingency tables.

The Seven Countries Study has had a unique opportunity to compare risk functions derived from populations differing in geography, culture, risk factor levels and burden of morbid and fatal events that started with the 5-year follow-up data (5). Moreover, it was the first study to produce the back application of risk functions from one population to risk factor distributions of another, and to evaluate the precision and force of different risk estimates – absolute vs. relative.

With the prolongation of the Seven Countries Study follow-up period beyond 10-15 years, it became necessary to use the Cox proportional hazards model (6), which is based on life table principles. In fact, the multiple logistic function does not take into account the time elapsed between measurement of risk factors and events and the same weight is given to persons who die early or late after the measurement of the risk factors. When the follow-up period is prolonged, the number of subjects with events not related to the one explored in the analysis increases largely. The problem is what to do with these events. If these cases are excluded from the computation, the structure of the population is crippled, and if they are left in the model, the predictive power of risk factors can be distorted (usually diluted) if they are also associated with events of primary interest. The Cox proportional hazard model requires the date for each event, and assumes that the risk is proportionate for different levels of risk factors. Tests are performed to show that this assumption is met, and the shape of the function is non-parametric, since no parameters are included to describe the function itself.

Most recently, attempts have been made to use the accelerated failure-time model, that is, a log-linear model incorporating the Weibull distribution (7), which includes parameters defining the shape of the risk function. This model allows us to follow with time the possibly changing shape and acceleration (or deceleration), of the hazard. An example of this model is given in the chapter on mortality. In this chapter an overview will be given of the results of multivariate analyses in predicting CHD risk performed during the course of the follow-up.

MULTIVARIATE ANALYSES ON 5-YEAR FOLLOW-UP DATA

After 5 years of follow-up, the logistic function was used to analyze the relationships between risk factors and CHD incidence and mortality (5). However, risk functions were not produced, while tests were made using a solution derived from the Framingham Study. The approach was to have a balance, applying the coefficients of the multiple logistic function derived from the Framingham Study to the risk factor distribution of the different cohorts. Thus, the estimated absolute risk for CHD incidence in different cultures could be compared with the absolute risk measured. This analysis was, however, approximate, since the Framingham Study used different criteria in defining endpoints (e.g. CHD incidence), measured different risk factors and employed different lengths of follow-up.

The comparison of predicted versus observed rates in the Seven Countries Study, based on the application of the Framingham coefficients, led to an underestimate of CHD incidence for the Finnish and the U.S. railroad cohorts, and to a systematic overestimate of CHD incidence for all other European population groups. When an analysis was done using the ratio of incidence for hard criteria CHD and angina pectoris for Framingham men compared to the rate for U.S. railroad men (the population thought to be most similar to Framingham), the correlation coefficient between observed and expected cases in the 13 European cohorts was good ($r = 0.83$). This approximate approach prompted the need to produce risk functions based on the true experience of the populations in different Seven Countries Study populations.

In a subsequent paper published in 1972, systematic risk functions were produced using the multiple logistic function separately for the U.S. railroad cohort and for the pool of the 13 European cohorts (8). This grouping was needed because of the small number of events in the first 5 years of follow-up. Separate functions were solved for two endpoints, hard CHD events (coronary death and definite myocardial infarction) and any CHD events (any coronary manifestation including hard events and possible myocardial infarction, angina pectoris, etc). Risk factors considered in the analysis were age, systolic blood pressure, serum cholesterol, smoking habits, and Body Mass Index (BMI). In general, all the risk factors were significantly related to CHD, except for BMI. Moreover, in Europe, smoking habits were of borderline significance in relation to CHD. The strength of the association was larger for the severe cases classified as hard CHD events than for the group of any CHD events that also included "softer events". Solutions for hard CHD events are reported in Table 1. Coefficients for the same risk factor in the U.S. railroad cohort are similar to those in the pool of the European cohorts; for none of the pairs were statistically significant differences detected. The magnitude of the intercepts suggested a larger absolute risk in the U.S. railroad, everything else being equal. A statistical comparison could not be made for the intercept since standard errors were not available.

The next step in this analysis was to re-apply the intercept and the coefficients to the risk factor levels of the same populations to rank the estimated risk from the lowest to the highest, to divide the distribution into decile classes, and to compare estimated cases with observed cases. The correlation coefficients were high between observed and expected cases in the decile classes; the proportion of observed cases in the top decile was always elevated (for hard CHD events, 29.5% in the U.S. railroad, and 34.6 % in the European pool). The ratio (relative risk) between observed cases in the top quintile and the bottom quintile of the distribution of estimated risk was 19.0

Table 1. Solutions of the multiple logistic function predicting hard CHD in 5 years, as a function of five risk factors in CHD-free men at entry examination. Reconstructed and modified from reference 8.

Risk factor	U.S. railroad Denominator=2404 Events=78		European pool Denominator=8728 Events=136		Difference between coefficients
	Coeff.	*t*-test	Coeff.	*t*-test	*t*-test
Age (y)	0.063	3.00	0.078	4.88	-0.57
Systolic BP (mm Hg)	0.025	4.17	0.020	4.00	0.64
Cholesterol (mg/dl)	0.009	3.00	0.010	5.00	-0.28
Smoking habits[a]	0.230	3.38	0.103	1.94	1.47
BMI (kg/m^2)	-0.023	-0.62	0.016	0.62	-0.86
Constant	-13.132	-	-14.203	-	-

a = Never-smoker =3; ex-smoker = 4; current smoker < 5 cigarettes per day = 5; current smoker 5-9 cigarettes per day = 6; current smoker 10-19 cigarettes per day = 6; current smoker 20-29 cigarettes per day = 7; current smoker 30 + cigarettes per day = 8.

for hard CHD and 6.5 for any CHD in the U.S. railroad cohort, and 15.0 for hard CHD and 8.2 for any CHD in the European pool. These few data suggested a satisfactory fit to the model in both groups, and good distinction between cases and non-cases (actually between high and low risk subgroups, as estimated by the model).

The most interesting section of this analysis for the investigators dealt with the crossover of multivariate solutions with risk factor distributions of other groups in an attempt to estimate the predictive power of one population experience versus others. Despite some differences, relative risk was estimated satisfactorily when a solution derived from a different population was used, whereas the absolute risk was grossly over- or underestimated. In this particular case, solutions from the U.S. population overestimated CHD risk in European populations.

Similar computations were made using the four-pool population employed in the U.S. Coronary Pooling Project (populations from Framingham, Albany, and two Chicago population studies) (9). In this case, overestimation of absolute risk was 1.41 for the U.S. railroad and 2.14 for the European pool, still providing, however, a satisfactory estimate of relative risk.

MULTIVARIATE ANALYSIS OF 10- AND 15-YEAR FOLLOW-UP DATA

The analysis of the 10-year follow-up data confirmed the first 5-year experience (10). However, larger numbers of events allowed more refined groupings of populations and sharper conclusions. A comparison between solutions of the multiple logistic function derived from the northern and southern European areas in the prediction of any CHD events (as a function of six risk factors, see Table 2) suggests that major risk factors were significantly related to events in both areas (except smoking habits in southern Europe). Again, the coefficients were not statistically different between the two areas despite the large difference in absolute risk and average risk factor levels. The ratios of expected versus observed cases in decile classes, obtained by applying the solution of one area to the risk factor distribution of the other, again produced an overestimated incidence when the northern European solution was

Table 2. Solutions of the multiple logistic function predicting any CHD in 10 years, as a function of six risk factors in CHD-free men at entry examination. Derived and modified from reference 10.

Risk factor	N.European pool		S.European pool		Diff coeff
	Coeff	*t*-test	Coeff	*t*-test	*t*-test
Age (y)	0.0979	6.08	0.0585	6.63	1.73
Systolic BP (mm Hg)	0.0202	5.18	0.0113	2.97	1.63
Cholesterol (mg/dl)	0.0054	3.60	0.0041	2.16	0.54
Smoking habits[a]	0.1322	2.60	0.0063	0.13	1.80
Heart rate (b/min)	0.0017	0.27	0.0109	1.98	-1.09
Physical activity[b]	-0.0759	-0.67	-0.0683	-0.62	-0.05
Constant	-12.2715	-9.91	-9.3925	8.47	-1.73

a = Never-smoker =3; ex-smoker = 4; current smoker < 5 cigarettes per day = 5; current smoker 5-9 cigarettes per day = 6; current smoker 10-19 cigarettes per day = 6; current smoker 20-29 cigarettes per day = 7; current smoker 30 + cigarettes per day = 8.
b = sedentary = 1; moderately active = 2; very active = 3

applied to the southern European risk. On the other hand, a solution for CHD mortality obtained from the U.S. railroad cohort applied to the northern European risk factor levels was associated with a ratio very close to one.

The analysis of the 10-year prediction of incidence in the northern and southern European areas showed a crude risk ratio of about 2.69 for hard CHD events between the two areas. However, this became about 1.5 when the northern European models were applied to the southern European cohorts (11). About 56% of the difference in incidence is "due to" the difference in the main risk factor levels, since the magnitude of multivariate coefficients was similar in the two areas. More information on this will be given in the chapter on " Risk factors as predictors of global coronary risk in preventive and clinical cardiology". Similar conclusions were reached, with an estimate of about 50% (12), in a previous analysis done according to the method of Lee (13). This produces covariance adjustment of rates based on the multiple logistic regression model.

A systematic inter-area comparison was made using the multiple logistic function and six risk factors as predictors (age, systolic blood pressure, serum cholesterol, smoking habits, BMI and physical activity), and the 15-year CHD mortality data (14). Table 3 shows that:

- solutions from northern Europe and the U.S. overestimate absolute risk in southern Europe and Japan;
- solutions from southern Europe and Japan strongly underestimate the risk in northern Europe and the U.S.;
- solutions from southern Europe overestimate the risk in Japan;
- solutions from Japan underestimate risk in the other three areas;
- solutions from northern Europe produce a good estimate of risk in the U.S.;
- solutions from U.S. produce a good estimate or risk in northern Europe.

Table 3. Summary of cross- application of multiple logistic solutions for CHD deaths to risk factor levels of different populations based on 15-year follow-up data. Derived from reference 14.

Solution from	Predicting CHD deaths in	Expected / observed ratio
U.S.A.	Northern Europe	1.04
U.S.A.	Southern Europe	1.92
U.S.A.	Japan	4.54
Northern Europe	U.S.A.	0.99
Northern Europe	Southern Europe	1.89
Northern Europe	Japan	4.54
Southern Europe	U.S.A.	0.76
Southern Europe	Northern Europe	0.53
Southern Europe	Japan	2.17
Japan	U.S.A.	0.09
Japan	Northern Europe	0.06
Japan	Southern Europe	0.20

It should be noted that the solution from Japan was unstable since it was based on only 10 CHD deaths in 15 years, and none of the risk factors was significantly associated with CHD risk.

The 15-year mortality data on CHD in northern and southern Europe were also used for a complex logistic model providing information on age, period, area, prevalence of CHD at entry and some interaction terms (12). "Area" stands for northern or southern Europe (codes 1 and 0); "period 1" is the first 5 years of follow-up (reference), "period 2" the second 5 years and "period 3" the third 5 years of follow-up. "Prevalence" is the presence of any cardiovascular manifestation at the start of each period, and "age" was expressed in years at the beginning of each 5-year period. Some interaction terms were also considered (e.g. cholesterol∗age, prevalence∗period, age∗area, systolic blood pressure∗area, smoking habits∗period, smoking habits∗age). Altogether 7,163 subjects entered in the analysis produced 406 CHD deaths during the three periods, corresponding to a total of 18,548 person-periods.

The following results were obtained:

- serum cholesterol and systolic blood pressure were strongly associated with risk, despite the presence of interaction terms;
- smoking habits were not associated with risk when the interaction terms smoking∗period and smoking∗age were included in the model;
- area, age, and prevalence, but not period, were individually associated with risk;
- people in northern Europe were at higher risk than those in southern Europe for similar levels of risk factors;
- older people were at higher risk than younger people;
- people with prevalent cardiovascular manifestations at entry ran a higher risk than initially healthy subjects, but this risk decreased with the period;
- risk increased with age, but more in northern Europe than in southern Europe;
- risk associated with cholesterol decreased with increasing age in both northern and southern Europe, despite the increasing levels of serum cholesterol;

218

- risk associated with smoking habits decreased with increasing age, but to be a smoker in the second and third period implies a greater risk than in the first period;
- blood pressure was likely a more important risk factor in southern Europe than in northern Europe, although the interaction term systolic blood pressure*area had a p-value of 0.10.

The previously mentioned model was preceded by the construction of a basic model, followed by a step-wise inclusion of interaction terms. Practically at each step, there was an improvement of the global chi-square, although not always statistically significant. Coefficients for serum cholesterol and systolic blood pressure became larger in the final model, compared to the basic one, despite the entry of interaction terms involving the same factors.

MULTIVARIATE ANALYSIS OF THE 25-YEAR FOLLOW-UP DATA

The availability of 20-year (15) and 25-year (16) follow-up data on mortality for all the cohorts coincided with the widespread use of the Cox proportional hazard model that came to be preferred for studies with a long follow-up period. A systematic analysis on 25-year CHD mortality for all the available data and four major risk factors (age, cholesterol, systolic blood pressure, and cigarette consumption) using this model was conducted for each country, pooling cohorts of the same country (17). Eight entities instead of seven countries were considered, since

Table 4. Solutions for the multivariate Cox proportional hazards model predicting 25-year CHD mortality in eight entities. Derived from reference 17.

Country	Age (y) RR	Cholesterol (mg/dl) RR	Systolic BP (mm Hg) RR	Cigarettes (No/day) RR
U.S.A.	1.27	1.31	1.35	1.38
95%CI	1.16 – 1.40	1.21 – 1.41	1.23 – 1.47	1.25 – 1.53
Finland	1.33	1.22	1.45	1.26
95%CI	1.21 –1.48	1.13 – 1.32	1.30 – 1.61	1.14 – 1.38
Netherlands	1.60	1.19	1.40	1.13
95%CI	1.35 – 1.89	1.03 – 1.37	1.02 – 1.60	0.94 – 1.36
Italy	1.49	1.26	1.46	1.17
95%CI	1.28 – 1.74	1.10 – 1.45	1.22 – 1.67	1.02 – 1.34
Croatia	1.19	1.20	1.25	1.17
95%CI	0.97 – 1.46	0.98 – 1.45	1.02 – 1.53	0.95 – 1.44
Serbia	1.19	1.20	1.21	1.11
95%CI	1.01 – 1.40	1.01 – 1.43	0.99 – 1.46	0.97 – 1.27
Greece	1.42	1.67	1.21	1.25
95%CI	1.05 – 1.93	1.30 – 2.16	0.89 – 1.65	0.98 – 1.59
Japan	1.15	1.04	1.55	1.70
95%CI	0.80 – 1.65	0.65 – 1.56	1.19 – 2.01	1.23 – 2.35

RR is relative risk expressed as hazard ratio for the following differences in risk factor levels: 5 years for age; 40 mg/dl for cholesterol; 20 mm Hg for systolic blood pressure; 10 cigarettes smoked per day. CI = Confidence interval former Yugoslavia was split into Croatia and Serbia. Attention was focused on the comparison of multivariate coefficients for the different entities. A summary is presented in Table 4.

Most risk ratios were statistically significant for each entity. A systematic comparison among all possible pairs of coefficients revealed significant differences in 4 out of 28 cases for age (usually the coefficient for the Netherlands was greater than in other areas); in 5 out 28 cases for serum cholesterol (the coefficient for Greece was larger than for the majority of the other areas), and in 4 out of 28 cases for cigarette smoking (usually the coefficient for Japan was greater than for other areas). However, in not one case out of 28 were the coefficients for systolic blood pressure statistically different. This overall situation was confirmed by a test of heterogeneity on the coefficients, using the technique of Dyer (18). The hypothesis that all coefficients were similar could not be rejected, with the exception of smoking. When Japan was excluded, the coefficients for smoking were homogeneous. Similar conclusions were reached using the test of log-likelihood in a model with interaction terms (factor＊entity). In this analysis (with 8 statistical units corresponding to the 8 entities) there was no statistically significant correlation between the magnitude of each multivariate coefficient, and the 25-year CHD death rate. This means that these two variables are independent of each other.

Table 5. Solution of the Cox proportional hazards model predicting CHD death in 25 years in 5 areas of 3 countries, as a function of 12 risk factors and a dummy variable identifying the countries. Reconstructed and modified from reference 19.

Factors	Coeff.	SE	*t*-value
Age (y)	0.0818	0.0074	11.02
Mean blood pressure (mm Hg)[a]	0.0273	0.0026	10.29
Serum cholesterol (mg/dl)	0.0050	0.0007	6.93
Cigarettes (no. per day)	0.0181	0.0036	5.09
Physical activity[b]	-0.1814	0.0589	-3.08
Mid-arm muscle circumference (cm)[c]	-0.0480	0.0240	-2.00
Shoulder / pelvis shape (ratio of diameters)[d]	-0.0086	0.0049	-1.74
Trunk/height ratio[e]	0.0429	0.0262	1.64
Heart rate (beats per min)	0.0042	0.0029	1.46
Laterality – linearity index (ratio)[f]	0.0350	0.0252	1.39
Body Mass Index (kg/m$^{2)}$	0.0085	0.0243	0.35
Sum of two skinfold thicknesses (mm) [g]	-0.0047	0.0063	-0.74
Physical activity (score of 3 levels)	-0.1814	0.0589	-3.08
Dummy Italy vs. Finland	-0.4371	0.1063	-4.11
Dummy The Netherlands vs. Finland	-0.3235	0.1172	-2.76

a = Diastolic + 1/3 (systolic – diastolic)
b = sedentary = 1; moderately active = 2; very active = 3
c = circumference minus the contribution of skin and subcutaneous tissue.
d = Ratio of bi-acromial over bi-cristal diameter
e = Height of trunk (taken in sitting position) over height taken in standing position
f = Sum of bi-acromial and bi-cristal diameters / height * 100
g = Tricipital and subscapular skinfold thickness

Systematic and comparable analyses were carried out on 25-year CHD deaths, calculated with the Cox proportional hazards model and employing many more risk factors. These analyses were reserved for the pool of the Finnish areas (rural Finland), the Dutch cohort of Zutphen, and the pool of the two rural Italian areas (rural Italy) (19). Despite disparities in solutions dealing with single cohorts or single countries, a pooled solution was published, as reconstructed in Table 5. Beyond the traditional predictors, such as age, blood pressure (average blood pressure in this case), serum cholesterol and smoking habits, other risk factors were tested. Among them, only job-related physical activity and right-arm muscle circumference were statistically significant, both with a negative sign, suggesting a protective role in the occurrence of CHD death. BMI, skinfold thicknesses, three composite anthropometric indices, and resting heart rate were not significantly related to events. In this solution, the dummy variables identifying the countries involved provided another tool for the estimate of differences in absolute CHD risk, everything else being equal. In particular, belonging to an Italian cohort, as estimated by the exponential of the dummy coefficient, means carrying a risk of 0.65, compared to the Finland reference of 1.0, while belonging to the Dutch cohort means carrying a risk of 0.72 compared to Finland. Both Italian and Dutch men were "protected" from CHD fatal events in comparison with the Finnish men, everything else being equal.

MULTIVARIATE PREDICTION OF 10-YEAR CHD DEATH IN THE ELDERLY

Data from five cohorts of three European countries, with men aged 65 to 84 years at baseline, were used to study the relationship between risk factors and CHD death in the elderly. Men with prevalent heart disease, or those on anti-hypertensive medication, identified by dichotomic codes, were kept in the model, since both conditions are common at that age. The endpoint was CHD death during the next 10 years of follow-up. The multiple logistic model was used, taking competing causes of death in account (20). This risk function was developed for physicians to predict risk of individual patients.

The final model suggests a complex situation (Table 6). Out of nine risk factors or conditions, age, serum total cholesterol, left ventricular hypertrophy, and CHD prevalence were the only factors significantly associated with CHD mortality. HDL cholesterol, systolic blood pressure, smoking habits, diabetes, and the use of anti-hypertensive medication were not significantly associated. For the Italian elderly men unexplained interactions were found, that is, a positive interaction with anti-hypertensive medication (which therefore seems harmful) and a negative interaction with prevalent CHD present at entry (being protective). Finally, the dummy variables identifying the countries suggest protection in the Netherlands and in Italy, compared to Finland as reference. All this reiterates the usual picture when comparing different cultures within Europe, but poses the problem of the lower predictive power of some risk factors when measured in the elderly, with the increasing role of morbid pre-existing conditions such as CHD or common ECG abnormalities (left ventricular hypertrophy).

Table 6. Solution of the multiple logistic model for the prediction of CHD deaths in 10 years in elderly men aged 65-84 years at entry from Finland, Italy, and the Netherlands. Modified from reference (20).

Factor	Coefficient	Relative risk	95 % CI
Age (1 year)	0.0682	1.07	1.04–1.10
Total cholesterol (1 mmol / l)	0.2146	1.24	1.11–1.38
HDL cholesterol (1 mmol / l)	-0.1842	0.83	0.54–1.27
Systolic blood pressure (10 mm Hg)	0.0014	1.01	0.94–1.07
Smoking habits (no / yes)	0.2140	1.24	0.91–1.69
Diabetes (no / yes)	0.0765	1.08	0.67–1.74
Left ventricular hypertrophy (no / yes)	0.6842	1.98	1.30–3.02
Anti-hypertensive medication (no / yes)	-0.0515	0.95	0.63–1.42
Anti-hypertensive medication*Italy (no/yes)	1.2741	3.58	1.72–7.43
Prevalent case (no/yes)	1.4291	4.18	3.05–5.71
Prevalent case*Italy (no/yes)	-1.1495	0.32	0.13–0.77
Dummy The Netherlands (no/yes)	-0.6264	0.53	0.40–0.72
Dummy Italy (no/yes)	-1.2469	0.29	0.16–0.50
Dummy Finland (Reference)	-	-	-
Constant	-7.9578	-	-

CONFOUNDING VARIABLES AND THE "SATURATION EFFECT" IN MULTIVARIATE PREDICTION

In several multivariate approaches it was shown that some risk factors, i.e. BMI and skinfold thickness, were not significantly predictive of CHD events when other major risk factors, such as age, blood pressure, serum cholesterol, and smoking habits were included in the model (10,21). For example, the coefficients for BMI were never statistically significant. Nor did the addition of this variable in the model produce change in discrimination between observed and expected cases in decile classes of estimated risk. Conversely, the deletion of this variable from the model did not decrease the coefficient of the major risk factors. This suggested that the association between BMI and CHD was confounded by the presence of other variables, such as blood pressure, cholesterol, and smoking. This meant, in turn, that the weak association of elevated levels of BMI seen in univariate analysis was simply a reflection of elevated levels of other factors, whose levels are associated with BMI.

This explanation probably applies to many potential risk factors whose independent role in prediction is marginal. Another example is the addition of diastolic blood pressure in a model already containing systolic blood pressure. In that case, diastolic blood pressure contributed nothing to the prediction of CHD, simply because the extra information carried by diastolic blood pressure is already contained in systolic blood pressure. In fact, the correlation coefficient between systolic and diastolic blood pressure is usually around $0.6 - 0.7$.

A specific analysis inspecting this problem was carried out using 5-year CHD incidence data of the rural cohorts of Finland and Italy (22). The analysis anticipated principles of backward stepwise procedures before they became available in commercial statistical packages. Multiple logistic models were computed separately for the two areas and four endpoints (CHD deaths, hard CHD, soft CHD, any CHD) with 14 risk factors as possible predictors. For each area-endpoint group, 14 different solutions were computed, starting with 14 risk factors, moving to 13, etc, deleting each time the factor that was weakest in prediction, based on the t-value of the coefficient. The use of empirical indicators of discrimination showed that the presence in the models of more than about eight risk factors was not associated with a better discrimination. There was a clear indication that among factors available in this study, there is no advantage in using more than eight properly selected risk factors in order to obtain the best possible discrimination.

COMMENTS

The main findings of multivariate analysis in the Seven Countries Study are similar to those of other population studies, but add knowledge on the cross-application of predictive functions from one population to another. Relative risks for major risk factors were found to be similar, but the absolute risks differed and were high in U.S.A. and northern Europe compared with southern Europe and Japan.

Multivariate analysis confirmed the powerful and independent role of those characteristics, usually called major risk factors (age, blood pressure, serum cholesterol, and smoking habits). This was basically true in all cultures and cohorts, although the small numbers involved, even in the 25-year follow-up data, probably prevented some coefficients from becoming statistically significant in smaller cohorts. The magnitude and significance of multivariate coefficients were stronger for the harder endpoints. The strongest associations were observed for CHD deaths, intermediate for hard CHD events, and the weakest for any CHD events.

Through the use of the multiple logistic function, the fit of the data to the models was satisfactory when judged according to the levels of log-likelihood ratios and the high correlation between observed and expected cases in decile classes of estimated risk. The relative risks between decile 10 and decile 1 were high (sometimes even around 10), as well as the relative risk between quintile 5 and quintile 1 of the estimated risk. These relative risks were larger for most severe CHD manifestations than for the softer, less severe CHD manifestations, reflecting the magnitude and significance of the multivariate coefficients.

Among risk factors other than the four major ones, a few emerged as independent predictors. However, this was only true in some analyses, or in some areas, or for some endpoints; it was not necessarily universal. An independent inverse predictive role was frequently, if not always, seen for job-related physical activity, physical fitness (resting heart rate), and mid-arm circumference. Prevalent cases showing cardiovascular disease at the entry examination had an increased risk from CHD during different periods of follow-up. The relative risk of the risk factors measured in elderly men was lower than in middle-aged men. The use of more than 6 or 8 risk factors failed to improve the discrimination of cases versus non-cases.

The issue that was almost unique in the early analysis of the Seven Countries Study was the discovery that the magnitude of multivariate coefficients was practically the same in all cultures, entities, and cohorts. The magnitude of coefficients was not correlated with population levels of risk factors, or with incidence of and mortality from CHD. This suggests a universal biological rule for the relationship between risk factor levels and the risk of CHD events in populations. Despite this, different populations have different levels of *absolute* risk for the same levels of risk factors, suggesting the existence of unmeasured or unknown factors explaining the residual difference. All this means is that applying a risk function from one population to risk-factor distributions of another produces good estimates of relative risk, but usually poor estimates of absolute risk. This introduces an overestimation of CHD risk using the northern European or North American risk functions in the southern European or Japanese populations.

Direct comparisons of multivariate functions derived from this study with those from others suffer the usual limitations of the different measurement techniques for the risk factors, different age ranges, length of follow-up, and diagnostic criteria. However, the similarity in the magnitude of multivariate coefficients is noted in comparing the four-pool populations of the U.S. Pooling Project (9). Incidentally, within the U.S. population samples studied in this project, the cross application of multivariate risk functions produced satisfactory estimates of both relative and absolute risk.

In a review paper from 1990 (23), risk functions for CHD derived in many studies from all over the world were compared, including those from the Seven Countries Study. The authors have reached the conclusion, although with much caution and uncertainty, that these models are similar, producing similar coefficients for the main risk factors and similar relative risks, while absolute risks are different.

SUMMARY AND CONCLUSIONS

Multivariate analyses have frequently been used in the Seven Countries Study, starting from simple cross-classifications, and then, depending on the length of follow-up analyzed time by time, moving on to the use of the multiple logistic function, the Cox proportional hazards model, and the accelerated failure-time model. These analyses showed that universal risk factors such as age, blood pressure, serum cholesterol, and smoking habits, are strong predictors of CHD in all cultures explored in the study. Other factors, such as job-related physical activity, resting heart rate, and mid-arm circumference, played a lesser role, usually only in some cultures. The combination of a few risk factors in multivariate models established large differences in relative risks between subgroups with high and low levels of risk factors. The Seven Countries Study showed that the strength of the association of risk factors with CHD incidence and death is similar in all populations, probably reflecting a universal rule in linking risk factors levels to disease. On the other hand, for the same levels of major risk factors, actual incidence and mortality differed largely among cultures, suggesting the existence of unmeasured or unknown factors to explain the residual difference. Unfortunately, some potential factors to explain part of this difference, such as dietary habits, could not be used in multivariate analyses, since individual information on diet was not universally available. Risk functions derived from North American and northern European cohorts overestimated the risk in southern Europe and Japan; solutions from southern European and Japanese cohorts underestimated the actual risk in northern Europe and North America.

REFERENCES

1. Mantel N. Chi-square test with one degree of freedom: extensions of the Mantel-Haenszel procedure. J Am Stat Assoc 1963; 58: 690-700.
2. Truett J, Cornfield J, Kannel W. A multivariate analysis of the risk of coronary heart disease in Framingham. J Chron Dis 1967; 20: 511-524.

3. Walker SH, Duncan DB. Estimation of the probability of an event as a function of several independent variables. Biometrika 1967; 54: 167-179.

4. Gordon T, Kannel WB, Halperin M. Predictability of coronary heart disease. J Chron Dis 1979; 32: 427-440.

5. Keys A (Ed). Coronary heart disease in seven countries. Circulation 1970; 41 Suppl 1: 1-211.

6. Cox DR. Regression models and life tables. J Roy Stat Soc 1972; B43: 187-220.

7. Afifi AA, Clark V. Computer aided multivariate analysis. Van Nostrand Reinhold Co. New York, 1990:1-505.

8. Keys A, Aravanis C, Blackburn H, Van Buchem FSP, Buzina R, Djordjevic BS, Fidanza F, Karvonen M, Menotti A, Puddu V, Taylor HL. Probability of middle aged men developing coronary heart disease in five years. Circulation 1972;45: 815-828.

9. Pooling Project Research Group. Relationship of blood pressure, serum cholesterol, smoking habits, relative body weight and ECG abnormalities to incidence of major coronary events. Final Report of the Pooling Project. J Chron Dis 1978;31:201-306.

10. Keys A, Aravanis C, Blackburn H, Buzina R, Djordjevic BS, Dontas AS, Fidanza F, Karvonen MJ, Kimura N, Menotti A, Mohacek I, Nedeljkovic S, Puddu V, Punsar S, Taylor HL, Van Buchem FSP. Seven Countries. A multivariate analysis of death and coronary heart disease. Harvard University Press, Cambridge MA 1980:1-381.

11. Menotti A, Lanti M, Puddu PE, Kromhout D. Coronary heart disease incidence in northern and southern European populations: a reanalysis of the Seven Countries Study for a European coronary risk chart. Heart 2000; 84: 238-244.

12. Mariotti S, Capocaccia R, Farchi G, Menotti A, Verdecchia A, Keys A. Age, period, cohort and geographical areas effects of the relationship between risk factors and coronary heart disease mortality. 15-year follow-up of the European cohorts of the Seven Countries Study. J Chron Dis 1986; 39: 229-242.

13. Lee J. Covariance adjustment of rates based on the multiple logistic regression model. J Chron Dis 1981; 34: 415-426.

14. Keys A,. Menotti A, Aravanis C, Blackburn H, Djordjevic BS, Buzina R, Dontas A, Fidanza F, Karvonen MJ, Kimura N, Mohacek I, Nedeljkovic S, Puddu V, Punsar S, Taylor HL, Conti S, Kromhout D, Toshima H. The Seven Countries Study: 2289 deaths in 15 years. Prev Med 1984, 13 : 141-154.

15. Menotti A, Keys A, Aravanis C, Blackburn H, Dontas A, Fidanza F, Karvonen MJ, Kromhout D, Nedeljkovic S, Nissinen A, Pekkanen J, Punsar S, Seccareccia F, Toshima H. Seven Countries Study. First 20 year mortality data in 12 cohorts of the Seven Countries. Ann Med 1989, 21: 175-179.

16. Menotti A, Keys A, Kromhout D, Blackburn H, Aravanis C, Bloemberg B, Buzina R, Dontas A, Fidanza F, Giampaoli S, Karvonen M, Lanti M, Pekkanen J, Punsar S, Seccareccia F, Toshima H. Inter-cohort differences in coronary heart disease mortality in the 25-year follow-up of the Seven Countries Study. Eur J Epidemiol 1993, 9: 527-536.

17. Menotti A, Keys A, Blackburn H, Kromhout D, Karvonen M, Nissinen A, Pekkanen J, Punsar S, Fidanza F, Giampaoli S, Seccareccia F, Buzina R, Mohacek I, Nedeljkovic S, Aravanis C, Dontas A, Toshima H, Lanti M. Comparison of multivariate predictive power of major risk factors for coronary heart disease in different countries: results from eight nations of the Seven Countries Study, 25-year follow-up. J Cardiov Risk 1996; 3: 69-75.

18. Dyer AR. A method for combining results from several prospective epidemiologial studies. Stat Med 1986; 5: 303-317.

19. Menotti A, Keys A, Kromhout D, Nissinen A, Blackburn H, Fidanza F, Giampaoli S, Karvonen M, Pekkanen J, Punsar S, Seccareccia F. Twenty-five year mortality from coronary heart disease and its prediction in five cohorts of middle aged men in Finland, the Netherlands and Italy. Prev Med 1990;19: 270-278.

20. Houterman S, Boshuizen HC, Verschuren WM, Giampaoli S, Nissinen A, Menotti A, Kromhout D. Predicting cardiovascular risk in the elderly in different European countries. Eur Heart J 2002;23:294-300.

21. Keys A, Aravanis C, Blackburn H, Van Buchem FSP, Buzina R, Djordjevic BS, Fidanza F, Karvonen MJ, Menotti A, Puddu V, Taylor HL. Coronary heart disease: overweight and obesity as risk factors. Ann Int Med 1972, 77: 15-27.
22. Menotti A, Capocaccia R, Conti S, Farchi G, Mariotti S, Verdecchia A, Keys A, Karvonen MJ, Punsar S. Identifying subsets of major risk factors in multivariate estimation of coronary risk. J Chron Dis 1977, 30: 557-565.
23. Chambless L, Dobson AJ, Patterson CC, Raines B. On the use of a logistic risk score in predicting risk of coronary heart disease. Stat Med 1990; 9: 385-396.

PART IV: IMPLICATIONS OF FINDINGS OF THE SEVEN COUNTRIES STUDY

CHAPTER 4.1

RISK FACTORS FOR GLOBAL CORONARY RISK IN PREVENTIVE AND CLINICAL CARDIOLOGY

Alessandro Menotti, Daan Kromhout

Epidemiological studies made clear by the late 1950s that blood cholesterol, blood pressure, and cigarette smoking were major risk factors for CHD. When firmly established in the 1970s, this led to the publication of the coronary risk handbook for the American Heart Association based on the Framingham Study risk chart (1), providing an aid for risk factor treatment in practice. However, we were into the 1990s before the concept of global risk based on multiple risk factors instead of single risk factors was widely accepted by the medical community and cardiologists. This was stimulated mainly by positive results of drug trials in primary and secondary prevention of CHD using statins for lowering cholesterol (2).

In this period, guidelines on treatment of risk factors were widely distributed in the U.S.A., Europe, and elsewhere (3-12). The European Guidelines were produced by a Task Force of three Societies (Cardiology, Hypertension, and Arteriosclerosis) (6,7) and they incorporated a chart for estimating coronary risk as a function of several risk factors. The so-called European chart was not based on a risk function derived from European populations, but on the Framingham Study risk function (13). In the 1990s many other tools, rulers, charts, PC software, and programs for Internet use were created and distributed (14-22). Older tools, risk manuals, had already become available in the 1970s and the 1980s in the U.S.A., Israel, and Italy (1,23,24). An Italian manual, published in 1980, exploited 10-year follow-up data from the Italian areas of the Seven Countries Study.

GLOBAL CORONARY RISK IN THE SEVEN COUNTRIES STUDY

The Seven Countries Study showed that large differences in diet, lifestyle, and personal characteristics (resulting in different population levels of risk factors) led to large differences in prevalence, incidence, and mortality from CHD. It was shown that these characteristics could explain two-thirds or more of the difference in incidence and mortality among cohorts. Moreover, it was confirmed that within populations, the

Figure 1. Risk for first major CHD events in 25 years (288 CHD cases) as a function of serum cholesterol levels among 1620 middle-aged men in the rural Italian areas (25).

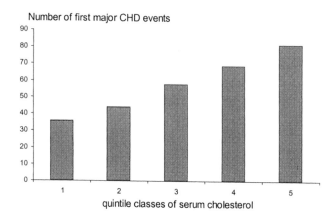

Figure 2. Risk for first major CHD events in 25 years (288 CHD cases) as a function of five risk factors (age, serum cholesterol, systolic blood pressure, and cigarette smoking and BMI) included in a multivariate model among 1620 middle-aged men in the rural Italian areas (25).

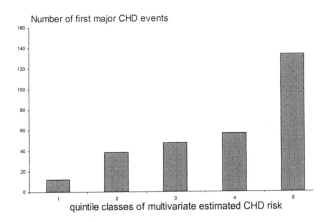

Number of first major CHD events

quintile classes of multivariate estimated CHD risk

Table 1. Risk of first major coronary events in 25 years in three hypothetical subjects. Estimate derived from a multivariate model based on Italian rural cohorts, as described in reference 25.

Risk factors	Mister A	Mister B	Mister C
Age (y)	50	50	50
Body mass index (kg/m$^{2)}$	25	25	25
Serum cholesterol (mmol/l)	8.3	4.7	5.7
Systolic BP (mm Hg)	115	170	145
Cigarettes (no. per day)	0	0	10
Risk for first major CHD event per 100 in 25 years	21	21	21

levels of some major risk factors such as age, serum cholesterol, blood pressure and smoking habits, were associated, at the individual level, with different absolute risks for future events.

Another contribution of the Seven Countries Study, which was shared with other studies, was that the evaluation of coronary risk is improved if several factors were considered simultaneously instead of focusing on single factors. Figure 1 shows the graded nature of a single (strong) risk factor, serum cholesterol, in relation to the first major CHD event. Figure 2 shows that an even stronger discrimination of CHD risk can be obtained when more risk factors are considered (25). This represents the basis for what we call "global coronary risk ."

Multivariate risk is understood from Table 1, where three individuals, free from coronary disease are characterized by different combinations of risk factor level yet have the same overall risk. This is based on a risk function derived from the rural Italian groups of the Seven Countries Study (25). Most clinicians are alerted by the situation in Mister A, or even Mister B, because of their very high respective serum cholesterol and high blood pressure. The obvious approach relied on treating them vigorously using specific drugs. On the other hand, there would be less attention paid to Mister C, whose risk factor levels were individually considered "normal," or at least very common. In fact, his risk was as high as that of the other two. Even when this situation was understood, the long and tiring approach of treating Mister C through diet and lifestyle change ("physiological hygiene") was usually neglected and often disliked by practicing physicians. Subjects with the characteristics of Mister A or even Mister B are, however, rare, whereas subjects similar to Mister C are common and represent the major source of CHD events in the general population. Until physicians and cardiologists started to act on these points, the results in primary prevention were poor.

The Seven Countries Study also demonstrated that the magnitude of the multivariate coefficients for the major risk factors is similar across cultures, as shown in the chapters on blood pressure, serum cholesterol, and multivariate analysis. The strength of the association between given risk factor levels and the risk of a coronary event is universally similar, so that risk functions or charts from different populations and cultures perform equally well in estimating relative risk. However, for the same levels of major risk factors, single or combined, the absolute risk is different among populations, owing to differences in duration of exposure or to unexplored or unknown factors. This concept was not known, or was disregarded when, in the 1990s, a number of tools to estimate global coronary risk were spread across Europe. This did not take into account that most risk functions originated from the North American or northern European experience and tended to overestimate actual risk in southern Europe and elsewhere (26).

GLOBAL CORONARY RISK IN NORTHERN AND SOUTHERN EUROPE

This neglect of the difference in absolute CHD risk, at the same risk factor levels, between northern and southern Europe, prompted us to conduct a systematic re-analysis of CHD prediction. We used 10-year CHD incidence events in northern European (Finland and the Netherlands) and southern European (Italy, Croatia, Serbia, and Greece) cohorts of the Seven Countries Study, specifically targeted toward elaboration of these concepts (27). Three endpoints were considered: CHD deaths, hard CHD events (deaths plus non-fatal definite myocardial infarction) and any CHD events (hard CHD plus possible myocardial infarction, plus definite angina pectoris). Risk factors were age, systolic blood pressure, cholesterol level, and smoking habits (yes/no). Entry cases of CHD were excluded, while the statistical model chosen was the multiple logistic function. Event rates were higher in northern Europe than in southern Europe, with practically equal ratios between north and south when considering CHD deaths (2.68), hard CHD (2.69) and any CHD (2.64). The ratio between CHD death and hard CHD incidence was 0.59 in both areas, and the ratio between CHD death and any CHD incidence was 0.28 in both areas. The ratio between hard CHD and any CHD incidence was 0.49 in northern Europe and 0.48 in southern Europe.

Analyses were made separately for the three endpoints, the two areas, and the two areas combined with a dummy variable identifying areas. All solutions showed similar coefficients for the two areas for each endpoint, with larger coefficients for CHD death, intermediate coefficients for hard-CHD and lowest coefficients for any CHD. No significant differences were found between pairs of coefficients for any risk

Table 2. Prediction of hard CHD events in 10 years in northern and southern European cohorts, based on the multiple logistic function. Derived from reference 27.

Factor		N. Europe	S. Europe
Age	Coefficient	0.0740	0.0576
	t-value	4.91	3.95
Systolic B.P.	Coefficient	0.0228	0.0149
	t-value	6.47	4.44
Cholesterol[a]	Coefficient	0.2552	0.2475
	t-value	4.40	4.00
Smoker	Coefficient	0.4497	0.2475
	t-value	2.57	3.12
Intercept	Coefficient	-11.48	-9.99
	t-value	11.3	11.5
Relative risk[b]		6.7	6.5

a = in mmol/l
b = Between observed cases in quintile 5 and quintile 1 of the distribution of the estimated risk

factor, and for any endpoint, comparing the northern with the southern European experience. An example dealing with hard CHD incidence is reported in Table 2. The proportion of cases observed in the top quintile of the distribution of estimated risk was similar in the two areas. However, those proportions were larger for CHD deaths, intermediate for hard CHD, and lower for any CHD. An example is reported in Table 2.

When the solutions were applied from one area to another, the estimate of relative risk, as suggested by the distribution of observed cases in quintile classes of estimated risk, was almost the same as when the original solution for each area was used (Figs. 3 and 4). This suggests that the relationship of risk factor levels to incidence will have roughly the same shape in the two areas. On the other hand, the estimate of absolute risk was underestimated in northern Europe and over-estimated in southern Europe. These estimates are given in Table 3. Overall, the over-estimates ranged from 1.47 to 1.78, and the under-estimates from 0.51 to 0.61.

An example of the similarity of coefficients between northern and southern European areas is given in Fig. 4, where the relationship of serum cholesterol levels to 10-year hard CHD incidence is graphically presented. The two curves have the same slope, but are located at different levels on the ordinate scale. They refer to two pools where the average cholesterol levels were about 6.5 mmol /l and 5 mmol (everything else being equal) as adjusted by the models. The distance between the two curves represents the gap in absolute risk, unexplained by serum cholesterol levels or by the other risk factors considered.

Figure 3. Distribution of observed cases in quintile classes of estimated risk derived from multiple logistic functions in the prediction of 10-year hard CHD events as a function of five risk factors. Data from northern Europe applying its own coefficients and those from southern Europe. Data derived from the multiple logistic functions presented in Table 2. Reconstructed from reference 27.

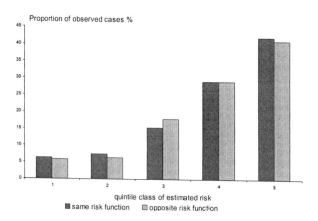

Table 3. Back application of coefficients to the opposite population in the prediction of CHD incidence in 10-year follow-up. Reconstructed and modified from reference 27.

Endpoint	Procedure	Expected cases (E)	Observed cases (O)	E / O ratio
CHD deaths	Coefficients of NE Applied to SE	166.2	113	1.47
CHD deaths	Coefficients of SE Applied to NE	70.0	114	0.61
Hard CHD	Coefficients of NE Applied to SE	316.6	192	1.65
Hard CHD	Coefficients of SE Applied to NE	113.4	190	0.60
Any CHD	Coefficients of NE Applied to SE	703.5	395	1.78
Any CHD	Coefficients of SE Applied to NE	201.0	391	0.51

NE = northern Europe   SE = southern Europe

Figure 4. Relationship between levels of serum total cholesterol and hard CHD events in pools of the northern and southern European cohorts. Derived from the coefficients of the multiple logistic functions presented in Table 2, other risk factors being equal.

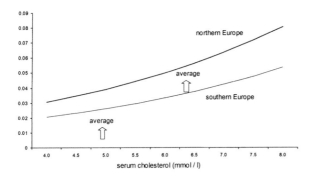

Figure 5. Risk chart for the prediction of hard-CHD events, derived from data presented in Table 2 (27).

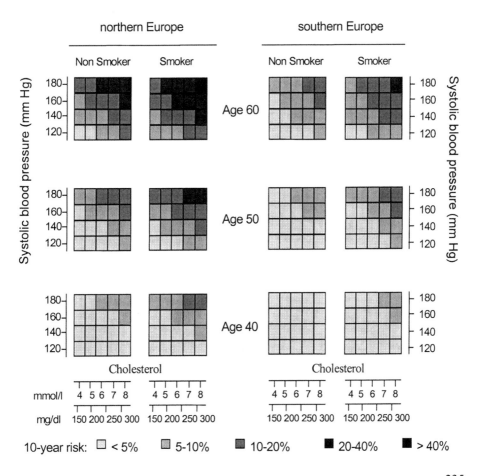

Further analyses derived from the solutions for hard CHD suggest that the crude ratio of northern to southern Europe incidence is 2.69; for similar levels of risk factors the ratio becomes 1.60; whereas the difference in realizing a ratio of 1 (a full explanation of differences) remains unexplained, presumably due to unmeasured or unknown factors. Among these are probably genetics, lifestyle, and dietary habits, and differences in other physiological measurements. The different levels and distribution of the three major risk factors (systolic blood pressure, serum cholesterol, and smoking habits) explain a large part of the crude ratio between northern and southern European incidence, roughly corresponding to 55-60% of the difference. This proportion is similar to that obtained when, using an ecological approach, average population levels of risk factors are plotted against incidence rates of single cohorts of the Seven Countries Study through multiple regression.

With the use of the above solutions in the Seven Countries Study, experimental risk charts were produced for each area and for each endpoint, filling 120 cells derived from age into three classes, smoking habits into 2 classes, and serum cholesterol and systolic blood pressure into 5 classes each (Fig. 6). The same level of risk factors revealed striking differences between the two areas. For example, out of 120 cells, those with a risk greater than 100/1000 in 10 years were, for CHD deaths, 20 in northern Europe and 5 in southern Europe; for hard CHD, 43 and 15, respectively; for any CHD, 92 and 49, respectively. Everything else being equal, the ratios of exact risk for northern to southern Europe (adjusted for age and smoking habits) range between 1.32 and 1.50 for CHD deaths, 1.43 and 1.96 for hard CHD, and 1.68 and 1.95 for any CHD.

Another comparison has been made recently between the European chart, derived from a Framingham risk function, and a similar chart using the experience of the rural Italian areas of the Seven Countries Study. The same procedure was followed in selection of risk factors, endpoint (any CHD event), length of follow-up, and type of statistical model (28). The net result was that the Framingham-derived risk chart was not applicable to Italy. In fact, of the 120 cells of the 2 charts, the cells with a 10-year CHD risk of 20 per 100 or greater numbered 4 in the Italian chart and 44 in the Framingham-based chart. This finding is parallel to that described in the re-analyses of the Seven Countries Study, where we compared the crossed use of models produced for northern and southern Europe.

IMPLICATIONS FOR PREVENTIVE AND CLINICAL CARDIOLOGY

It took decades of observational epidemiology and clinical trials for the importance of the global risk concept to be accepted by the medical profession. Traditionally, prevention and treatment were based on single risk factors, such as hypercholesterolemia and hypertension. In fact, coronary risk is determined by the combined effect of several risk factors. It is therefore necessary to base prevention and treatment decisions on absolute risk derived from multivariate risk estimates.

If the level of absolute risk is crucial for taking action in prevention and treatment of CHD, it is also necessary to differentiate between primary and secondary prevention. Serum cholesterol and blood pressure are related to coronary risk in persons free from CHD, and as well in cardiac patients (29, 30), while the relative risk of these risk factors for a coronary event is similar. The absolute risk for a coronary event is higher in cardiac patients than in CHD-free persons at the same level of serum cholesterol and blood pressure. However, CHD-free persons with elevated levels of several risk factors may have the same absolute risk as cardiac patients with lower risk factor levels. Absolute risk based on multiple risk factors and disease status is therefore the appropriate measure for rational treatment decisions.

A separate but important issue is the difference among cultures in absolute risk for similar combined risk factor levels. If absolute risk is the measure on which to base treatment decisions, should treatment not take place at a lower level of risk factors in northern Europe than in southern Europe (because at the same risk factor level the absolute risk in northern Europe is higher than in southern Europe)? Currently, the situation for blood pressure treatment is the reverse. Hypertensive patients are more frequently treated in Italy than in the Netherlands (31). By concepts of global CHD risk, it should be the other way round.

The global risk concept also raises the question of which risk factor – of several elevated ones – should be treated first in an individual patient. Mister A in Table 1 should be treated for hypercholesterolemia and Mister B for hypertension. Possibly the best advice for Mister C would be to stop smoking first and achieve as much as possible a lower serum cholesterol and blood pressure through changes in diet and lifestyle. Stopping smoking is always the most effective measure to decrease health risk, because it not only lowers the risk of CHD, but also the risk of other vascular diseases, cancer, and chronic obstructive pulmonary disease. The Dutch Cholesterol Consensus showed that only 25% of all persons free from CHD, with elevated serum cholesterol levels and a high absolute risk for CHD, needed treatment with statins if the smokers decided to stop smoking (32). Because of stopping smoking, the absolute risk for CHD was lowered so much that cholesterol-lowering by statins was no longer cost-effective.

In conclusion, an integrated approach is needed to lower coronary risk in cardiac patients and in high-risk persons. Substantial risk reductions can be obtained by stopping smoking and improving dietary and physical activity levels. For patients with substantially elevated levels of blood cholesterol and blood pressure this is not enough, however. They may require drug treatment.

SUMMARY AND CONCLUSIONS

The concept of global coronary risk was developed on the basis of evidence from observational epidemiology and from clinical trials. Consequently, decisions on prevention and treatment are based on absolute risk of a CHD event, derived from multivariate risk functions. The results of the Seven Countries Study showed the strength of associations between the major risk factors (serum cholesterol and blood pressure) and CHD risk to be similar in different cultures, with a great difference in absolute risk. Northern Europe and the U.S.A. are characterized by high absolute risk and southern Europe, and Japan by low risk. If these results are taken into account in medical practice, more persons should be treated in northern Europe and the United States for the same elevated levels of risk factors than in southern Europe and Japan. Smoking is a very important contributor to CHD risk. If smokers with a mildly elevated serum cholesterol and blood pressure level, and a high absolute risk for CHD, stop smoking, they may not need drug treatment for lowering cholesterol and blood pressure. This illustrates the importance of an integrated "global" approach to the prevention and treatment of CHD.

237

REFERENCES

1. American Heart Association. Coronary risk handbook: estimating the risk of coronary heart disease in daily practice. Dallas, AHA, 1973:1-35.
2. Pitt B, Julian D, Pocock S (Eds). Clinical trials in cardiology. W B Saunders Co Ltd.1997.
3. Grundy SM, Balady GJ, Criqui MH, Fletcher G, Greenland P, Hiratska LF, Houston-Miller N, Kris-Etherton P, Krumholz HM, LaRosa J, Ockene ISA, Pearson TA, Reed J, Washington R, Smith SC, Guide to primary prevention of cardiovascular diseases. A statement for healthcare professionals from the Task Force on risk reduction. Circulation 1997; 95: 2329-2331.
4. Grundy SM, Pasternak R, Greenland P, Smith S, Fuster V. Assessment of cardiovascular risk by use of multiple-risk-factor assessment equations. A statement for healthcare professionals from the American Heart Association and the American College of Cardiology. J Am Coll Cardiol 1999; 34: 1348-1359.
5. Expert Panel on Detection, Evaluation and Treatment of High Blood Cholesterol in Adults: Executive summary of the third report of the National Cholesterol Education Program (NCEP) Expert Panel on Detection, Evaluation and Treatment of High Blood Cholesterol, in Adults (Adult Treatment Panel III). JAMA 2001; 285: 2486-2696.
6. Prevention of coronary heart disease in clinical practice. Recommendations of the Task Force of the European Society of Cardiology, European Atherosclerosis Society and European Society of Hypertension. Eur Heart J 1994;15:1300-31.
7. Prevention of coronary heart disease in clinical practice. Recommendations of the Second Joint Task Force of European and other Societies on coronary prevention. Eur Heart J 1998;19:1434-503.
8. The International Task Force for Prevention of Coronary Heart Disease: Coronary Heart Disease: reducing the risk. Nutr Metab Cardiovasc Dis 1998; 8: 205-271.
9. Jackson R, Barham P, Bills J, Birch T, McLennan L, McMahon S, Maling T. The management of raised blood pressure in New Zealand. BMJ 1993; 307: 127-110.
10. Mann JI, Crooke M, Fear H, Hay DR, Jackson RT, Neutze JM, White HD. Guidelines for detection and management of dyslipidemia. NZ Med J 1993; 106: 133-142.
11. Joint British recommendations on prevention of coronary heart disease in clinical practice. British Cardiac Society, British Hyperlipidaemia Association, British Hypertension Society, endorsed by the British Diabetic Association. Heart 1998; 80, Suppl 2: S1-29.
12. Joint British recommendations on prevention of coronary heart disease in clinical practice. British Cardiac Society, British Hyperlipidaemia Association, British Hypertension Society, British Diabetic Association. BMJ 2000; 320: 705-708.
13. Anderson KM, Wilson PWF, Odell PM, Kannel WB. An updated coronary risk profile. A statement for health professionals. Circulation 1991;83:356-62.
14. Dyslipidaemia Advisory Committee. 1996 National Heart Foundation clinical guidelines for the assessment and management of dyslipidaemia. NZ Med J 1996; 109:224-232.
15. National Health Committee. Guidelines for the management of mildly raised blood pressure in New Zealand. Wellington. Ministry of Health, 1995.
16. Tunstall-Pedoe H. The Dundee coronary risk-disk for management of change in risk factors. Br Med J 1991; 303: 744-47.
17. American Heart Association: Internet Site www.amhrt.org. Health Risk Awareness. June 2000.
18. Internet Site www.CHD-Taskforce.de/Calculator. PROCAM risk calculator. June 2001
19. Assmann G, Schulte H, von Eckardstein A. Hypertriglyceridemia and elevated lipoprotein(a) are risk factors for major coronary events in middle-aged men. Am J Cardiol 1996; 77: 1179-1184.
20. Cardiac Risk Assessment. V.98.02. Program for PC. Copyright University of Manchester. UK.,1 1998.
21. Thomsen T. Prediction and prevention of cardiovascular diseases. Precard.©. Thesis at the University of Copenhagen, 2000.

22. Riscor-1998. Software for prediction of coronary events. Cardioricerca, Rome, Italy, 1998.

23. Medalie JH, Goldbourt U. Estimated probabilities of men aged 40 and over developing a first myocardial infarction in five years. Ministry of Health of Israel and the Hadassah Medical Organization, Israel 1973:1-26.

24. Manuale del Rischio Coronarico. Per stimare il rischio coronarico nella pratica medica. Udine, Associazione Nazionale Centri per le Malattie Cardiovascolari, 1980:1-36.

25. Menotti A, Seccareccia F, Lanti M, Giampaoli S, Dima F. Time changes in predictability of coronary heart disease in an Italian aging population. Cardiology 1993, 82: 172-180.

26. Haq IU, Ramsay LE, Yeo WW, Jackson PR, Wallis EJ. Is the Framingham risk function valid for northern European populations? A comparison of methods for estimating absolute coronary risk in high risk men. Heart 1999; 81: 40-46.

27. Menotti A, Lanti M, Puddu PE, Kromhout D. Coronary heart disease incidence in Northern and Southern European populations: a reanalysis of the Seven Countries Study for a European coronary risk chart. Heart 2000; 84: 238-244.

28. Menotti A , Lanti M. Puddu PE. Comparison of the Framingham risk function-based coronary chart with risk function from an Italian population study. Eur Heart J 2000; 21: 365-370.

29. Pekkanen J, Linn S, Heiss G, Suchindran CM, Leon A, Rifkind BM, Tyroler HA. Ten-year mortality from cardiovascular disease in relation to cholesterol level among men with and without pre-existing cardiovascular disease. N Engl J Med 1990;322:1700-7.

30. Browner WS, Hulley SB. Effect of risk status on treatment criteria. Implications for hypertension trials. Hypertension 1989;13 Suppl 1: 151-156.

31. Van den Hoogen PCW, Seidell JC, Feskens EJM, Nissinen A, Menotti A, Kromhout D. Systolic, diastolic and pulse pressure and 10-year cardiovascular mortality among elderly men in Finland, Italy and the Netherlands. Submitted.

32. Jukema JW, Simoons ML. Treatment and prevention of coronary heart disease by lowering serum cholesterol: from the pioneer work of C.D. de Langen to the third "Dutch Consensus on Cholesterol." Acta Cardiol 1999;54:163-168.

CHAPTER 4.2

DIET, LIFESTYLE AND PREVENTION OF CORONARY HEART DISEASE
THE INTEGRATION OF OBSERVATIONAL AND EXPERIMENTAL EVIDENCE

Daan Kromhout, Bennie Bloemberg, Alessandro Menotti

Epidemiological studies, including the Seven Countries Study, have provided substantial evidence that diet is involved in the etiology of CHD. Observational epidemiology and controlled dietary intervention studies have shown that for prevention of CHD, fatty acid composition of the diet is of primary importance. A healthy diet should be low in saturated and *trans* fatty acids and should have an adequate amount of N-3 polyunsaturated fatty acids, and a balance between N-3 and N-6 polyunsaturated fatty acids. Dietary antioxidants and dietary fiber may be important, however, evidence for these factors is less impressive than that for fatty acids.

Selected nutrients or food groups have been extensively studied in relation to coronary risk. However, the content of nutrients in diets is often strongly intercorrelated. It is therefore more practical to study dietary *patterns* in relation to coronary risk. Dietary patterns also provide the possibility to evaluate the health effects of adherence to recommended dietary guidelines.

Dietary patterns are related to other lifestyle factors such as cigarette smoking. In European populations smokers, for example, have a lower intake of polyunsaturated fatty acids, dietary antioxidants and dietary fiber, consume more alcohol and are less frequently involved in heavy physical activity (1,2). Different aspects of diet and lifestyle are intercorrelated. Thus, it is important to study the *combined* effect of diet and lifestyle on CHD risk. We will summarize the results of major studies, both observational and experimental, on the effect of diet and lifestyle and their combination on coronary risk. Finally, we will make recommendations on diet and lifestyle for prevention of CHD.

DIET, LIFESTYLE, AND CARDIOVASCULAR MORTALITY IN OBSERVATIONAL STUDIES

Many national organizations have formulated dietary recommendations for prevention of CHD or for chronic diseases, in general, as has WHO. We developed a healthy diet indicator based on the WHO guidelines (3). A dichotomous variable was generated for each nutrient or food group (Table 1). When a person's intake was within the recommended range, this variable was coded 1; otherwise, it was coded 0. The healthy diet indicator was the sum of all the dichotomous variables.

We applied this healthy diet indicator to the dietary data of Finnish, Dutch, and Italian cohorts of the Seven Countries Study, data collected in 3,045 men aged 50-69 in 1970, who were followed for 20 years (4). In total, 1,796 men (59%) died. In each country the healthy diet indicator was inversely related to all-causes mortality (Table 2). The pooled estimate for the three countries showed that in the group with the healthiest diet indicator, compared with the least healthy, the adjusted relative risk was 0.87 (95%CI 0.77-0.98). The largest risk reduction was observed for cardiovascular disease mortality (18%, p < 0.05). Individual components of the healthy diet indicator were not consistently related to either all-causes or cardiovascular disease mortality.

These results suggest that the whole dietary pattern is more important to mortality from all-causes and cardiovascular diseases than are the individual dietary components. This points to the importance of a well-balanced diet of foods and nutrients. The results also showed that the lowest mortality risk in all countries was observed for those with the best diet.

Table 1. Criteria used for the healthy diet indicator (dichotomous values) based on dietary guidelines for the prevention of chronic diseases, with values as percentage of energy intake unless indicated otherwise (3,4)

Nutrient or food group (daily intake)	Dichotomous values	
	1.	0
Saturated fatty acids (%E)	0-10	>10
Polyunsaturated fatty acids (%E)	3-7	<3 or >7
Monosaccharides and disaccharides(%E)	0-10	>10
Protein (%E)	10-15	<10 or >15
Complex carbohydrates (%E)	50-70	<50 or >70
Dietary fiber (g)	27-40	<27 or >40
Fruits and vegetables (g)	>400	<400
Legumes, nuts, seeds (g)	>30	<30
Cholesterol (mg)	0-300	>300

Table 2. Adjusted relative risk (RR, 95%CI) for 20-year all-causes mortality by healthy diet indicator among 3,045 men aged 50-69 aged 50-69 at baseline (4).

	Healthy diet indicator (HDI)			
	Low	Medium	High	p-trend
		Finland		
Mean HDI	0.9	2.0	3.1	
Adjusted RR	1.00	0.97	0.90	0.31
95%CI		0.83-1.12	0.73-1.10	
		Netherlands		
Mean HDI	0.9	2.0	3.4	
Adjusted RR	1.00	0.91	0.75	0.09
95%CI		0.91-1.16	0.53-1.05	
		Italy		
Mean HDI	1.6	3.4	5.5	
Adjusted RR	1.00	1.04	0.89	0.23
95%CI		0.86-1.26	0.72-1.09	
		Pooled		
Mean HDI	0.9	2.0	4.0	
Adjusted RR	1.00	0.99	0.87	0.03
95%CI		0.87-1.11	0.77-0.98	

Adjusted for age, cigarette smoking and alcohol consumption.   CI = Confidence interval

The relationship of different lifestyle factors to the risk for cardiovascular diseases and diabetes was investigated in the British Regional Heart Study (5). In total, 7,142 men aged 40-59 were followed for 15 years. During the follow-up period, 1,064 men died, 770 developed a major fatal or non-fatal myocardial infarction, 247 developed a fatal or non-fatal stroke, and 252 developed diabetes. These combined endpoints were related to smoking, physical activity and Body Mass Index (BMI), an indicator of energy balance.

Smoking and physical activity were related to those combined endpoints in a dose-response manner. Men who smoked more than 20 cigarettes per day had a relative risk of 2.50 (95%CI 2.12-2.94) compared with never-smokers. For those who exercised vigorously compared with inactive men, the relative risk was 0.64 (95%CI 0.50-0.83). A BMI $\geq$30 kg/m^2 compared with a BMI of > 20-21.9 kg/m^2 was associated with a relative risk of 2.11 (95%CI 1.71-2.62). This study also showed the large impact of combined risk factors. The probability of surviving 15 years free of major cardiovascular events and diabetes in a man aged 50 years ranged from 89% in an active man with BMI levels of 20 to 24 kg/m^2 (a never-smoker) to 42% in an inactive smoker with BMI levels of 30 kg/m^2 or higher.

The effect on CHD of a healthy diet in combination with a healthy lifestyle was tested in the Nurses Health Study, in which 84,129 women aged 30-55 were enrolled and followed for 14 years (6). A healthy lifestyle was defined as no smoking, consuming at least half a drink of an alcoholic beverage per day, engagement in moderate to vigorous physical activity for at least 30 minutes per day and a BMI below 25 kg/m^2. A healthy diet was defined as the highest 40% of the cohort for consumption of cereal fiber, marine N-3 polyunsaturated fatty acids, folate, ratio of polyunsaturated to saturated fatty acids and low in *trans* fatty acids, and glycemic load, which reflects the extent to which diet raises blood glucose levels. These lifestyle and dietary factors were related to 14-year CHD incidence.

The strongest association with CHD was observed for smoking: RR = 5.48 (95% CI 4.67-6.42) for nurses who smoked more than 12 cigarettes per day, compared with never smokers. For alcohol consumption, exercise, BMI, and diet score, the risk ratios varied between 1.41 and 1.90. Women who had a BMI below 25 kg/m^2, a diet score in the upper 2 quintiles, and who exercised moderately to vigorously, drank more than 4 g alcohol per day, and did not smoke, had a risk ratio of 0.17 (95%CI 0.07-0.41) and a population attributable risk of 82% (95%CI 58 –93), compared with women at higher risk. A dose-response relationship was also observed. The more low-risk factors present, the greater the "prevention" of CHD. In non-smokers, a substantial effect was also observed of the other lifestyle factors and diet. The 4% of non-smoking nurses who also had low values for the other four risk factors had a risk ratio of 0.25 (95%CI 0.10-0.60) for CHD, compared to the other non-smoking nurses.

The results of these prospective cohort studies suggest that CHD and cardiovascular diseases mortality are low in middle-aged men and women if a healthy diet and lifestyle are practiced. These results are in accordance with those of the Seven Countries Study, which showed that CHD mortality rates were low in populations characterized by a healthy diet and low smoking rates (7).

DIET, LIFESTYLE, CORONARY AND ALL-CAUSES MORTALITY IN EXPERIMENTAL STUDIES

Comprehensive trials have not been carried out on diet and lifestyle in relation to coronary risk. Trials intervening on diet and smoking performed in Norway and Finland (8-10) obtained substantial changes in serum total cholesterol level. In the 1960s and 1970s these countries were characterized by a high intake of saturated fatty acids and a high prevalence of smokers, thus potentially large reductions in risk factor levels could be obtained. In addition, large changes occurred in risk factors for CHD in the Finnish population (11,12). Finally, Finland was a participant in the Seven Countries Study, which provided the possibility to compare changes in diet and smoking in relation to coronary and all-causes mortality in both experimental and observational studies.

At the beginning of the Seven Countries Study, the intake of saturated fatty acids and the prevalence of smokers were high. In West Finland, for example, the average population intake of saturated fatty acids among men aged 40-59 was 19.3% of energy and the prevalence of smokers, 57%. This is similar to the average saturated fatty acid intake and smoking prevalence of Finnish men aged 35-64 in 1972, and to the average values of the control groups in the Finnish Mental Hospital Study carried out in the 1959-1971 period, and the Oslo Study carried out in 1972-1981 (8-12). In the Seven Countries Study, the associations were studied between average population nutrient intake, prevalence of smokers, and 25-year CHD and all-causes mortality (7,13). The regression equations of these analyses provide estimates of the expected difference in mortality from CHD and all-causes, based on differences in average nutrient intake and prevalence of smokers. Differences in CHD and all-causes mortality rates were calculated for the changes that occurred in saturated fatty acid intake, and the prevalence of smokers in the Finnish population between 1972 and 1992. Calculations were also made for the difference in saturated fatty acid intake and the prevalence of smokers in the experimental group, compared with the control group in the Finnish Mental Hospital Study. The estimated differences in CHD and all-causes mortality rates in the three experimental studies were similar to the observed differences (Table 3). These results indicate that differences in mortality rates can be predicted effectively from population differences in saturated fatty acid intake and prevalence of smokers.

Table 3. Observed and expected differences in mortality rates in observational and experimental studies in Finland and Norway (7-13).

	Finland		FMHS		Oslo Study	
Age (y)	35 - 64		34 - 64		40 - 49	
Risk factor/endpoint	1992	1972	E	C	E	C
Saturated fat (%E)	15.6	20.5	8.7	17.4	8.2	18.3
Cig. smokers (%)	37	53	65	69	55	63
CHD diff. Obs. (%)	- 55		-51		- 55	
CHD diff. Exp. (%)	- 50		-48		- 61	
AC diff. Obs. (%)	- 38		-12		- 32	
AC diff. Exp. (%)	- 27		-21		- 28	

FMHS = Finnish Mental Hospital Study   CHD = Coronary heart disease mortality
E = Experimental group   AC = All-causes mortality
C = Control group
Exp = Expected mortality based on the regression equations for CHD and all-causes mortality in the Seven Countries Study (7,13)

Saturated fatty acid intake and the prevalence of smokers in the studies from Finland and Norway varied between 8 and 21% of energy for saturated fatty acid intake, and 37 and 69% in the prevalence of smokers. These differences are within the known limits of average population intake of saturated fatty acids, and the prevalence of smokers in the Seven Countries Study. The question, however, is whether the results for saturated fatty acids can also be extrapolated to populations with a low prevalence of smokers. An example is formed by the health professionals from the U.S., examined for the first time in 1986 (14). Their prevalence rate of smokers was 9% and average intake of saturated fatty acids 11% of energy. In this almost non-smoking population the adjusted relative risk for CHD mortality in men with a high intake of saturated fatty acids (median = 14.8% of energy), compared to those with a low intake (median = 7.2% of energy), was 1.72 (95%CI 1.01-2.90). These are comparable with the risk ratio observed in the Seven Countries Study for populations with similar intakes of saturated fatty acids (RR = 1.62). These results suggest that the relative differences observed in CHD mortality, based on differences in saturated fatty acid intake observed in cohorts with a high prevalence of smokers, can also be used for estimations in population groups with a low prevalence of smokers.

We conclude that changes in diet and prevalence of smokers are good predictors of changes in CHD and all-causes mortality, observed both in populations and in experimental studies. These associations are therefore likely to be causal.

Intervention trials have not been carried out on diet, smoking, and physical activity simultaneously. Secondary prevention, clinical trials have intervened on diet and physical activity and using angiographic endpoints in small groups (15-17). The effect of a low-fat vegetarian diet, moderate exercise, and stress management was tested in a randomized controlled trial of 48 patients in the so-called Lifestyle Heart Trial (15). The diet of the experimental group contained 8% of energy from fat compared with 30% of energy in the control group. Time spent on exercise was 38 min per day in the experimental group and 21 min per day in the control group. The time spent on stress reduction was more than an hour per day in the experimental group, and about 5 min per day in the control group. No lipid-lowering drugs were used.

These differences in diet and lifestyle led, in the course of one year, to a reduction of 10 kg in body weight in the experimental group and no weight change in the control group. In the experimental group, serum total cholesterol fell by 24% and LDL cholesterol by 37%. No change was observed in HDL cholesterol. In the control group the different cholesterol fractions did not change. The average percentage diameter stenosis of coronary vessels regressed from 40.0 (SD 16.9)% to 37.8 (16.5)% in the experimental group, and progressed from 42.7 (15.5)% to 46.1 (18.5)% in the control group.

The Lifestyle Heart Trial was continued for another four years (16). After 5 years, the differences in intervention measures between the two groups were smaller than after one year. For dietary fat these were 9 vs. 25% of energy, for exercise 31 vs. 25 min per day and for stress management 49 vs. 8 min per day. After 5 years, weight loss was 6 kg in the experimental group, with little change from baseline in the control group. LDL cholesterol levels were about 20% lower in both groups after five years, compared with baseline. Lack of difference between the two groups was due to the fact that 60% of the members of the control group took lipid-lowering drugs between year 1 and 5 of the study. HDL cholesterol levels did not differ between the two groups.

Despite the fact that differences between the experimental and control groups became smaller during the 5-year intervention period, substantial differences were observed in angiographic endpoints. After 5 years, a relative improvement of 7.5%

246

was noted in the experimental group, compared with a relative worsening of 11.8% in the control group (p = 0.001). The risk ratio for any cardiac event in the control compared with the experimental group was 2.47 (95% CI 1.48 –4.20). Adherence to the lifestyle intervention was strongly related to changes in diameter stenosis, the better the adherence the more regression (Fig.1).

Figure 1. Changes in percentage diameter stenosis by 5-year adherence tertiles for the experimental group (16)

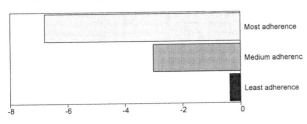

change diameter stenosis (%)

The changes in diet and lifestyle in the Lifestyle Heart Trial were drastic. It is therefore of interest to know what the effect of less dramatic changes in diet and lifestyle may be. This was studied in a secondary prevention trial carried out in Germany (17). In total, 113 cardiac patients were randomized. The experimental group was advised to use a low-fat diet and to exercise daily for at least 30 minutes. The control group got similar instructions, but adherence to the guidelines was left to their own initiative. No lipid-lowering drugs were used.

Total fat consumed by the experimental group was 26% of energy compared with 34% in the control group. Of the experimental group, 68% of patients attended exercise sessions. During the year-long intervention period body weight was reduced by 4 kg in the experimental group, compared with no change in the control group. Total and LDL cholesterol levels decreased in the experimental group by 10%. No change was observed in HDL cholesterol level. In the control group blood lipid changes were not observed. Physical work capacity improved by 23% in the experimental group. After one year of intervention, 7% of patients in the experimental group and 12% of the patients in the control group smoked cigarettes.

Evaluation on a per lesion basis showed no change in lesion diameter in the experimental group, compared to a significant increase in the control group. In the experimental group, 23% of the patients showed progression, 45% showed no change, and 32% showed regression in lesion diameter. For the control group, these percentages were 48%, 35% and 17%, respectively. The changes were significantly different between groups. This trial shows that the course of coronary artery disease can be influenced by dietary intervention and regular exercise. As could be expected, because of the less drastic changes in diet and exercise, this study showed smaller changes in angiographic endpoints between the experimental and control group than in the Lifestyle Heart Trial.

The clinical trials reviewed showed that interventions on diet and exercise may favorably influence angiographic endpoints, the effect is dependent on the intensity of the diet and lifestyle changes. There is a clear dose-response relationship between adherence to dietary and lifestyle interventions and the effect on angiographic endpoints. The results of different intervention studies showed that beneficial effects on different cardiac endpoints may be obtained in both high-risk persons and cardiac patients.

A question remaining is whether the interventions used so far are the best ones, based on currently available evidence. The diets used in the trials described were either low or moderate in total fat and low in saturated fatty acids. These diets did not have an ideal fatty acid composition and paid no attention to the content of N-3 polyunsaturated fatty acids or to the balance in N-3 and N-6 polyunsaturated fatty acids. If this is done, substantial reductions in CHD and all-causes mortality can be obtained, as shown in the Lyon Diet Heart Study (18,19). In that trial, much attention was paid to the fatty acid composition of the diet, that is, a well-balanced diet with respect to fatty acids, and rich in dietary antioxidants and fiber. This diet reduced both coronary and all-causes mortality by 70%. In combination with regular exercise and non-smoking this diet will apparently result in a very low risk for CHD and all-causes mortality.

The results of the clinical trails reviewed provide evidence that adherence to a healthy diet and lifestyle can substantially lower the risk for CHD and all-causes mortality. A disadvantage of the trials carried out so far is their open design. Because of the great potential of these interventions there is an urgent need to replicate these trials under better controlled conditions. With respect to dietary interventions this can be done by the use of functional foods designed to contain different amounts of active compounds that lower coronary risk compared to traditional foods.

SUMMARY AND CONCLUSIONS

Based on the currently available evidence from observational epidemiology and controlled intervention studies, we conclude that a healthy diet and lifestyle will reduce coronary risk in both primary and secondary prevention. This can be accomplished by adhering to the relatively simple guidelines formulated by the Task Force Report of the European Society of Cardiology on "Prevention of Coronary Heart Disease in Clinical Practice" (20), the Dietary Guidelines of the American Heart Association (21) and the National Cholesterol Education Program (22). The recommendations on lifestyle are:

- don't smoke
- if you use alcohol, do so in moderation
- be moderate – to – vigorously physically active (e.g. brisk walking, biking, gardening) at least 30 minutes per day

The recommendations on diet are:

- keep energy balance so that BMI is below 25 kg/m^2
- keep energy from saturated fat to less than 10%
- keep energy from *trans* fat to less than 2%
- eat (fatty) fish at least once a week
- eat at least 400 g per day of vegetables and fruits
- limit salt consumption to less than 6 g per day

If these recommendations are followed, coronary heart disease can, to a large extent, be eliminated in the population below 70 years of age.

REFERENCES

1. Margetts BM, Jackson AA. Interactions between people's diet and their smoking habits: the dietary and nutritional survey of British adults. BMJ 1993; 307:1381-1384.
2. Bijnen FCH, Feskens EJM, Caspersen CJ, Giampaoli S, Nissinen AM, Menotti A, Mosterd WL, Kromhout D. Physical activity and cardiovascular risk factors in elderly men in Finland, Italy and the Netherlands. Am J Epidemiol 1996;143:553-561.
3. World Health Organisation. Diet, nutrition and the prevention of chronic diseases. Report of a WHO Study Group. Geneva: World Health Organisation, (WHO Technical Report Series No 797) 1990:1-203.
4. Huijbregts P, Feskens E, Räsänen L, Fidanza F, Nissinen A, Menotti A, Kromhout D. Dietary pattern and 20 year mortality in elderly men in Finland, Italy, and the Netherlands: Longitudinal cohort study. BMJ 1997; 315:13-17.
5. Wannamethee SG, Shaper GA, Walker M, Ebrahim S. Lifestyle and 15-year survival free of heart attack, stroke and diabetes in middle-aged British men. Arch Intern Med 1998; 158:2433-2440.
6. Stampfer MJ, Hu FB, Manson JE, Rimm, EB, Willett WC. Primary prevention on coronary heart disease in women through diet and lifestyle. N Engl J Med 2000; 343:16-22.
7. Hertog MGL, Kromhout D, Aravanis C, Blackburn H, Buzina R, Fidanza F, Giampaoli S, Jansen A, Menotti A, Nedeljkovic S, Pekkarinen M, Simic BS, Toshima H, Feskens EJM, Hollman PCH, Katan MB. Flavonoid intake and long-term risk of coronary heart disease and cancer in the Seven Countries Study. Arch Intern Med 1995;155:381-386.
8. Hjermann I, Byre KV, Holme I, Leren P. Effect of diet and smoking intervention on incidence of coronary heart disease. Report from the Oslo Study Group of a randomized trial in healthy men. Lancet 1981; ii:1303-1310.
9. Miettinen M, Turpeinen O, Karvonen MJ, Elosuo R, Paavilainen E. Effect of cholesterol – lowering diet on mortality from coronary heart disease and other causes. A twelve-year clinical trial in men and women. Lancet 1972;ii:835-838.
10. Turpeinen O, Karvonen MJ, Pekkarinen M, Miettinen M, Eluoso R, Paavilainen E. Dietary prevention of coronary heart disease: The Finnish Mental Hospital Study. Int J Epidemiol 1979;8:99-118.
11. Vartiainen E, Puska P, Pekkanen J, Tuomilehto J, Jousilahti P. Changes in risk factors explain changes in mortality from ischaemic heart disease in Finland. BMJ 1994;309:23-27.
12. Pietinen P, Vartiainen E, Seppänen R, Aro A, Puska P. Changes in diet in Finland from 1972 to 1992. Impact on coronary heart disease risk. Prev Med 1996;25:243-250.
13. Kromhout D, Bloemberg B, Feskens E, Menotti A, Nissinen A for the Seven Countries Study Group. Saturated fat, vitamin C and smoking predict long-term all-cause mortality rates in the Seven Countries Study. Int J Epidemiol 2000;29:260-265.
14. Ascherio A, Rimm EB, Giovannucci EL, Spiegelman D, Stampfer MJ, Willett WC. Dietary fat and risk of coronary heart disease in men: cohort follow-up study in the United States. BMJ 1996; 313:84-90.
15. Ornish D, Brown SE, Scherwirtz LW, Billings JH, Armstrong WT, Ports TA, McLanahan SM, Kirkeeide RL, Brand RJ, Gould KL. Can lifestyle changes reverse coronary heart disease? The Lifestyle Heart Trial. Lancet 1990;336:129-133.
16. Ornish D, Scherwitz LW, Billings JH Gould L, Merritt TA, Sparler S, Armstrong WT, Ports TA, Kirkeeide RL, Hogeboom C, Brand RJ. Intensive lifestyle changes for reversal of coronary heart disease. JAMA 1998;280:2001-2007.
17. Schuler G, Hambrecht R, Schlierf R, Niebauer J, Hauer K, Neumann J, Hoberg E, Drinkmann A, Bacher F, Grunze M. Regular physical exercise and a low-fat diet. Effects on progression of coronary artery disease. Circulation 1992;86:1-11.
18. De Logeril M, Renaud S, Mamelle N, Salen P, Martin JL, Monjaud I, Guidollet J, Touboul P, Delaye J. Mediterranean alpha-linolenic acid rich diet in secondary prevention of coronary heart disease. Lancet 1994;343:1454-1459.

249

19. Renaud S, De Lorgeril M, Delaye J, Guidollet J, Jacquard F, Mamelle N, Martin JL, Monjaud I, Salen P, Toubol P. Cretan Mediterranean diet for prevention of coronary heart disease. Am J Clin Nutr 1995;61 Suppl:1360S-1367S.
20. Wood D, De Backer G, Faergeman O, Graham I, Mancia G, Pyörälä K. Task Force Report "Prevention of Coronary Heart Disease in Clinical Practice. Eur Heart J 1998;19:1434-1503.
21. AHA Scientific Statement. AHA Dietary Guidelines. Revision 2000: A statement for health care professionals from the Nutrition Committee of the American Heart Association. Circulation 2000;102:2284-2299.
22. Expert Panel on Detection, Evaluation, and Treatment of High Blood Cholesterol in Adults (Adults Treatment Panel III). Executive Summary of the Third Report of the National Cholesterol Education Program (NCEP). JAMA 2001;285:2486-2497.

CHAPTER 4.3

EPILOGUE FOR THE SEVEN COUNTRIES STUDY

Henry Blackburn

The Seven Countries Study was the first to establish credible data on incidence and death rates of CHD and stroke in contrasting cultures. Differences were found on the order of 5 -fold in 25-year CHD mortality rates, along with measurable trends in rates over as little as a decade. Thus, whole populations and cultures are at relatively high or low risk and their risk and disease rates may change rapidly in historical terms. Such findings can only be explained by the operation of powerful sociocultural influences. These may include changes in health behaviors, in risk factor levels and in medical care. The public health implications for prevention are clear and profound.

The study was the first to document population differences in average levels and distributions of coronary risk factors. It also demonstrated large differences in composition of the diet in otherwise similar, stable, rural agricultural or pastoral populations, varying from 3% to 22% of energy for saturated fatty acids, and 9% to 40% for total fat. Diet and cigarette smoking explained most of the differences in population CHD risk, while changes in serum cholesterol and blood pressure between entry and 25-year follow-up examinations explained much of the change in population CHD death rates.

In consequence, the major overall influence of the Seven Countries Study has been to strengthen the concept of population causes, that is, the mass phenomena involved in the genesis of CHD and stroke. It has contributed powerfully to the idea that we are concerned with mass cultural phenomena that influence an already widespread individual and species susceptibility. Where environments are unfavorable, the result is a maximal exhibition of risk and a heavy population burden of disease. Where they are favorable, individual (genetic) susceptibility is attenuated. And where the environment, behavior, and risk factor levels change, the population risk and death rates can change or be changed in a decade or less and either toward or away from epidemics.

These findings and the resulting concepts have played a central role in the wider population strategy of prevention and health promotion, complementing the traditional medical strategies used among patients and susceptible individuals. The findings have stimulated greater research on population-wide causes and community-wide preventive strategies, which now characterize much ongoing research and programs in epidemiology and prevention of heart and blood vessel diseases. They have also resulted in international efforts to monitor the trends in cardiovascular diseases and their risk factors, as well as the relative impact of medical care and health promotion on them. All this has provided a sound scientific basis for public health policy and programs on prevention. Finally, the medical, public health, and nutrition community, as well as agri-business internationally, have been profoundly influenced by the Seven Countries Study in their recommendations, and their production, distribution, promotion, and sales approaches toward more healthy eating patterns.

The Seven Countries Study was the first to investigate simultaneously the influence of population and individual levels of risk factors on subsequent risk and rates of disease. It therefore confirmed the results of the Framingham Study and the numerous other longitudinal studies of cardiovascular disease risk carried out internationally, in which individual values of major risk factors universally predicted individual risk of CHD and stroke. Thus, the major modifiable risk factors were established as "universals," applicable to preventive strategies in any clinical setting. Though prediction of excess relative risk is demonstrably universal, cultures as well as individuals were found to differ greatly in their absolute risk of a coronary event at any given single or combined risk factor level or risk score. This is due presumably to different durations of risk exposure, to different gene–environment interactions, and to factors not yet known that apparently raise or lower risk. Intervention strategy is therefore best determined globally by the rational and the more relevant issue of absolute risk.

Seven Countries Study findings of multivariate high or low risk confirm the widely demonstrated importance of *combined* risk factors, a concept particularly useful to the clinician in practice. For example, combined modest risk factor elevations, easily ignored, may convey equivalent risk to the more obvious excess risk from pathological elevations of a single risk factor, and they may require combined intervention strategies.

The Seven Countries Study and other epidemiological studies have been useful to preventive and clinical practice in other respects by demonstrating:

- that serum cholesterol and systolic blood pressure levels are reliable and valid predictors of coronary risk;
- that precision and prediction of an individual's coronary risk is substantially improved by taking multiple and repeated risk factor measurements;
- that the frequency and duration of cigarette smoking are strongly related to coronary risk in populations and individuals;
- that physical activity is an important determinant of body fatness and diabetes type 2 in both individuals and populations and of coronary heart disease in individuals;
- that the Mediterranean habit of taking a couple of glasses of wine with meals is associated with a lower coronary risk compared to non-drinking;
- that traditional eating patterns, especially Mediterranean and Asian cuisine, are the more attractive, tried-and-true approaches to healthy eating patterns than are the low-fat, dietetic modifications of Western food products and cuisine. They also contain greater nutrient value and have more variety and satiety;
- that emphasis on whole grains, fish, fruits and vegetables, and the quality of fats and oils is justified, based on Seven Countries-derived evidence about the effects of specific fatty acids, anti-oxidants, fiber, and whole foods;
- that clinical prevention for the individual is facilitated by its integration with family, community, and culture-wide efforts at health promotion.

In sum, the Seven Countries Study has, in these many ways, influenced profoundly the concepts and the practice of prevention in cardiovascular diseases, as well as public policy and strategies of prevention and health promotion.

APPENDIX

ABBREVIATIONS OF THE 16 COHORTS OF THE SEVEN COUNTRIES STUDY

A   U.S. Railroad, U.S.A.
B   Belgrade, Serbia, former Yugoslavia
C   Crevalcore, Italy
D   Dalmatia, Croatia, former Yugoslavia
E   East Finland
G   Corfu, Greece
K   Crete, Greece
M   Montegiorgio, Italy
N   Zutphen, Netherlands
R   Rome, Italy
S   Slavonia, Croatia, former Yugoslavia
T   Tanushimaru, Japan
U   Ushibuka, Japan
V   Velika Krsna, Serbia, former Yugoslavia
W   West Finland
Z   Zrenjanin, Serbia, former Yugoslavia

INDEX